Case Studies in Adult Intensive Care Medicine

T0201479

Case Studies in Adult Intensive Care Medicine

Edited by

Daniele Bryden
Honorary Senior Lecturer, University of Sheffield; Regional Advisor for Intensive Care Medicine in South Yorkshire, Sheffield Teaching Hospitals NHS Foundation Trust, Sheffield, UK.

Andrew Temple
Honorary Senior Lecturer, University of Sheffield; Former Training Programme Director for Intensive Care Medicine in South Yorkshire, Sheffield Teaching Hospitals NHS Foundation Trust, Sheffield, UK.

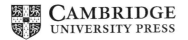

CAMBRIDGE
UNIVERSITY PRESS

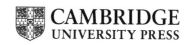

Shaftesbury Road, Cambridge CB2 8EA, United Kingdom

One Liberty Plaza, 20th Floor, New York, NY 10006, USA

477 Williamstown Road, Port Melbourne, VIC 3207, Australia

314–321, 3rd Floor, Plot 3, Splendor Forum, Jasola District Centre, New Delhi – 110025, India

103 Penang Road, #05–06/07, Visioncrest Commercial, Singapore 238467

Cambridge University Press is part of Cambridge University Press & Assessment, a department of the University of Cambridge.

We share the University's mission to contribute to society through the pursuit of education, learning and research at the highest international levels of excellence.

www.cambridge.org
Information on this title: www.cambridge.org/9781107423374

First published 2017 (version 4, March 2023)

Printed in the United Kingdom by Print on Demand, World Wide

A catalogue record for this publication is available from the British Library

Library of Congress Cataloging-in-Publication data
Names: Bryden, Daniele, editor. | Temple, Andrew (Training programme director for intensive care medicine), editor.
Title: Case studies in adult intensive care medicine / edited by Daniele Bryden, Andrew Temple.
Description: Cambridge, United Kingdom ; New York : Cambridge University Press, 2017. | Includes bibliographical references and index.
Identifiers: LCCN 2016040383 | ISBN 9781107423374 (Pbk. : alk. paper)
Subjects: | MESH: Critical Care–methods | Adult | Case Reports
Classification: LCC RC86.8 | NLM WX 218 | DDC 616.02/8–dc23
LC record available at https://lccn.loc.gov/2016040383

ISBN   978-1-107-42337-4   Paperback

. . . .

Contents

The color plates appear between pages 206 and 207.

Contributors

Ahmed Al-Mukhtar
Consultant in Hepatobiliary Surgery, Sheffield Teaching Hospitals NHS Foundation Trust

Peter Andrews
Professor, Department of Anaesthesia and Critical Care, University of Edinburgh and Western General Hospital, Edinburgh

Michael Athanassacopoulos
Consultant Spinal Surgeon, Sheffield Teaching Hospitals NHS Foundation Trust

Vicky Banks
Consultant in ICM/Anaesthesia, Nottingham University Hospitals NHS Foundation Trust

Julian Barker
Consultant in Cardiothoracic Critical Care and Cardiothoracic Anaesthesia, University Hospital of South Manchester, Manchester

James Beck
Consultant in Anaesthesia and Intensive Care Medicine, Leeds Teaching Hospitals NHS Trust

Thearina de Beer
Consultant in ICM/Anaesthesia, Nottingham University Hospitals NHS Foundation Trust

Richard Bourne
Consultant Pharmacist, Critical Care, Sheffield Teaching Hospitals NHS Foundation Trust

Daniele Bryden
Consultant in Intensive Care Medicine/ Anaesthesia, Sheffield Teaching Hospitals NHS Foundation Trust

Steven Cantellow
Consultant in ICM/Anaesthesia, Nottingham University Hospitals NHS Foundation Trust

Aylwin J Chick
Consultant Physician in Acute Medicine, Northumbria Healthcare NHS Foundation Trust

Neil Chiverton
Consultant Spinal Surgeon, Sheffield Teaching Hospitals NHS Foundation Trust

Gordon Craig
Consultant in Intensive Care Medicine and Anaesthesia, Portsmouth Hospitals NHS Foundation Trust

Jane Cunningham
Trainee in Microbiology, South Yorkshire Microbiology rotation

Philip Docherty
Intensive Care Medicine Specialist Registrar, Edinburgh Royal Infirmary, Edinburgh

Helen Ellis
Consultant in Intensive Care Medicine/ Anaesthesia, Sheffield Teaching Hospitals NHS Foundation Trust

Ingi Elsayed
Consultant in ICM/Renal Medicine, Royal Stoke University Hospital

Emma England
Intensive Care Clinical Fellow, St Helens and Knowsley Teaching Hospitals NHS Trust

Martin J Feat
Consultant in Anaesthesia, Sheffield Teaching Hospitals NHS Foundation Trust

Miguel Garcia
Clinical Fellow, Cardiothoracic Critical Care, University Hospital of South Manchester, Manchester

Dermot Gleeson
Professor o Hepatology and Consultant in Hepatology, Sheffield Teaching Hospitals NHS Foundation Trust

Alastair J Glossop
Consultant in Intensive Care Medicine/Anaesthesia, Sheffield Teaching Hospitals NHS Foundation Trust

Zhe Hui Hui
NIHR Doctoral Research Fellow Department of Design, Trials and Statistics, ScHARR, The University of Sheffield

Sarah Irving
Consultant in Intensive Care Medicine/Anaesthesia, Sheffield Teaching Hospitals NHS Foundation Trust

Phil Jackson
Consultant in Anaesthesia and Intensive Care Medicine, Leeds Teaching Hospitals NHS Trust

Qaiser Jalal
Fellow in Hepatobiliary Surgery, Sheffield Teaching Hospitals NHS Foundation Trust

John Jameson
Consultant Colorectal Surgeon, University Hospitals of Leicester NHS Trust

Aditya Krishan Kapoor
Trainee in Intensive Care Medicine and Anaesthesia, South Yorkshire rotation

James Keegan
Trainee in Anaesthesia/ICM, Wessex Regional Rotation

Andrew Klein
Consultant in Cardiothoracic Anaesthesia and Intensive Care, Papworth Hospital NHS Foundation Trust

Andrew Leeson
Consultant in Anaesthesia and Intensive Care Medicine, Barnsley Hospital NHS Foundation Trust

Sarah Linford
Advanced Trainee in Anaesthetics and ICM, East Midlands Rotation

Steven Lobaz
Consultant in Anaesthesia and Intensive Care Medicine, Barnsley Hospital NHS Foundation Trust

Ne-Hooi Will Loh
Consultant in Anaesthesia and Intensive Care, National University Hospital, Singapore

Gerry Lynch
Consultant in Intensive Care Medicine/Anaesthesia, Rotherham NHS Foundation Trust

Tushar Mahambrey
Consultant Intensivist, St Helens and Knowsley Teaching Hospitals NHS Trust

Samir Matloob
Trainee in Neurosurgery, North Thames (London) Rotation

Gregor McNeill
Consultant in Critical Care and Acute Medicine, Royal Infirmary, Edinburgh

Tim Meekings
Consultant in Anaesthesia/Intensive Care
Medicine, Chesterfield Royal Hospital NHS
Foundation Trust

Gary H Mills
Professor of Intensive Care Medicine,
University of Sheffield, Consultant in
Intensive Care Medicine/Anaesthesia,
Sheffield Teaching Hospitals NHS
Foundation Trust

Alastair James Morgan
Consultant in Intensive Care Medicine/
Anaesthesia, Sheffield Teaching Hospitals
NHS Foundation Trust

Nick Morgan-Hughes
Consultant in Cardiac Anaesthesia/
Intensive Care Medicine, Sheffield
Teaching Hospitals NHS Foundation
Trust

Graeme Nimmo
Consultant Physician in Intensive Care
Medicine and Clinical Education, Western
General Hospital, Edinburgh

Dave Partridge
Consultant in Medical Microbiology,
Sheffield Teaching Hospitals NHS
Foundation Trust

Nicola Pawley
Consultant in Anaesthesia/Intensive Care
Medicine, Chesterfield Royal Hospital NHS
Foundation Trust

Omar Pirzada
Consultant in Respiratory Medicine,
Sheffield Teaching Hospitals NHS
Foundation Trust

Richard Porter
Consultant in Intensive Care Medicine,
University Hospitals of Leicester NHS
Trust

Ajay H Raithatha
Consultant in Intensive Care Medicine/
Anaesthesia, Sheffield Teaching Hospitals
NHS Foundation Trust

Jonathan H Rosser
Consultant in Cardiac Anaesthesia/
Intensive Care Medicine, Sheffield
Teaching Hospitals NHS Foundation
Trust

David Rowney
Lead Retrieval Consultant, Royal Hospital
for Sick Children, Edinburgh

Jochen Seidel
Consultant in Intensive Care Medicine/
Anaesthesia, Doncaster and Bassetlaw NHS
Foundation Trust

Martin Smith
Professor, University College London,
Consultant in Neuroanaesthesia and
Neurocritical Care, National Hospital for
Neurology and Neurosurgery, University
College London Hospitals

Andrew Temple
Consultant in Intensive Care Medicine/
Anaesthesia, Sheffield Teaching Hospitals
NHS Foundation Trust

Chris Thorpe
Consultant in Anaesthesia/Intensive Care,
Ysbyty Gwynedd Hospital, Bangor

Ascanio Tridente
Consultant Intensivist and Physician,
St Helens and Knowsley Teaching
Hospitals

Alex Trotman
Postgraduate Office, The Chancellor's
Building, 49 Little France Crescent,
National Hospital for Neurology and
Neurosurgery, University College London
Hospitals, Edinburgh

Bevan Vickery
Consultant, Department of Adult Anaesthesia, Auckland City Hospital, Auckland, New Zealand

Rachel Wadsworth
Consultant in Intensive Care Medicine/ Anaesthesia, Sheffield Teaching Hospitals NHS Foundation Trust

Stephen Webber
Consultant in Intensive Care Medicine/ Anaesthesia, Sheffield Teaching Hospitals NHS Foundation Trust

Timothy Wenham
Consultant in Anaesthesia and Intensive Care Medicine, Barnsley Hospital NHS Foundation Trust

Paul Whiting
Consultant in Intensive Care Medicine/ Anaesthesia, Sheffield Teaching Hospitals NHS Foundation Trust

James Wigfull
Consultant in Intensive Care Medicine/ Anaesthesia, Sheffield Teaching Hospitals NHS Foundation Trust

Matthew Wiles
Consultant in Neuroanaesthesia and Neurocritical Care, Sheffield Teaching Hospitals NHS Foundation Trust

Elizabeth Wilson
Consultant in Critical Care Medicine and Anaesthesia, Royal Infirmary, Edinburgh

Lin Lee Wong
Specialty Registrar in Gastroenterology and Hepatology, Royal Hallamshire Hospital, Sheffield

Preface

Case-based discussion is an integral part of critical care teaching and training.

Although the specialty is a relatively young branch of medicine, in addition to its own specific knowledge base, it requires a detailed background knowledge of surgery, medicine and trauma across all age ranges.

In creating this book, we have approached knowledgeable and enthusiastic trainers in their subject fields to discuss an interesting or illustrative case. The aim was to create a number of discrete small chapters that could be used as the basis for individual general reading, group tutorials or as a starting point for further exploration around a topic area. This is not intended to be a definitive text but contains a mixture of core knowledge and detailed background information so that there is material of interest to everyone looking after critically ill patients.

The cases chosen have all been mapped to the UK Faculty of Intensive Care Medicine FFICM exam and the European Society of Intensive Care Medicine EDIC exam so we hope it will provide alternative reading for those studying for those exams.

We have enjoyed reading and editing the cases and have learnt from the expertise of the authors. We hope you will too.

Levels of Evidence

(adapted from the Centre for Evidence Based Medicine, Oxford)

1a Systematic reviews (with homogeneity) of randomised controlled trials

1b Individual randomised controlled trials (with narrow confidence intervals)

1c 'All or none' randomised controlled trials (i.e., when all patients died before the treatment became available, but some now survive on it; or when some patients died before the treatment became available, but none now die on it)

2a Systematic reviews (with homogeneity) of cohort studies

2b Individual cohort study or low quality randomised controlled trials (e.g., <80% follow-up)

2c "Outcomes" Research

3a Systematic review (with homogeneity) of case-control studies

3b Individual case-control study

4   Case-series (and poor quality cohort and case-control studies)

5   Expert opinion without explicit critical appraisal, or based on physiology, bench research or "first principles"

Abbreviations Referred to in Case Discussions

AAA	abdominal aortic aneurysm
AAGBI	Association of Anaesthetists of Great Britain and Ireland
ABGs	arterial blood gas(es)
ABI	acute brain injury
ACE	angiotensin converting enzyme
ACS	abdominal compartment syndrome
ACTH	adrenocorticotrophic hormone
ADH	antidiuretic hormone
AF	atrial fibrillation
AGNB	aerobic gram negative bacilli
AIH	autoimmune hepatitis
AIP	acute interstitial pneumonitis
AIS	acute ischaemic stroke abbreviated injury scale
AKI	acute kidney injury
ALD	alcoholic liver disease
ALT	alanine transaminase
ANP	advanced nurse practitioner
APACHE	acute physiology and chronic health evaluation
APP	abdominal perfusion pressure
APPT	activated partial thromboplastin time
APRV	airway pressure release ventilation
ARDS	adult respiratory distress syndrome
ARF	acute respiratory failure
aSAH	aneurysmal subarachnoid haemorrhage
ASB	assisted spontaneous breathing
ASPEN	American Society for Parenteral and Enteral Nutrition
AST	aspartate aminotransferase
ATC	acute traumatic coagulopathy
ATN	acute tubular nephropathy
ATP	adenosine triphosphate
ATS	American Thoracic Society
AU	absorbance units
BAL	bronchoalveolar lavage
BIPAP	biphasic positive airway pressure
BIS	bispectral index
BMI	body mass index
BP	blood pressure
bpm	beats per minute
BSI	blood stream infection
BTF	brain trauma foundation
BTS	British Thoracic Society
BURP	backwards, upwards and rightwards pressure on the thyroid cartilage
CA	cerebral autoregulation
CAM-ICU	Confusion Assessment Method for the Intensive Care Unit
CAP	community acquired pneumonia
CBF	cerebral blood flow
CBG	capillary blood gases
CBV	cerebral blood volume
CFA	crytpogenic fibrosing alveolitis
CFAM	cerebral function analysing monitor
CFU	colony forming units

CHO	carbohydrate
CI	cardiac index
CK	creatine kinase
CLA-BSI	central line associated blood stream infection
CMRO2	cerebral metabolic rate for oxygen
COMT	catchyl-0-methyltransferase
COP	cryptogenic organising pneumonia
COPD	chronic obstructive pulmonary disease
CPAP	continuous positive airway pressure
CPC	cerebral performance category
CPIS	Clinical Pulmonary Infection Score
CPK	creatine phosphokinase
CPM	central pontine myelinloysis
CPP	cerebral perfusion pressure
CPS	Child Pugh Score
CR-BSI	catheter related blood stream infection
CRP	C-reactive protein
CRT	capillary refill time
CRRT	continuous renal replacement therapy
CSW	cerebral salt wasting syndrome
CT	computed tomography
CTA	CT angiography
CTEPH	chronic thromboembolic pulmonary hypertension
CTPA	CT pulmonary angiogram
CVC	central venous catheter
CVST	cerebral venous and sinus thrombosis
CVVH	continuous venovenous haemofiltration
CVVHD	continuous venovenous haemodiafiltration
DAS	Difficult Airway Society
DBD	donation after brainstem death
DC	direct current
DCCV	direct current cardioversion
DCD	donation after circulatory death
DCI	delayed ischaemic deficit/ delayed cerebral ischaemia
DGH	district general hospital
DHI	dynamic hyperinflation
DIC	disseminated intravascular coagulation
DKA	diabetic ketoacidosis
DSA	digital subtraction angiography
DVT	deep venous thrombosis
EBIC	European Brain Injury Consortium
E-CPR	extra-corporeal support during cardiopulmonary resuscitation
ED	emergency department
EEG	electroencephalogram
ERCP	endoscopic retrograde cholangio pancreatography
ESPEN	European Society for Clinical Nutrition and Metabolism
ESBL	extended spectrum beta lactamases
EWS	early warning score
FBC	full blood count
FEV1	forced expiratory volume in 1 second
FiO_2	fraction of inspired oxygen
FRC	functional residual capacity
FV	flow velocity
GAS	group A streptococcus
GCS	Glasgow Coma Scale
GDC	Guglielmi detachable coil

GEB	gum elastic bougie
GGS	Group G beta-haemolytic streptococcus
GMC	general medical council
GP	General Practitioner
G6PD	glucose 6 phosphate deyhdrogenase
HCAI	healthcare associated infection
HELLP	Haemolysis, Elevated Liver enzymes, Low Platelets syndrome
HR	heart rate
HAART	highly active antiretroviral therapy
HAP	hospital acquired pneumonia
HASU	hyperacute stroke unit
HDU	high dependency unit (level 2 unit)
HELICS	Hospitals in Europe Link for Infection Control through Surveillance
HES	hydroxy ethyl starch
HFOV	high frequency oscillatory ventilation
HHS	hyperosmolar hyperglycaemic state
HPB	hepatobiliary
HRCT	high resolution CT chest
HRS	hepatorenal syndrome
IABP	intra aortic balloon pump
IAP	intra abdominal pressure
IAH	intra abdominal hypertension
IBW	ideal body weight
ICD	implantable cardiac defibrillator
ICDSC	Intensive Care Delirium Screening Checklist
ICNARC	Intensive Care National Audit and Research Centre
ICP	intracranial pressure
ICU	intensive care unit (level 3 unit)
ID	infectious diseases
IE	infective endocarditis
IMV	intermittent mandatory ventilation
INR	international normalised ratio
IO	intraosseous
iv/IV	intravenous
IVIG	intravenous immunoglobulin
ILCOR	International Liaison Committee on Resuscitation
ILD	interstitial lung disease
IPF	idiopathic pulmonary fibrosis
ISAT	International Subarachnoid Aneurysm Trial
ISS	injury severity score
LDH	lactate dehydrogenase
LFTs	liver function tests
LMA	laryngeal mask airway
LP	lumbar puncture
L-VAD	left ventricular assist device
MAO	monoamine oxidase inhibitors
MAP	mean arterial pressure
MCF	mean clot firmness
MD	microdialysis (usually cerebral)
MDR	multi-drug resistant
MH	malignant hyperpyrexia
MIC	mean inhibitory concentration
MCA	middle cerebral artery
MDR	multidrug resistance
MELD	model for end stage liver disease
mmHG	millimetres of mercury

MODS	multiorgan dysfunction syndrome
MRA	magnetic resonance angiography
MRCP	magnetic resonance cholangiopancreatogram
MRI	magnetic resonance imaging
MUST	malnutrition universal screening test
MV	mechanical ventilation
NAC	N-acetylcysteine
NAP4	4th National Anaesthesia Project Audit Report
NBA	net bilirubin absorbance
NHSBT	NHS blood and transplant
NIBP	non invasive blood pressure
NICE	National Institute for Health and Care Excellence
NIRS	near infrared spectroscopy
NIV	non invasive ventilation
NJ	naso-jejunal
NMB	neuromuscular blocking agent
NMS	neuroleptic malignant syndrome
NOA	net oxyhaemoglobin absorbance
NPE	neurogenic pulmonary oedema
NPIS	national poisons information service
NPPV	noninvasive positive pressure ventilation
NPSA	National Patient Safety Agency
NPWT	negative pressure wound therapy
NSAIDs	non steroidal anti-inflammatory drugs
NSE	neurone specific enolase
NSIP	non specific interstitial pneumonitis
NTSP	national tracheostomy safety project
OELM	optimal external laryngeal manipulation
OHCA	out of hospital cardiac arrest
PAC	pulmonary artery catheter
PAOP	pulmonary artery occlusion pressure
PaO_2	partial pressure of oxygen in arterial blood
$PaCO_2$	partial pressure of carbon dioxide in arterial blood
$PbtO_2$	partial pressure of oxygen in brain tissue
PCP	pneumocystis jirovecii pneumonia
PCR	polymerase chain reaction
PDT	percutaneous dilational trachesotomy
PEA	pulseless electrical activity or pulmonary endarterectomy
PEEP	positive end expiratory pressure
PHE	Public Health England
PI	pulsatility index
PICC	peripherally inserted central catheter
PICCO	pulse index contour cardiac output
PICU	paediatric intensive care unit
PF	(ratio) of arterial oxygen concentration as PaO2 to the fraction of inspired oxygen
p MDI	pressurised metered dose inhaler
PRx	pressure reactivity index
PSA	prostate-specific antigen
PSB	protected specimen brush
PSI	pneumonia severity index
PT	prothrombin time
PTE	pulmonary thromboembolism
$PtiO_2$	brain tissue oxygen tension
PTr	prothrombin time ratio
PVL	Panton-Valentine leukocidin
PVR	pulmonary vascular resistance

QTc	corrected QT interval
RCT	randomised controlled trial
ROS	reactive oxygen species
ROSC	return of spontaneous circulation
ROTEM	thromboelastometry
RR	respiratory rate
RRT	renal replacement therapy
rRNA	ribosmal ribonucleic acid
RRT	renal replacement therapy
SaO$_2$	arterial oxygen saturation
SBP	systolic blood pressure
SBP	spontaneous bacterial peritonitis
SBT	spontaneous breathing trial
SDD	selective decontamination of the digestive tract
SIADH	syndrome of inappropriate ADH
SIGN	Scottish Intercollegiate Guideline Network
SIRS	systemic inflammatory response syndrome
SNOD	specialist nurse for organ donation
SOD	selective oral decontamination
SOFA	sequential organ failure assessment
SpO2	oxygen saturation (via pulse oximetry)
SSEP	somatosensory evoked potentials
STEMI	ST elevation myocardial infarction
SVRI	systemic vascular resistance index
TACI	total anterior circulation infarct
TAPSE	Tricuspid Annular Plane Systolic Excursion
TARN	trauma audit and research network
TB	tuberculosis
TBI	traumatic brain injury
TCA	tricyclic antidepressant
TCD	transcranial doppler ultrasonography
TEG	thromboelastography
TIPS	Transjugular Intrahepatic Portosystemic Shunt
TNF-α	tumour necrosis factor alpha
TOE	transoesophageal echocardiogram
tPA	tissue plasminogen activator
TPG	transpulmonary gradient
TPN	total parenteral nutrition
TPMT	thiopurine methyl transferase
TRALI	transfusion associated lung injury
TTM	targeted temperature management
UIP	usual interstitial pneumonitis
UKDEC	UK Donor Ethics Committee
VAC	vacuum assisted closure
VA-ECMO	venous-arterial extracorporeal membrane oxygenation
VAP	ventilator associated pneumonia
VATS	video-assisted thoracoscopic surgery
VF	ventricular fibrillation
Vt	(as part of GCS) not assessed verbal score due to presence of tracheostomy
WCC	white cell count
WSACS	World Society of the Abdominal Compartment Syndrome

Chapter 1

Cardiac Arrest: Post Resuscitation Management

Richard Porter and Andrew Temple

Introduction

Every year in the United Kingdom (UK) approximately 50,000 people suffer an out-of-hospital cardiac arrest (OHCA). Historically, of these arrests, only approximately 6,250 people are admitted to UK intensive care units (ICU) for post cardiac arrest care. Despite improving resuscitation practices, mortality for those who suffer an OHCA is greater than 90 percent, with many survivors being left with severe neurological impairment. However, in the last few years, there has been a major change in the way OHCAs are managed with signs of improved overall mortality and morbidity. This case will summarise the latest advances in OHCA care.

Case

A 58-year-old man was admitted to Accident and Emergency after sustaining an OHCA. He had collapsed at home in front of his wife, who performed cardiopulmonary resuscitation immediately after calling for an ambulance. It took five minutes for the paramedic rapid response car to arrive, at which point the rhythm was noted to be ventricular fibrillation (VF). He required two biphasic DC shocks and 1 dose of 1 mg of adrenaline to restore circulation. His estimated downtime prior to return of spontaneous circulation (ROSC) was a total of 12 minutes. He was intubated on the scene by the paramedics. On arrival in hospital, 20 minutes later, he was making agonal gasping respirations which were being assisted with manual ventilation. He was maintaining a blood pressure of 135/60 mmHg with a pulse rate of 95 bpm, confirmed to be sinus rhythm on cardiac monitoring. A 12 lead electrocardiogram (ECG) revealed significant ST elevation in the anterior chest leads. He was deeply unconscious with a Glasgow Coma Scale of 3 out of 15.

No exclusions to targeted temperature management were present and this was commenced shortly after arrival to the emergency department, using cold intravenous fluids and application of a cooling helmet and vest. Sedation was maintained with propofol and alfentanil. Given the history and ECG findings, a computerised tomography (CT) scan of the head was not performed, as a neurological cause for the arrest was not suspected.

Cardiology review was urgently sought and he was subsequently transferred to the cardiac angiography suite. It was discovered that his proximal left anterior descending coronary artery was blocked and this was stented with excellent results. He was transferred to ICU, where he completed 24 hours of targeted temperature management, with a core body temperature maintained between 32 and 36°C.

Following slow passive rewarming of no greater than 0.5°C per hour, there was no recovery of consciousness with a persistent GCS of 3/15. At 72 hours post arrest, an electroencephalogram (EEG) showed burst suppression. Subsequent somatosensory evoked potentials (SSEP) revealed bilateral absence at the N20 level. Following discussion with the family, active therapy was withdrawn as the neurological prognosis was considered hopeless.

Discussion

ROSC is just the preliminary step in attaining complete recovery after cardiac arrest. Of those subsequently admitted to ICU, as many as 40–50 percent survive to hospital discharge, often with good neurological outcome, although many will have subtle cognitive impairments that are not immediately obvious on ICU discharge.

Complex pathophysiological processes occur during the cardiac arrest when the body is in an ischaemic (limited blood flow) state, and after ROSC when there is increased cellular activity due to reperfusion. These processes have been termed the post-cardiac arrest syndrome. The syndrome comprises: the precipitating pathology which may still persist; post-cardiac arrest brain injury; post-cardiac arrest myocardial dysfunction; and the systemic ischaemia/ reperfusion response. The severity of the syndrome is extremely variable depending on length and cause of cardiac arrest. Some patients have a very brief post-cardiac arrest syndrome and regain consciousness rapidly. Others manifest, in the first few days, signs of cardiac failure and multi-organ failure, which has many features in common with sepsis and confers significant risk of mortality. The remainder exhibit varying degrees of neurological dysfunction (seizures, myoclonus, cognitive memory impairments, coma, cortical brain death and brainstem death). Prognosticated bad neurological outcome often leads to withdrawal of active life sustaining therapy (WLST) and is consequently a late cause of death in patients.

Post-cardiac arrest comatose patients have multiple treatment requirements which often need to be instigated at the scene of ROSC outside the ICU. All hospitals should follow a post-resuscitation care algorithm similar to the one outlined in Figure 1.1.

The specific requirements for targeted temperature management, coronary angiography, mechanical support and neurological prognostication will be discussed in more detail below.

Targeted Temperature Management

Following the publication of two landmark papers in 2002, therapeutic hypothermia (32 to 34°C) became the treatment of choice for comatose patients following OHCA when the underlying rhythm was VF.[1,2] The study by Bernard et al. involved 4 Australian centres and enrolled 77 patients; the European study recruited in 9 centres across 5 European countries and enrolled 275 patients. The Australian study used alternate day randomisation, a technique which is subject to operator bias. In the European group, the control group who received normothermia actually became hyperthermia, so the perceived benefit from hypothermia may have been biased by the potential harm caused by hyperthermia. An additional criticism of both studies is that the clinicians could not be blinded to the separate treatment arms. Despite this, widespread adoption of therapeutic hypothermia occurred within the critical care community after publication of the trials.

The mechanism of the action of cooling is thought to suppress many of the pathways leading to cell death. Hypothermia decreases the cerebral metabolic rate for oxygen by

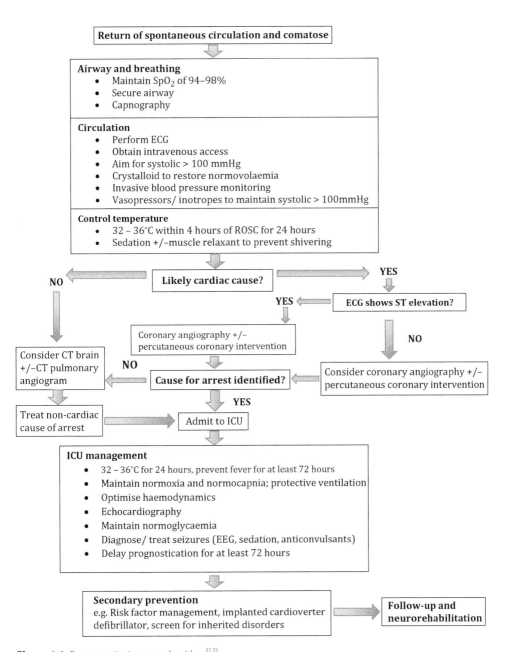

Figure 1.1 Post-resuscitation care algorithm.[12]

approximately 6 per cent for every 1°C drop in core temperature and this may reduce the inflammatory cytokine response associated with the post-cardiac arrest syndrome.

The use of therapeutic hypothermia in non-VF arrests (i.e., asystole and pulseless electrical activity (PEA)) and in hospital cardiac arrests has remained more contentious. However in 2010, the International Liaison Committee on Resuscitation (ILCOR), although accepting of the lower evidence strength, advocated the use of therapeutic hypothermia in comatose patients following both 'shockable – VF/VT' and 'non-shockable – PEA/ Asystole' cardiac arrests.[3]

The publication of the 'Targeted Temperature Management at 33°C versus 36°C after Cardiac Arrest' (TTM) study looked at 950 all rhythm OHCA patients. The study showed no difference in survival and neurological outcome between those cooled to 33°C and those cooled to 36°C.[4] While the implications of this are still to be fully realised, the term *targeted temperature management* or *temperature control* is now preferred over the previous term *therapeutic hypothermia*. The optimal duration of targeted temperature management is unknown, but a period of 24 hours is most commonly chosen.

ILCOR has subsequently produced new guidelines in 2015 which now recommend maintaining a constant target temperature between 32 to 36°C for those patients in whom temperature control is used. TTM is recommended for adults after OHCA with an initial shockable rhythm who remain unresponsive after ROSC (strong recommendation, low quality evidence). However, TTM is suggested in adults after OHCA with an initial non-shockable rhythm and in adults after in hospital cardiac arrests with any initial rhythm (weak recommendation, very low quality evidence). Whether or not certain subpopulations of cardiac arrest patients may benefit from lower or higher temperatures remains unknown; further research is required.

At present, it is unclear what target temperature individual centres will choose to adopt. There is concern that controlling temperature at 36°C will run the risk of temperature overshoot, leading to hyperthermia, which is known to be deleterious. It is likely that most centres will aim for a target temperature of 32 to 36°C for 24 hours post-ROSC in the first instance. However, if there are contra-indications to cooling e.g., arrhythmias, pre-existing medical coagulopathy (fibrinolytic therapy is not a contra-indication), electrolyte disturbance or sepsis, or direct complications that occur due to cooling at 32 to 36°C, then it is probable controlled normothermia will be attained. Hyperthermia must be meticulously avoided for 72 hours following the arrest and cooling devices may be required to achieve this. Rebound hyperthermia is common after targeted temperature management and can be difficult to control.

In this case, it was felt that a VF arrest with cardiac aetiology gave a strong indication to cool. It is very important after the cooling period not to increase the temperature too quickly. Passive rewarming at between 0.25 to 0.5°C per hour is recommended to avoid rebound hyperthermia, vasodilatation and hypotension which can lead to coronary ischaemia and deleterious effects on the heart.

Coronary Angiography

Should we perform coronary angiography and intervention following successful resuscitation after cardiac arrest?

At present we have no trials to answer this question. The large trials looking at coronary angiography following ST elevation myocardial infarction (STEMI) specifically exclude post-cardiac arrest patients. However, case series of patients post arrest with STEMIs show 60% survival to hospital discharge thus indicating that these patients could benefit from urgent angiography.[5] In the non-STEMI population approximately 25% have acute coronary lesions.[6] It would appear that the post-cardiac arrest ECG does not accurately predict the presence, or more importantly the absence, of occluded coronary arteries.

This has led the 2010 International Consensus on Cardiopulmonary Resuscitation and Emergency Cardiovascular Care Science with Treatment Recommendations to state:

> It is reasonable to perform early angiography and primary percutaneous coronary intervention in selected patients despite the absence of ST-segment elevation on the ECG or prior clinical findings, such as chest pain, if coronary ischaemia is considered the likely cause on clinical grounds.[5]

Therapeutic hypothermia does not preclude the use of urgent coronary intervention.

The European Association for Percutaneous Cardiovascular Interventions (EAPCI) has also recently produced a consensus statement that states coronary angiography should be immediately performed in the presence of ST elevation on an ECG in OHCA patients and considered within two hours in other patients in the absence of a non-coronary cause, particularly if there is haemodynamic instability.

It would therefore seem reasonable to perform urgent coronary angiography in OHCA patients where a cardiac cause is suspected.

Mechanical Support

The recent clinical IABP-Shock II trial of the intra-aortic balloon pump (IABP) in cardiogenic shock from acute myocardial infarction has shown that the insertion of this device does not lead to an improvement in 30 day mortality.[7] In this trial, the mortality for those in whom an IABP was inserted is 39.7% and 41.3% in the control group managed conventionally, giving a P value of 0.69. Extrapolating this data to post-cardiac arrest patients may be difficult as reversible myocardial stunning could be contributing to the cardiogenic failure. In patients with post-cardiac arrest myocardial stunning, IABP can be considered as rescue therapy but it may be unlikely to improve overall outcome.

Neurological Prognostication

Predicting the neurological outcome in a comatose cardiac arrest survivor can be very difficult. It is important that poor outcome is clearly defined. The majority of studies use Cerebral Performance Category (CPC) grades of 3 or more as poor outcome (see Table 1.1).

Multiple modalities are now used to aid this prognostication: clinical; electrophysiological; radiological and biochemical (see Table 1.2).

Table 1.1 Cerebral performance categories (CPC) and outcome class

CPC	Activity level	Outcome class
1 – Good cerebral performance	Conscious. Can lead normal life and work. May have minor deficits.	Good
2 – Moderate cerebral disability	Conscious. Cerebral function adequate for part-time work in sheltered environment or independent activities of daily living.	Good
3 – Severe cerebral disability	Conscious. Dependent on others for daily support because of neurological deficit.	Poor
4 – Coma, vegetative state	Not conscious. No interaction with environment.	Poor
5 – Dead	Brainstem dead or dead by conventional criteria	Poor

Table 1.2 Prognostic factors false positive rate (FPR) in comatose survivors 72 hours post arrest, unless stated, by application of targeted temperature management (TTM) post arrest. 24 to 72 hours post arrest

Prognostic factor	FPR - No TTM	FPR - TTM
Corneal reflexes	0	0.05
Pupillary reflexes	0	0.04
Motor score M1 or M2	0	0.05
Myoclonic status (<72 hours)	0	0.05
Serum NSE >33 mcg/ml	0.09	0.12
Unfavourable EEG	0.03	0.10
Bilateral absence N20 SSEP	0.07	0.06

In the pre-targeted temperature era, the following clinical signs predicted poor neurological signs with a false positive rate (FPR) of zero, if present 72 hours post-cardiac arrest: absent pupillary or corneal reflexes and extensor or absent motor reflex.[8,9] Myoclonic status from 24 hours onwards, in patients who have not suffered cardiac arrest secondary to respiratory causes and who have not been cooled, has been associated with a hopeless neurological prognosis.[9] However, caution in diagnosis is essential as this condition closely mimics Lance–Adams syndrome, a voluntary myoclonic syndrome, which has a good prognosis.[10] There are many other case reports that describe early onset of prolonged and generalised myoclonus which disappears on sedation holds and subsequent recovery of consciousness. If any diagnostic uncertainty is present, expert neurological opinion should be considered.

In the targeted temperature era, no clinical signs are associated with a FPR of zero. After 72 hours, pupillary reflex has the lowest FPR of 0.04, followed by corneal reflex and absent or extensor motor reflex with a FPR of 0.05. Myoclonic status after day 1 has a FPR of 0.05 after TTM.[11]

Clinical examination is inexpensive and easy to perform but can lead to bias and variability in interpretation of findings which can potentially influence management and lead to a self-fulfilling prophecy. Using clinical signs as the sole method of prognostication cannot be recommended.

Unfavourable EEG results are defined as any of the following patterns: generalised suppression; burst suppression; status epilepticus; suppression or unreactive pattern. These patterns are invariably associated with a poor outcome with a FPR of 0.1 following TTM 72 hours after the arrest.[11] EEG requires expert interpretation, which may limit availability in many hospitals.

SSEP involves monitoring brain response to electrical stimulation of peripheral nerves and specifically looks at cerebral cortical function. At time zero the median nerve is stimulated, responses are looked for at 9 to 10 ms at the brachial plexus (N9/10), 13 ms at the dorsal nerve root (N13), and 20 ms (N20) at the somatosensory cortex. Bilateral loss of the N20 response indicates cortical cell death, assuming response is seen at both the N9/10 and N13 points indicating intact peripheral nerves.

In the pre-TTM era, bilateral absence of SSEP was associated with a FPR of 0.07 up to 72 hours post-cardiac arrest. With the introduction of TTM, bilateral absence of SSEP is associated with a FPR of 0.06, 72 hours post-cardiac arrest.[11] SSEP has been adopted in some large treatment centres and is a useful test in establishing cerebral cortical death. SSEP is frequently a criterion investigation for deciding on WLST however, it requires expert interpretation and is prone to artefact (electrical interference from muscle artefacts or the ICU environment).

Radiological techniques are useful to exclude intracerebral catastrophe in the early stages. However, as a prognostication tool, radiological findings are not reliable enough to predict neurological outcome in the early stages. The radiological CT finding of loss of grey white matter differentiation is commonly seen immediately after ROSC and is not reliable enough to prognosticate with in the initial stages. Extreme caution must be exhibited in interpretation of the initial head CT immediately after ROSC. However, CT becomes more beneficial as a prognostic tool a few days after ROSC. The grey–white matter interface can be quantitatively measured as a ratio between grey matter and white matter (GWR). The GWR threshold for prediction of poor outcome with FPR of zero ranged between 1.10 and 1.22 but the methods for GWR calculation were inconsistent amongst studies.[12]

MRI changes after global anoxic ischaemic injury due to cardiac arrest appear as hyperintensity signals in cortical areas or basal ganglia on diffusion weighted imaging sequences. MRI is more sensitive in identifying ischaemic brain injury compared with CT and often reveals extensive abnormalities when SSEP is normal. MRI is a potentially useful investigation 4 to 5 days after ROSC but is a more lengthy procedure than CT which often precludes use in haemodynamically unstable patients.[12]

Raised levels of an enzyme neurone specific enolase (NSE) have been used as a predictor of poor neurological outcome. Levels greater than 33 mcg/l following cardiac arrest are associated with poor neurological outcome with a false positive rate of 0.12.[11] However, the NSE thresholds vary in TTM treated and non-TTM treated patients. The measurement techniques are extremely heterogeneous due to variation among different analysers and an incomplete understanding of the kinetics of NSE blood concentration in the first few days after ROSC. NSE measurement is still not commonly used in clinical practice and is largely confined to the research setting.

Various algorithms for neurological prognostication exist, but some of the investigations are expensive and require expert interpretation which leads to variable uptake. This, in addition to the increasing requirement for coronary angiography and the need for implanted cardiac defibrillators after subsequent survival from cardiac arrest, has led to the view that post–cardiac arrest care should be regionalised in a similar manner to care for major trauma. Whether this centralisation of care will occur in the future remains to be seen.

Conclusion

Cardiac arrest is a potentially devastating condition with overall poor survival. In patients in whom there is ROSC, various treatment strategies including targeted temperature management and early revascularisation can be used which may improve physiological survival.

Neurological prognostication has become less certain in the targeted temperature era with a requirement of ideally 72 hours post-ROSC to elapse before prognostication can reliably be attempted. Neurological prognostication immediately after cardiac arrest is unreliable and cannot be recommended as a reason not to admit a patient to critical care. All escalation decisions should be based purely on pre-morbidity and frailty assessment. Neurological prognostication becomes clearer in the ensuing days after the cardiac arrest.

Key Learning Points

- Targeted temperature management (target of 36°C) is at least as effective as therapeutic hypothermia. The ILCOR guidelines in 2015 recommend to maintain a temperature between 32 to 36°C. Active normothermia for 72 hours and avoidance of hyperthermia is very important.

- Consideration should be given to performing coronary angiography and intervention in patients in whom a cardiac cause is suspected regardless of ECG findings.
- Mechanical support with IABP does not improve cardiogenic shock survival in patients with acute myocardial infarction. The role of post-cardiac arrest is unclear; however it is likely to have a role in rescue therapy.
- No clinical or electrophysiological markers predict poor neurological outcome with a false positive rate of zero following targeted temperature management.
- A period of 72 hours should elapse post-cardiac arrest before prognostication is attempted in the targeted-temperature managed patient, unless there is clinical evidence of brainstem death.

References

1. Bernard SA, Gray TW, Buist MD et al. Treatment of comatose survivors of out-of-hospital cardiac arrest with induced hypothermia. *N Engl J Med* 2002 21 Feb;346(8):557–63.

2. Hypothermia after Cardiac Arrest Study Group. Mild therapeutic hypothermia to improve the neurologic outcome after cardiac arrest. *N Engl J Med* 2002 21 Feb;346(8):549–56.

3. Nolan JP, Soar J, Zideman DA et al. European Resuscitation Council Guidelines for Resuscitation 2010 Section 1. Executive summary. Resuscitation. *Elsevier* 2010 Oct;81(10):1219–76.

4. Nielsen N, Wetterslev J, Cronberg T et al. Targeted temperature management at 33°C versus 36°C after cardiac arrest. *N Engl J Med* 2013 5 Dec;369(23): 2197–206.

5. Kern KB. Optimal treatment of patients surviving out-of-hospital cardiac arrest. *JACC Cardiovasc Interv* 2012 Jun;5(6): 597–605.

6. Radsel P, Knafelj R, Kocjancic S, Noc M. Angiographic characteristics of coronary disease and postresuscitation electrocardiograms in patients with aborted cardiac arrest outside a hospital. *Am J Cardiol* 2011 Sep;108(5): 634–8.

7. Thiele H, Zeymer U, Neumann F-J et al. Intraaortic balloon support for myocardial infarction with cardiogenic shock. *N Engl J Med* 2012 4 Oct;367(14):1287–96.

8. Zandbergen EG, de Haan RJ, Hidjra A. Systematic review of prediction of poor outcome in anoxic-ischaemic coma with biochemical markers of brain damage. *Intensive Care Med* 2001 1 Oct;27(10): 1661–7.

9. Wijdicks EFM, Hijdra A, Young GB, Bassetti CL, Wiebe S. Practice parameter: Prediction of outcome in comatose survivors after cardiopulmonary resuscitation (an evidence-based review): Report of the quality standards subcommittee of the American Academy of Neurology. *Neurology* 2006 24 Jul;67(2): 203–10.

10. English WA, Giffin NJ, Nolan JP. Myoclonus after cardiac arrest: pitfalls in diagnosis and prognosis. *Anaesthesia* 2009 Aug;64(8):908–11.

11. Golan E, Barrett K, Alali AS et al. Predicting neurologic outcome after targeted temperature management for cardiac arrest: systematic review and meta-analysis. *Critical Care Medicine* 2014 Aug;42(8):1919–30.

12. Nolan JP, Soar J, Cariou A, Cronberg T, Moulaert V et al. European Resuscitation Council and European Society of Intensive Care Guidelines for Post-resuscitation Care 2015. Section 5 of the European Resuscitation Council Guidelines for Resuscitation 2015. *Resuscitation* 2015;95:202–22.

Chapter 2

Initial Management of the Polytrauma Patient

Nicola Pawley and Paul Whiting

Introduction

Trauma is the leading cause of death worldwide in people under the age of 40. In England and Scotland there are an estimated 21,000 cases of major trauma each year, with a resultant 5,400 deaths.[1] The vast majority of cases, this trauma is blunt, with the most common mechanisms of injury being related to road traffic accidents and falls.

The definition and use of the term polytrauma currently remains inconsistent in academic and clinical settings. According to international consensus opinion, both anatomical and physiological parameters should be included in the definition. Recent work has demonstrated that the involvement of two body regions, with an Abbreviated Injury Scale (AIS) >2, is a good indicator of polytrauma, in preference to the Injury Severity Score (ISS) which could be elevated in monotrauma. Physiological parameters will most likely be descriptors of tissue hypoxia and coagulopathy.[2] For the purposes of this chapter polytrauma refers to any patient who has been subjected to multiple traumatic injuries.

In polytrauma uncontrolled haemorrhage accounts for a third of deaths and traumatic brain injury is common, proving fatal in approximately 40 per cent of cases where it occurs.[3]

It is imperative that when patients have sustained polytrauma, they are 'transferred to the right place at the right time'. Evidence from the United States, Germany and Australia has demonstrated improved survival and outcomes with centralised trauma care.[4,5] The National Audit office report in 2010 'Major trauma care in England' highlighted deficiencies in care provided to trauma victims in England and led to the establishment of major trauma centres in England in 2011.[1]

Survivors of significant polytrauma often face lengthy physical rehabilitation regimens and can suffer longterm physical, cognitive and psychological problems as a consequence.[6]

Case

A 50-year-old male presented to the Emergency Department (ED), having been knocked over at a crossing point by a car travelling at 50 mph. At the scene, his Glasgow Coma Score (GCS) was reduced and he was cardiovascularly compromised. As part of his initial management, 1 g of tranexamic acid was administered and a pelvic binder applied at the scene.

On hid arrival to the ED, his cervical spine continued to be immobilised and he was maintaining his own airway. His oxygen saturations were 98 per cent on 15l of oxygen (O_2) delivered via a non-rebreathe mask. There was obvious right-sided chest wall deformity with ipsilateral diminished air entry and his trachea remained central. On examination, of his cardiovascular system, his blood pressure (BP) was 95/58 mmHg, his pulse was 120 beats per minute and he had a regular and a reduced capillary refill time of 3 seconds centrally. He was noted to have a cool and pulseless right arm. His GCS was calculated as 9 (E1, V2, M6), his blood glucose 6.6 mmol/l and both pupils were equal and reactive.

His abdomen was firm and tender in the right loin. He was also noted to have a dislocated right knee and remained hypothermic with a core body temperature of 34.5°C.

Initial concurrent management included large bore intravenous cannulae, blood sampling and the administration of two units of O-negative blood via a fluid warmer. Following the primary survey, a right-sided chest drain was inserted, and the patient was intubated using a modified rapid sequence technique with alfentanil, ketamine and rocuronium. He was then transferred for a triple-contrast whole body CT scan (non-contrast head; contrast enhanced thorax, abdomen and pelvis)

The CT scan demonstrated a possible basal ganglia contusional haemorrhage; right-sided lung contusion and haemopneumothorax with fractures to ribs 2 to 9; a right axillary artery dissection with an associated large haematoma and a right renal laceration with associated haematoma.

From the CT scan, the patient was taken to theatre for exploration of the axillary artery. The patient's right knee was relocated and immobilised and following discussions with urology and neurosurgery, his other injuries were managed conservatively.

Throughout the initial resuscitation period, normotensive fluid resuscitation was performed in view of the associated traumatic brain injury. As a consequence he received 2 units of O-negative blood, 3 bags of fresh frozen plasma, 2 bags of cryoprecipitate, 1 bag of platelets and 500 mls of crystalloid (Hartmann's solution). In addition, he received a further 1 g of tranexamic acid and 20 mls of calcium gluconate.

Following a prolonged theatre, stay he was taken to the intensive care unit for ongoing management.

Case Discussion

This case illustrates the challenging nature of the polytrauma patient and demonstrates the multidisciplinary team approach required during the initial resuscitation and stabilisation of the patient. Decision processes are complex, and are aided by protocolised care and timely interventions. Guidelines exist, but vary in their evidence base, and as a consequence the intensivist needs to be appraised of the controversies and guidance that exist with regards to initial management.

Airway Control: When to Intubate?; What Induction Agent to Use?

Indications for definitive airway control with an endotracheal tube in the polytrauma patient include:

- Airway obstruction
- Hypoventilation
- GCS of <8
- An inability to maintain saturations of >90 per cent with supplemental oxygen
- Haemorrhagic cardiac arrest
- Severe maxillo-facial injury
- Facial and upper airway burns

Although in this case the patient's GCS was 9, the addition of likely chest injuries made securing the airway a priority. Evidence is accumulating that delaying intubation in an otherwise stable patient can adversely affect mortality. A retrospective review of 239 moderately injured (ISS <20), but initially stable patients, showed a significant increase in mortality (11.8% vs 1.8%; P = 0.045) in those patients who had delayed intubation defined as >25 minutes after arrival in the ED department.[7]

Ketamine was chosen as the induction agent of choice in this case, due to its more stable haemodynamic profile, as compared with either propofol or thiopentone, in the hypotensive shocked patient.[8,9] Historically, there have been concerns regarding a detrimental increase in intracranial pressure (ICP) associated with the use of ketamine in those patients with a Traumatic Brain Injury (TBI). These concerns were founded on a series of case-control studies performed in the 1970s in patients in whom ketamine sedation was administered for diagnostic pneumoventriculography.[10] Those patients with obstructed cerebrospinal fluid (CSF) flow demonstrated an increase in ICP; those without, did not.

Currently there is no strong evidence to suggest that ketamine causes harm in TBI. Ketamine has been shown to attenuate an increase in ICP in TBI patients undergoing procedures that may normally provoke a rise in ICP, e.g. suctioning.[11] Ketamine has been increasingly used in the pre-hospital setting where it has been demonstrated to be a safe induction agent that effectively facilitates endotracheal intubation,[12] and maintains mean arterial and cerebral perfusion pressure.

Another induction agent that is felt to have a favourable haemodynamic profile is etomidate. However, its use has been shown to suppress the functioning of the adrenal axis[13] and increase the incidence of Acute Respiratory Distress Syndrome (ARDS) and Multi Organ Dysfunction Syndrome (MODS).[14]

What MAP to Aim for? What Fluids to Use? How Much Fluid to Use?

In this case, the patient was hypotensive and tachycardic, signs consistent with ongoing haemorrhage. Following the primary survey, several potential sources were identified:

- Pulseless right arm
- Tender abdomen
- Haemothorax
- Pelvic fracture

Traditionally, haemorrhage in the polytrauma patient was treated with aggressive fluid resuscitation. Concerns arose, however, that excess fluid administration precipitated deleterious consequences such as;

- Worsening coagulopathy
- Excessive tissue oedema leading to complications such as abdominal compartment syndrome, acute respiratory distress syndrome and multi-organ failure.
- Excessive arterial pressure and flow that leads to clot disruption, attenuation of reflex vasoconstriction and further bleeding.

From this the concepts of 'hypotensive resuscitation' and 'low volume resuscitation' were developed. Studies from the early 1990s highlighted improved survival when low volume resuscitation was instigated before definitive treatment in theatre.[15] Retrospective reviews of the German Trauma Database demonstrated a worsening coagulopathy, compared with baseline, in those patients who received increasing volumes of resuscitation fluid (coagulopathy occurred in >40% of patients who had received >2000 ml, in >50% in patients who had received >3000 ml and >70% in patients who had received >4000 ml).[16]

Critics of hypotensive resuscitation question the methodology, and hence the general applicability of the evidence base which concentrates predominantly on penetrating rather than blunt trauma.[15] There are also concerns that 'permissive' hypotension can be deleterious in those patients who have a concurrent TBI. One single episode of hypotension (SBP<90 mmHg) in patients with a TBI has been shown to more than double mortality,[17] as an adequate cerebral perfusion pressure is vital to prevent secondary brain injury. The patient in this case had a GCS of 9 in the ED and a CT scan demonstrating a possible basal ganglial contusional haemorrhage. European guidelines updated in 2013 recommend that a mean arterial pressure of >80 mmHg is maintained in patients with combined haemorrhagic shock and severe TBI.[18] (Grade 1C)

With regards the choice of fluid to administer, there is no evidence to suggest the superiority of crystalloid over colloid in the trauma setting. The European guidelines[18] advocate the use of crystalloids in the resuscitative stage (evidence grade 1B), as a recent Cochrane review failed to demonstrate a survival advantage with colloids. Of note however, they recommend that hypotonic solutions, such as Ringer's lactate, are to be avoided in patients with severe head injury (Grade 1C). Colloid use, in particular hydroxyethyl starch (HES), in a recent meta-analysis, has been shown to increase the incidence of acute kidney injury AKI and coagulopathy.[19] As of April 2013, the UK's medicine's healthcare regulatory agency has suspended the license of HES for all indications.

When to Transfuse and What to Give?
Red Blood Cell Transfusion

Current European guidelines recommend transfusion to a target Haemoglobin (Hb) of at least 70 g/l.[16] These recommendations are based on the The Transfusion Requirements in Critical Care (TRICC) study,[20] which demonstrated no mortality difference in a liberal versus restrictive transfusion policy; i.e., a restrictive policy was just as safe. However the study looked at haemodynamically stable patients. When a subgroup analysis was performed on the 203 trauma patients within the study cohort, a similar conclusion was drawn for the trauma setting. Several studies have shown that excess transfusions are associated with increased morbidity and mortality: a RCT in patients with bleeding varices showed a significantly lower mortality at 45 days in the restrictive group (5%) as compared with the liberal group (9%) (P = 0.02)[21] Currently there are no prospective RCTs that address this practice in polytrauma patients or those who have sustained a traumatic brain injury.

Transfusion of Plasma and Platelets

Before hospital admission, approximately 25 per cent of severely injured trauma patients have an established coagulopathy, with an associated increase of multi-organ failure and death.[22] The concept of 'coagulopathy of trauma' has gained credibility and represents a situation whereby systemic anticoagulation and fibrinolysis are driven by severe haemorrhagic shock. When further dilution of endogenous clotting factors occurs, with red blood cell administration and liberal fluids but without exogenous coagulation factor administration, the coagulopathy worsens. The ideal ratio of packed red cells to fresh frozen plasma to platelets is yet to be determined. Recent combat military experience advocates a volume ratio of 1:1:1 as this most closely resembles whole blood. Retrospective reviews have demonstrated a reduced mortality in those polytrauma patients who received a higher plasma and platelet to RBC volume ratio (Mortality decreased from 66% to 19% following a decrease in the RBC:Plasma volume ratio from 8:1 to 2:1).[23] However these studies were retrospective and subject to significant survival bias. The prospective cohort PROMMITT study[24] demonstrated improved in-hospital mortality with RBC:plasma and RBC:platelet ratio <2:1 in the first 6 hours. Current UK guidelines state that FFP should be transfused in doses of 12 to 15ml/kg (at least 4 units in the average adult).[25]

European guidelines recommend that platelets be administered to maintain a count of >50 x 10^9/l and that this should increase to 100 x 10^9/l in patients with ongoing bleeding or TBI.[18] The evidence base supporting this threshold is drawn from a predominance of small observational studies, and there is still little understanding of the role that platelets play in traumatic coagulopathy.

Most hospitals in the United Kingdom have massive transfusion protocols, ensuring the immediate availability of blood and blood products. The benefit of routinely transfusing FFP and platelets in a fixed ratio to red cells ('shock Packs') in traumatic haemorrhage is still uncertain. In addition, the products are administered blindly, invariably without the availability of a patient's full blood count and coagulation profile. Future therapies will likely involve point-of-care testing where blood and blood product administration can be tailored to the individual patient needs.

Anti-fibrinolyitics

The patient in this case received 1 g of tranexamic acid in the pre-hospital setting and a further 1 g over the subsequent 8 hours. The CRASH-2 trial demonstrated that administration of this anti-fibrinolytic drug, within an hour of injury, significantly improved survival at 30 days compared with placebo.[26] Subsequently it has been incorporated into major haemorrhage protocols and is often administered in the pre-hospital setting.

Timing of the CT Scan

Following initial stabilisation of the patient in ED, he immediately underwent a whole body CT scan. A CT scan is now the investigation of choice for the polytrauma patient and is crucial in identifying injuries and planning targeted resuscitative treatment. A retrospective study from the German Trauma Society demonstrated a significantly increased rate of death in those patients with severe blunt trauma who did not have a whole body CT scan compared with those who did.[27]

The question of when to perform a scan and how much of the body to scan has also been debated. Traditional teaching stipulated that a patient needed to be stabilised before being transferred to the CT scanner, as treating an unstable patient in an isolated environment was likely to be fraught with difficulties and risk. With the advent of newer generation CT scans, comprehensive head, neck, thoracic and pelvic scans can now be acquired in a matter of minutes. Concerns regarding the ability of CT to detect hollow viscous injuries have been addressed with the administration of oral, rectal and intravenous contrast, with extravasation and bowel wall thickening signs that such an injury may have occurred.

The UK Trauma Audit and Research Network (TARN) has stated that the duration between a patients' arrival in ED and their CT scan being performed should no more than 30 minutes.

Damage Control Surgery and the Exploratory Laparotomy

The patient in the case above was expedited to theatre directly from the CT scanner for exploration of his axillary artery.

Damage control surgery has a role in the polytrauma patient;

- To control haemorrhage
- To achieve simple closure of a ruptured viscera
- To evacuate life threatening haematomas of the cranium and thorax
- To excise contaminated tissue and washout open fractures

Overall it is estimated that around 10 per cent of trauma patients would benefit from damage control surgery. Patient selection is crucial. Denying stable patients early definitive management of their injuries may lead to an increase in morbidity, mortality and additional avoidable interventions. However it can be lifesaving in unstable patients. Certain mechanisms and patterns of injury necessitate an exploratory laparotomy such as multiple penetrating injuries, high-energy blunt injuries to the torso, injuries across multiple compartments or combined vascular and visceral injuries.

Interventional radiological techniques can also be used to achieve rapid haemorrhage control, often with selective or unselective embolisation. This can be performed either prior to theatre to minimize further blood loss, or as an alternative to surgery. Short operating times aim to minimise the surgical insult, achieve physiological stability prior to transfer to the intensive care unit and necessitate further timely interventions.

Conclusion

Care of the polytrauma patient remains challenging. There is an evolving evidence base but it is clear that definitions need further consensus. Timely airway management, radiological assessment and intervention, along with optimal cardiovascular and haematological manipulation, have been demonstrated to improve outcome. This has been shown in the 2012/2013 TARN data which demonstrated a significant 19 per cent improvement in the probability of surviving trauma (ISS>8) in England,[6] evidence that the current structured approach to delivering care to the polytrauma patient is effective.

Key Learning Points

- Ketamine is a safe induction agent with a favourable haemodynamic profile and can be used in patients with a suspected traumatic brain injury.
- Caution should be exercised with permissive hypotension in the patient with a suspected traumatic brain injury. In this patient group, a MAP of at least 80 mmHg should be achieved.
- Early replacement of clotting products and platelets may attenuate the acute coagulopathy of trauma.
- Early use of tranexamic acid is safe and has been shown to improve 30-day survival.
- Aim for early transfer of the patient for definitive haemorrhage control to theatre or the angiography suite for damage control surgery.
- The ideal transfusion trigger in polytrauma patients is unknown but the evidence base available thus far supports a more restrictive approach.

References

1. National Audit Office: Major Trauma Care in the England 2010.

2. Butcher NE, Balogh ZJ. Update on the definition of Polytrauma. *European Journal of Trauma and Emergency Surgery* 2014; 40: 107–111.

3. Rosenfeld JV, Maas AI, Bragge P, Morganti-Kossmann MC, Manley GT, Gruen RL. Early management of severe traumatic brain injury. *Lancet* 2012; 380: 1088–98.

4. Kreis DJ, Plasencia G, Augenstein D et al. Preventable trauma deaths: Dade County, Florida. *J Trauma* 1986; 26: 649–54.

5. Cameron PA, Gabbe BJ, Cooper DJ et al. A statewide system of trauma care in Victoria: effect on patient survival. *Med J Aust* 2008; 10: 546–50.

6. McCullough AL, Haycock JC, Forward DP, Moran CG: Major trauma networks in England. *Br J Anaesth*. 2014; 113 (2): 202–6.

7. Miraflor E et al. Timing is everything: delayed intubation is associated with increased mortality in initially stable trauma patients. *Journal of Surgical Research* 2011; 170: 286–90.

8. Reich DL, Silvay G. Ketamine: an update on the first twenty-five years of clinical experience. *Canadian Journal of Anaesthesia* 1989; 36: 186–97.

9. Pandit JJ. Intravenous anaesthetic agents. *Anaesthesia and Intensive Care Medicine* 2008; 9: 154–9.

10. Hughes S. Towards evidence based emergency medicine: best BETs from the Manchester Royal Infirmary. BET 3: is ketamine a viable induction agent for the trauma patient with potential brain injury. *Emerg Med J*. 2011 Dec; 28 (12): 1076–7.

11. Bar-Joseph G, Guilburd Y, Guilburd J. Ketamine effectively prevents intracranial pressure elevations during endotracheal suctioning and other distressing interventions in patients with severe traumatic brain injury. *Crit Care Med* 2009; 37 (12 Suppl A402): 90–3493.

12. Sibley A, Mackenzie M, Bawden J, et al. A prospective review of the use of ketamine to facilitate endotracheal intubation in the helicopter emergency medical services (HEMS) setting. *Emerg Med J* 2011; 28: 521–5.

13. De Jong FH, Mallios C, Jansen C et al. Etomidate suppresses adrenocortical function by inhibition of 11 beta-hydroxylation. *J Clin Endocrinol Metab* 1984; 59: 1143–47.

14. Malerba G, Romano-Girard F, Cravoisy A, et al. Risk factors of relative adrenocortical deficiency in intensive care patients needing mechanical ventilation. *Intensive Care Med* 2005; 31: 388–92.

15. Bickell WH, Wall MJ, Pepe PE et al. Immediate versus delayed fluid resuscitation for hypotensive patients with penetrating torso injuries. *New England Journal of Medicine* 1994; 331: 1105–9.

16. Maegele M, Lefering R, Yucel N et al. Early coagulopathy in multiple injury: an analysis from the German Trauma Registry on 8724 patients. *Injury* 2007; 38(3): 298–304.

17. Wiles MD. Blood pressure management in trauma: from feast to famine? *Anaesthesia* 2013; 68: 445–52

18. Spahn et al. Management of bleeding and coagulopathy following major trauma: an updated European guideline. *Critical Care* 2013; 17: R76.

19. Zarychanski R et al. Association of hydorxyethyl starch administration with mortality and acute kidney injury in critically ill patients requiring volume resuscitation: a systemic review and meta-analysis. *JAMA* 2013; 309: 678–688.

20. Hebert PC, Wells G, Blajchman MA, Marshall J, Martic C, Pagilarello G, Tweedale M, Schweitzer I, Yetisir E. A multicenter, randomized, controlled clinical trial of transfusion requirements in critical care. Tranfusion requirements in the critical care trials group. *New England Journal of Medicine* 1999; 340(6): 409–17.

21. Villanueva C, Colomo A, Bosch A et al. Transfusion strategies for acute upper gastrointestinal haemorrhage. *New Enlgand Journal of Medicine* 2013; 368: 11–21.

22. Brohi K, Singh J, Heron M, Coats T. Acute traumatic coagulopathy. *J Trauma Injury Infect Crit Care* 2003; 54: 1127–30.

23. Borgman MA, Spinella PC, Perkins JG et al. The ratio of blood products transfused affects mortality in patients receiving massive transfusion at a combat support hospital. *J Trauma* 2007; 63: 805–13.

24. Holcomb JB, del Junco DJ, Fox EE, et al. The prospective, observational, multicenter, major trauma transfusion (PROMMITT) study: comparative effectiveness of a time-varying treatment with competing risks. *JAMA Surg* 2013; 148: 127–36.

25. Joint United Kingdom (UK) Blood Transfusion and Tissue Transplantaiton Services Professional Advisory Committee 2014.

26. The CRASH-2 collaborators. Effects of tranexamic acid on death, vascular occlusive events, and blood transfusion in trauma patients with significant haemorrhage (CRASH-2): a randomized placebo controlled trial. *Lancet* 2010; 376: 23–32.

27. Huber-Wagneer S, Lefering R, Qvick LM et al. Working group on polytrauma of the German trauma society. Effect of whole-body CT during trauma resuscitation on survival: a retrospective, multicenter study. *Lancet* 2009; 373: 1455–61.

Chapter 3

Management of Major Burns on the Intensive Care Unit

Tushar Mahambrey, Emma England and Will Loh

Introduction

Major burns are arguably the most devastating trauma an individual can suffer. They can precipitate a multi-system disorder and are often fatal. Survival comes with significant physical and psychological sequelae. It is estimated there are 250,000 cases of burns in the United Kingdom per annum, 175,000 of which involve individuals visiting the emergency department for treatment. Of those patients, around 13,000 are admitted to hospital and those needing ongoing major burns care or surgery will be transferred to one of 30 specialist UK burns units.[1]

There has been unprecedented progress in the care of burns patients over the past few decades with reductions in morbidity and mortality. Burns trauma represents major trauma and hence initial resuscitation and treatment should be based on standard guidelines e.g. the American College of Surgeons ATLS guidance.

This case outlines the evidence base behind current critical care management of major burns.

Case Study

A 19-year-old female sustained a 96 per cent thermal burns injury, mostly full thickness, during a road traffic accident. The patient was intubated at the scene and taken to the nearest hospital where a primary and secondary survey was undertaken. Her other injuries included rib fractures with pulmonary contusions and a kidney contusion.

Emergency fasciotomies were performed on all limbs. There was no clinical suggestion of major inhalational or lung injury although bronchoscopy could not be performed due to the small size 7 endotracheal tube used for intubation. Total fluid in the resuscitation period amounted to 44 litres as calculated with the Parkland formula and vasopressors were also required to sustain a perfusing mean arterial pressure (MAP). Feeding was started via a nasogastric tube and temperature was maintained, preventing hypothermia between dressing changes and aiming for an upper limit of a core temperature of 38.5 °C.

Following initial resuscitation and a four-day admission at the receiving hospital, she was transferred to the critical care unit at the specialist burns centre for tertiary level 3 care and further surgery.

Within the next 24 hours, she underwent debridement of chest and abdominal burns and implantation of cadaveric skin with skin biopsy for keratinocyte culture.

Peri-operatively she required a major transfusion with 10 units of packed red cells 4 units of fresh frozen plasma and 1 unit of platelets.

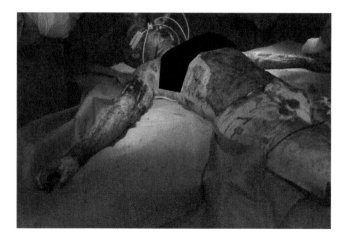

Figure 3.1 Image: intra-op wound debridement and grafting. A black and white version of this figure will appear in some formats. For the colour version, please refer to the plate section.

Sedation and analgesia were based on intravenous propofol with morphine and later midazolam with remifentanil for dressing changes, in addition to regular laxatives. Gabapentin via nasogastric tube was started early to reduce opioid requirements.

As facial swelling subsided, a larger endotracheal tube was placed and a dietician reviewed her for targeted calorie management at 35 Kcal/kg/day via nasogastric feeding. Swabs from wounds had grown Enterococcus, Group A streptococcus and Staph aureus that were treated with clindamycin. Central venous and arterial lines were replaced and meropenem and vancomycin were also continued. A selective digestive decontamination (SDD) regimen was started with 2 percent SDD paste containing amphotericin, colomycin and tobramycin.

In order to prevent muscle wasting, oxandrolone at 10 mg twice daily was given. Five days after transfer, a further trip to theatre comprised debridement and skin grafting to the neck in preparation for a tracheostomy and skin grafting of the abdomen. 6 units of red blood cells and 4 units of fresh frozen plasma were administered peri-operatively.

On day 10 the patient was immersed in the first of several baths in order to keep grafted skin clean and promote graft adherence and growth.

By day 11 a percutaneous tracheostomy was performed on the ICU and on day 12 a colostomy formed in theatre in order to prevent peri-anal, groin and buttock wound faecal contamination and aid in bowel management.

Whenever albumin levels dropped below 20 g/dl, 20 percent human albumin solution was used as colloid fluid replacement and when the haemoglobin fell to less than 80 g/l, the patient was transfused with packed red cells and on theatre days, a pre-operative haemoglobin of 120 g/l was the specified target.

A unified stepwise weaning programme was agreed upon with slow removal of sedation throughout the second month of admission, coupled with replacement of intravenous analgesics (opiates and clonidine) with enteral alternatives including methadone.

Burns nurse specialists had daily involvement with all over body dressings, including silver nitrate soaks. Ophthalmologists were regularly involved as eyelid grafting led to difficulty with closing the eyes and therefore corneal drying.

Daily microbiology ward rounds were critical to the patient's ongoing care. During admission, she developed a candidaemia and was colonised with pseudomonas and so long term antifungal therapy was prescribed along with anti-bacterial agents. Trans-thoracic echo showed no vegetations on the heart valves.

By the end of the second month of her admission, weaning progress was hampered by on-going sepsis and by a small pulmonary embolus mandating anticoagulation with low molecular weight heparin and specialist haematology input. Despite episodic complications, the patient progressed with weaning, resulting in tracheostomy de-cannulation three months following admission to the unit.

She had had multiple theatre trips, baths, constant multidisciplinary team (MDT) input with burns team and physiotherapy input and only days after decannulation, she left the intensive care unit for the burns high dependency unit. She is now back at home with regular outpatient follow up and ongoing surgical procedures to improve limb function and aesthetic outcome.

Discussion

The journey of any patient with major burns is usually long and complicated and thus needs a multi-disciplinary approach, ideally in a specialist intensive care unit. Estimation of the total burn surface area can be assessed using the rule of nines in adults (including only areas of partial and full thickness burn). This will give a rough guide to initial fluid resuscitation when using the Parkland formula and also guide decisions as to the severity of the burn and need for referral to a specialist centre.

Specialist considerations in critical care include:

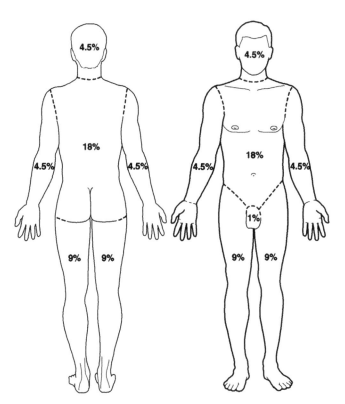

Figure 3.2 Rule of nines chart: adult burn assessment.

Ventilation

On admission to intensive care, the level 3 burn-injured patient should have strict ventilatory parameters set. The aim is to optimise oxygenation, recruiting healthy and affected lung whilst preventing secondary lung injury through over ventilation. Low tidal volume ventilation between 4–6 ml/kg, allowing permissive hypercapnia, has been shown to reduce the development of ventilator associated lung injury and improve outcomes.[2,3] Acute lung injury (ALI) and acute respiratory distress syndrome (ARDS) will often occur in major burns as a result of a general systemic inflammatory response or as a direct consequence of inhalational injury. Patho-physiological consequences are related to altered capillary permeability, leading to proteinaceous fluid leaking from the intra vascular compartment to the interstitial space, in turn leading to increase in intra pulmonary shunt, reduction in alveolar diffusing capacity and hypoxaemia.

Current management strategies therefore also still include prone positioning, high frequency percussive ventilation, high frequency oscillator ventilation (HFOV) and extracorporeal membrane oxygenation (ECMO) for refractory hypoxaemia.

Bronchoscopy

Lung injury resulting from smoke inhalation or chemical products of combustion continues to be associated with significant mortality and morbidity. Combined with cutaneous burns, inhalational injury increases fluid resuscitation requirements, the incidence of pulmonary complications and doubles the mortality of thermal injury. The mechanism for lung injury in the burn injured patient is multifactorial: both direct due to pulmonary and upper airway inhalational injury and indirect due to SIRS induced ARDS and then pneumonia and sepsis.[3]

The diagnosis of inhalational injury is a subjective assessment based largely on history of smoke exposure in an enclosed space. Physical findings – including facial injury, singed nasal hairs, soot in the proximal airways, carbonaceous sputum production and changes in voice – may help support the diagnosis. These findings can be confirmed by performing a fibre-optic bronchoscopy, typically within the first 24 hours.

Early bronchoscopy helps in assessing the extent of airway and direct lung injury as well as aiding in the clearance of secretions, carbon affected epithelium and epithelial sloughing.

Circulation

Improving fluid resuscitation techniques have been central to recent advances and prompt crystalloid transfusion is directed to prevent burns shock from hypovolaemia. Early fluid therapy cannot normalise the cardiovascular response to major burns but is aimed at damage limitation. In the first 24 hours and beyond, the aim is to replace massive fluid loss by replenishing intravascular volume and therefore improve organ perfusion. These aims are balanced against the risk of fluid overload, potential worsening of ALI and ARDS and compartment syndromes in various parts of the body.

Early balanced crystalloid resuscitation should begin according to recognised resuscitation formulae, e.g., the Parkland formula at 4 ml/kg/percent burn from the time of the burn: half the volume should be given in the first 8 hours and the other half should be given in the next 16 hours. Resuscitation is titrated to endpoints including urine output of

30–50 ml/hr and haemodynamic parameters.[4] The difficulty with fluid resuscitation in the burned patient is in the assessment of objective endpoints.

Currently, urine output and standard haemodynamic parameter measurement targets define our resuscitation endpoints despite the fact that an 'ideal' target urine output is ill-defined. The American Burn Association (ABA) guidelines target 0.5 ml/kg/hr urine output in adults in keeping with the parameters of the Parkland resuscitation formula and certainly a urine output below this is likely to represent inadequate crystalloid administration in the early stages of resuscitation. Again, ideal targets in terms of haemodynamic variables are likely to be patient dependent. A heart rate below 110 beats per minute with a MAP above 65 and targeted urine output of 0.5 ml/kg/hr can be combined with a low or reducing lactate and improving base deficit on arterial blood sample to give a fair assessment of the success of ongoing resuscitation. Recently, the increased use of sedation and analgesics, leading to vasodilatation, has also contributed to the increased fluid requirement in these patients.[3]

The current high volume resuscitation has shifted post-burn resuscitation complications from renal failure to pulmonary oedema and abdominal compartment syndrome leading to multi-organ failure also termed as 'fluid creep'.[5] Protein leak into the interstitial space is also part of the pathophysiology of shock in the burn-injured patient and previous volume resuscitation techniques have advocated the use of albumin. Intuitively this reduces the need for crystalloid use and potentially the overall fluid requirement, although use of albumin is currently still empirically based on maintaining a serum level above 20 g/dl as in this case.

Transfusion

Haemoglobin count will drop in the major burn-injured patient. This will depend on the extent and depth of burn and the number and extent of surgical interventions, along with regular phlebotomy on intensive care. Often the burn injured intensive care patient will need several blood transfusions during the course of their illness but the trigger for transfusion remains controversial.

Significant drops in haemoglobin with red blood cell destruction and haemodilution can impair oxygen carriage at a time when organs and surviving dermal tissues have high metabolic and therefore high oxygen requirements. In critically ill patients, the consensus has been for a restrictive transfusion strategy following the TRICC trial[6] although burn-injured patients were not included in this trial and a trial in this group is ongoing.[7] A multicenter study by Palmieri et al.,[7] found a 10 per cent increased risk of infection for every blood transfusion given outside the operating room and increased mortality in burns patients associated with blood transfusion. Thus there is a push to decrease blood transfusion in burns patients. Surgical interventions can predictably cause huge blood loss with or without haemodynamic instability. Common practice for such patients is to have a high haemoglobin target pre-operatively to allow for large haemoglobin drops peri-operatively, although there is no consensus over what that target should be in any given burn excision. This difference currently renders it difficult to translate results regarding liberal and conservative transfusion strategies into general critical care burns practice.

Nutrition

Severe burns induce a hyper-metabolic systemic inflammatory response syndrome-(SIRS) like state which could persist for up to one year following injury. This leads to an increase in protein catabolism and lipolysis, leading to reduced lean mass and poor wound healing with a weakened immune system. Severe burns can also lead to hypothalamic dysfunction and altered temperature regulation, along with increases in catecholamine production and release. Severe burns also pre-dispose the patient to sepsis and reduce the ability to sustain wound healing.

Providing adequate nutrition is a delicate balance between meeting the patient's metabolic demands and avoiding overfeeding. Measuring or estimating an individual patient's calorific demands, however, can be problematic. To counteract the hyper-metabolic state, most authors recommend prevention of infectious complications, adequate calorie intake via early enteral feeding, avoidance of overfeeding and early excision of full thickness burns[3] as in this patient.

Hyperglycaemia occurs in most major burns patients as a result of increased production and reduced utilisation of glucose with the stress response. It is strictly controlled using individual hospital protocols for insulin infusion. Enteral beta blockade with Propranolol has shown in various studies to aid glycaemic control, reduce peripheral lipolysis and enhance immune response to sepsis during severe burn injury by slowing the hyper-metabolic state.[9]

Anabolic Steroids

Major burns patients lose muscle mass in a hyper-catabolic state. Anabolic steroids like oxandrolone have been shown to help in promoting protein synthesis, nitrogen retention and therefore skeletal muscle growth. A multicentre randomised controlled trial in burns patients[8] showed enteral oxandrolone, a synthetic analogue and one twentieth the potency of testosterone, given at 10 mg/day twelve hourly, reduced hospital stay by 28 percent. However, its use still remains controversial and studies are ongoing to show a clear benefit.

Infective Complications

While mortality from burns shock has greatly improved, major burns patients are now surviving to suffer the consequences of hospital exposure to micro-organisms. Through burns wounds, prolonged ventilation, intra vascular lines and urinary catheterisation, the burn-injured patient is susceptible to infections and multi-resistant organisms without the benefit of the usual host defence mechanisms or a normal immune response. Diagnosis of infection is often clouded, as a high leucocyte count, pyrexia and tachycardia are expected responses to the burn, yet can also reflect newly developing sepsis and delay treatment.

Wound care remains vital in the prevention and treatment of cutaneous infection. Chlorhexidine or saline washes on a daily basis can reduce colonisation as can strict barrier nursing with careful hygiene precautions.

Common topical agents for wound care – including silver sulfadiazine, mafenide acetate and silver nitrate – all have a role in the effective management of colonised wounds; however, they have an array of side effects like reduction of epithelial healing, and require daily changes. Newer silver-impregnated dressings such as aquacel need less frequent changes and also provide anti-microbial coverage.

De La Cal[10] published a randomised controlled trial into the use of selective digestive tract decontamination (SDD) in the level 3 burn injured patient. The study used cefotaxime systemically compared with tobramycin, polymixin B and amphotericin enterally as solution or paste. The study demonstrated that for every five burns patients treated with SDD without any immediately obvious side effects, one patient could be saved. Since that study

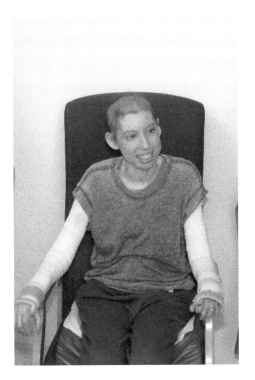

Figure 3.3 Image: patient attending for outpatient follow up. A black and white version of this figure will appear in some formats. For the colour version, please refer to the plate section.

55 randomised controlled trials and meta-analysis have likewise shown survival benefit. Clearly, in the future major burns patients will face the prospect of infection with new multi-resistant organisms.

Conclusion

Regional burn centres have developed to address resource requirements and the complexity of burn care. There have been significant improvements in survival outcomes following burn injuries and this can be attributed to advances in some key areas. Developments in fluid resuscitation strategies, wound care and early surgical intervention, nutritional support, control of the hyper-metabolic state and the diagnosis and treatment of infection have all contributed to improved burns care and outcomes. This case study is an example of the rapidly advancing quality of care delivered in tertiary centres for major burns patients.

Key Learning Points

- Progress in the care of burns patients has considerably improved outcomes with reductions in morbidity and mortality, but survival comes with significant physical and psychological sequelae
- Patients with significant burns or those with burns to key areas, e.g., face and hands, should be managed in a tertiary burns centre as soon as such a transfer is possible.
- Major burns can precipitate a multi-system disorder.
- MDT input is vital to manage both the initial injuries and complications that may develop.

References

1. NBCR, National Burn Care Review, Standards and Strategy for Burn Care in the British Isles. 2001, British Burns Association: Manchester. www .britishburnsassociation.org/downloads/ NBCR2001.pdf(Accessed June 2014).

2. The Acute Respiratory Distress Syndrome Network. Ventilation with lower tidal volumes as compared with traditional tidal volumes for acute lung injury. *N Engl J Med* 2000;342:1301–8.

3. Ipaktchi K, Arbabi S. Advances in burn critical care. *Critical Care Med* 2006;34(9): Suppl 239–44.

4. Pruit BA Jr. Fluid and electrolyte replacement in the burned patient. *Surg Clin N Am* 1978;58:1291–1312.

5. Pruitt BA. Protection from excessive resuscitation: 'Pushing the pendulum back'. *J Trauma* 2000;49:567–8.

6. Hébert PC, Wells G, Blajchman MA, et al. A multicenter, randomized, controlled clinical trial of transfusion requirements in critical care. Transfusion Requirements in Critical Care. *N Engl J Med* 1999; 340:409–17.

7. Palmeiri TL, Caruso DM, Foster KN et al. Impact of blood transfusion on outcome after major burn injury: a multicentre study. *Crit Care Med* 2006;34: 1602–7.

8. Wolf SE, Edelman LS, Kemalyan N et al. Effects of oxandrolone on outcome measures in the severely burned: a multicenter prospective randomized double-blind trial. *J Burn Care Res.* 2006; 27(2):131–9.

9. Norbury WB, Jeschke MG, Herndon DN. Metabolism modulation in sepsis: propranolol. *Crit Care Med* 2007;35(9 suppl):S616–20.

10. de La Cal MD, Cerdá E, García-Hierro P, et al. Survival benefit in critically ill burned patients receiving selective decontamination of the digestive tract a randomized, placebo-controlled, double-blind trial. *Ann Surg.* 2005;241(3): 424–30.

Management of Sepsis

Chris Thorpe

Introduction

Septic shock kills around 37,000 patients a year in the United Kingdom. Although attempts have been made to find specific treatments, evolving evidence has cast doubt on the effectiveness of many therapies that target the inflammatory response that characterises sepsis and septic shock. Current best practice therefore is based around prompt diagnosis, source control and early antibiotic administration, accompanied by attentive resuscitation and expert intensive care management of organ failure.

This case describes a patient managed along these lines and reviews the evidence base for some of the therapies.

Case Report

A 59-year-old man was admitted to the intensive care unit (ICU) following a laparotomy and subsequent colostomy for an anastomotic leak.

Two weeks after a sigmoid colectomy for carcinoma of the bowel, he developed abdominal pain, vomiting, tachycardia and pyrexia. He was started on antibiotics after blood cultures had been drawn, and a CT scan was ordered which showed significant free air in the abdomen along with pulmonary emboli in both lung bases. He was subsequently taken to the operating theatre where the surgeon found faecal peritonitis. During the operation, he developed hypotension and worsening acidosis and was started on noradrenaline, which reached a rate of 0.914 mcg/kg/min by the end of surgery.

On admission to the ICU he was intubated and ventilated, with sedation maintained by a propofol infusion. He had a right femoral arterial line and a right internal jugular central venous catheter in place. His temperature was 38.1°C, he had cool peripheries, a heart rate of 111 beats/minute, a blood pressure of 105/65 mmHg and a central venous pressure of 15 cm H_2O. Auscultation revealed vesicular breath sounds throughout and his gas exchange was acceptable with an inspired oxygen fraction of 0.4. He had passed an average of 20 ml/hour of urine while in theatre.

Blood results confirmed an acidosis, with a pH of 7.15 and a base deficit of −7.5 mmol/l. His lactate was 5.3 mmol/l. He had a haemoglobin concentration of 10.5 g/dl, a white cell count of 14.9 and a platelet count of 339. Electrolytes were within the normal range, his urea was 8mmol/l and he had an elevated creatinine of 121 µmol/l compared with a baseline of 94 µmol/l a week previously. An electrocardiograph showed ST elevation in leads I and aVL with ST depression in leads III and aVR. Serum Troponin T showed a significant rise in concentration from 7 on admission to 214 at 6 hours.

Ventilation was altered to deliver tidal volumes of 6 ml/kg and sedation was maintained with infusions of propofol and alfentanil. A pulse index contour cardiac output (PICCO) monitor was inserted in the left femoral artery and revealed an indexed cardiac output of 3.84 l/min/m^2 and a low indexed systemic vascular resistance. The decision tree accompanying the PICCO monitor was used to help guide fluid resuscitation and vasopressor use. Initially 4 per cent succinylated gelatin fluid boluses were administered on a background of a maintenance infusion of Hartmann's solution. Hydrocortisone was started as an infusion at 10 mg/hr. Lactate concentration was reduced to 2.4 mmol/l following initial resuscitation on the ICU.

Piperacillin/tazobactam and metronidazole had already been started prior to theatre and gentamicin was added to this. Stress ulcer prophylaxis was commenced with Omeprazole and Chlorhexidine mouthwash was started to help prevent ventilator-associated pneumonia. Prophylactic dose enoxaparin was administered 6 hours after surgery. Full anticoagulation to address the pulmonary emboli demonstrated on the CT scan was withheld in the immediate postoperative period to avoid increased bleeding risk and was begun on day 2. Total parenteral nutrition was started on day 1 and blood glucose was maintained below 10.0 mmol/l by an insulin infusion.

Over the next three days, vasopressor requirements remained high. Adrenaline was added to noradrenaline on day 2 to improve cardiac output and maintain a mean arterial pressure above 65 mmHg. The patient remained in an overall positive fluid balance and developed peripheral oedema. Renal function continued to deteriorate and continuous venovenous haemodiafiltration (CVVHD) was instituted on day 2. His lungs remained clear, with a PaO2 greater than 9 kPa on an inspired oxygen fraction of 0.4. Permissive hypercapnia as a result of low tidal volume ventilation led to PaCO2 levels between 6.1 kPa and 7.1 kPa.

By day 5 vasopressor requirements had reduced considerably, and the patient was receiving noradrenaline at 0.19 mcg/kg/min. Hydrocortisone was discontinued and the PICCO line was removed. By day 8 renal function had recovered enough for the CVVHD to be discontinued. Although gas exchange remained good, the patient developed a degree of neuromuscular weakness, and he was subsequently extubated on day 10. Bowel function returned and the stoma started to function around this time, with oral diet eventually established on day 12. He still had global neuromuscular weakness and had continued physiotherapy over the next two weeks.

He was eventually discharged home 32 days after his admission to the ICU, and was reviewed at an outpatient appointment two months later. He had continued to improve but was still housebound for the most part. Weakness and reduced appetite were the principle problems at this point.

Discussion

Epidemiology and Definitions of Sepsis

The incidence of sepsis has increased over recent years. It is uncertain to what extent this is due a genuine increase in the disease process in an increasingly elderly and vulnerable population or reflects at least in part an increased awareness and diagnosis by medical staff. In the United States the method of coding for insurance purposes has altered in this time, and this is thought to have been partially responsible.[1] Heightened awareness of sepsis has been reinforced by a variety of sepsis protocols and early warning scores aimed at improving outcome.

This patient had a known infective source with signs of SIRS and organ dysfunction and fulfilled the criteria for severe sepsis (Boxes 4.1 and 4.2).

Furthermore, his sepsis-induced hypotension persisted despite adequate fluid resuscitation, and therefore he had septic shock.[2] Appropriate antibiotics had already been commenced and resuscitation started at that point.

Care Bundles

Early diagnosis and better treatment of sepsis is an essential part of improving outcomes and the use of early warning scores and sepsis protocols have entered common practice. Care bundles have been developed to ensure that best evidence is translated into practice,

---

Box 4.1 Diagnostic criteria for sepsis (from the Surviving Sepsis Campaign[2])

Definition of Sepsis: Infection, documented or suspected, and some of the following:

General variables

Temperature >38.3 or <36°C
Heart rate >90 beats/min or more than two standard deviations above the normal value for age
Tachypnea
Altered mental status
Significant edema or positive fluid balance (>20 mL/kg over 24 hours)
Hyperglycemia (plasma glucose >140 mg/dL or 7.7 mmol/l) in the absence of diabetes

Inflammatory variables

Leukocytosis (WBC count >12,000 /mm^3) or leukopenia (WBC count <4000 mm^3)
Normal WBC count with greater than 10 percent immature forms
Plasma C-reactive protein more than two standard deviations above the normal value
Plasma procalcitonin more than two standard deviations above the normal value

Hemodynamic variables

Arterial hypotension: systolic blood pressure <90 mmHg, MAP <70 mmHg, or an systolic blood pressure decrease >40 mmHg in adults or less than two standard deviations below normal for age)

Organ dysfunction variables

Arterial hypoxemia (arterial oxygen tension [PaO2]/fraction of inspired oxygen [FiO2] <300)
Acute oliguria (urine output <0.5 mL/kg/hr for at least two hours despite adequate fluid resuscitation)
Creatinine increase >0.5 mg/dL or 44.2 µmol/L
Coagulation abnormalities (international normalized ratio [INR] >1.5 or activated partial thromboplastin time [aPTT] >60 seconds)
Ileus (absent bowel sounds)
Thrombocytopenia (platelet count <100,000/mm^3)
Hyperbilirubinemia (plasma total bilirubin >4 mg/dL or 70 µmol/L)
Tissue perfusion variables
Hyperlactatemia (>1 mmol/L)
Decreased capillary refill or mottling

Box 4.2 Severe sepsis criteria (from the Surviving Sepsis campaign[2]). Sepsis-induced hypotension is defined as a systolic blood pressure (SBP) <90 mmHg or mean arterial pressure (MAP) <70 mmHg or a SBP decrease >40 mmHg or less than two standard deviations below normal for age in the absence of other causes of hypotension

Severe sepsis refers to sepsis-induced tissue hypoperfusion or organ dysfunction with any of the following thought to be due to the infection:

Sepsis-induced hypotension
Lactate above upper limits of laboratory normal
Urine output <0.5 mL/kg/hr for more than two hours despite adequate fluid resuscitation
Acute lung injury with PaO2/FIO2 <250 in the absence of pneumonia as infection source
Acute lung injury with PaO2/FIO2 <200 in the presence of pneumonia as infection source
Creatinine >2 mg/dL (176.8 µmol/L)
Bilirubin >4 mg/dL (34.2 µmol/L)
Platelet count <100,000 /mm3
Coagulopathy (INR >1.5)

Box 4.3 Resuscitation bundles (from the Surviving Sepsis Campaign[2])

Surviving Sepsis 3-Hour Resuscitation Bundle to be completed within 3 hours of presentation with severe sepsis:

Measure lactate level
Obtain blood cultures prior to administration of antibiotics
Administer broad spectrum antibiotics
Administer 30 ml/kg crystalloid for hypotension or lactate ≥ 4 mmol/l

Surviving sepsis 6-Hour Resuscitation Bundle to be completed within 6 hours of presentation with severe sepsis:

Apply vasopressors (for hypotension that does not respond to initial fluid resuscitation to maintain a mean arterial pressure (MAP) ≥ 65mmHg
In the event of persistent arterial hypotension despite volume resuscitation or initial lactate ≥ 4 mmol/l:

Measure Central Venous Pressure: target ≥ 8 mmHg
Measure Central Venous Oxygen Saturation: target ≥ 70 per cent

Remeasure lactate if initial lactate was elevated

and the use of care bundles for sepsis have been championed by the Surviving Sepsis Campaign (Box 4.3).

One of the advantages of care bundles is that they can be easily adapted as new evidence becomes available. For example use of activated protein C has been removed and glycaemic control parameters adjusted in the light of new research since the sepsis care bundles were first developed.

Adherence to sepsis care bundles appears to impact patient survival. A study from the Netherlands demonstrated that implementation of a sepsis programme improved both sepsis bundle compliance and adjusted inpatient mortality in screened patients with severe sepsis and septic shock, with a reduction in absolute mortality equivalent to 5.8 percent when compared with non-participating hospitals.[3] The effectiveness of the bundles is inevitably linked to an appropriate diagnosis and a robust screening programme should be in place throughout the hospital to enable the early use of antibiotics once the diagnosis is made. Every hour delayed in first antibiotic administration increases mortality, and a linear relationship has been shown between mortality and time to first antibiotic over the first 6 hours, with adjusted mortality deteriorating from 24.6% at 0–1 hours to 33.1% at more than 6 hours.[4] Wherever possible, microbiological samples should be obtained prior to antibiotics being given, as in this case.

Not all prospective trials have shown a benefit for protocol driven care. In 2014 The PROCESS trial investigators compared protocol based early goal directed therapy (EGDT) against both protocol based non-EGDT and non-protocol based care and found no difference in outcome,[5] contradicting earlier findings by Rivers in 2001. Similarly early warning scores and rapid response teams should intuitively provide better outcomes but it has been difficult to provide evidence of benefit. Early resuscitation and antibiotic use remain, however, the cornerstone of successful treatment.

Shock

Initial management of the hypotensive septic patient commences with fluid resuscitation, and the patient had already received 4 l of saline and 1 l of 4% succinylated gelatin in theatre before arrival on the ICU.

The goal for mean arterial blood pressure (MAP) was set at >65 mmHg. The surviving sepsis campaign recommends maintaining a MAP of greater than 65 mmHg. Increasing this target to 80–85 mmHg has no impact on adjusted mortality, with higher target patients experiencing an increased incidence of atrial fibrillation (6.7% vs 2.8%). In patients with chronic hypertension, a higher blood pressure target was associated with shortened time needed for renal replacement therapy suggesting some protective effect on kidney function.[8]

The shock observed in severe sepsis can have more than one component and it is important to guard against missing other causes that may contribute to this. An ECG on admission to the ICU showed new ischaemic changes, which settled 18 hours later. The troponin T rise was considered non-specific and potentially related to sepsis, primary myocardial ischaemia or pulmonary emboli as reported on the CT scan, and therefore there was no indication for further treatment beyond the anticoagulation already in place.

Fluids in Sepsis

The choice of fluid for resuscitation has undergone considerable debate. Hydroxyethyl starch (HES) worsens outcome and should be avoided: HES 6% carries a 21% relative increase in the need for renal replacement therapy compared with saline. The use of gelatin as a fluid bolus in this patient reflected the practice of the hospital but is not supported by current evidence. Although there is uncertainty about the relative merits of gelatins and crystalloids, current opinion is that there is no clinical advantage of gelatins over crystalloids in volume expansion, and there is a lack of robust safety information available. These factors accompanied by the increased cost of gelatins make crystalloids the current resuscitation of choice. Albumin replacement in addition to crystalloids confers no advantage in survival and the use of blood products should be limited to those who are likely to breach the transfusion trigger. Overall there is no evidence to use any fluid in preference to crystalloids as a plasma expander. Although balanced salt solutions have a theoretical advantage in avoiding the hyperchloraemic acidosis associated with saline, there is no clear evidence that this affects long-term outcome. In practice the crystalloid chosen takes account of the patient's electrolyte and acid base profile.

Vasoactive Agents

Despite adequate fluid replacement, hypotension was still an issue in this case and nor-adrenaline therapy was commenced. The use of vasopressors and inotropes to maintain perfusion pressure in septic shock is universally accepted but there is no overwhelming evidence to guide us as to which drug to use. In general, vasopressors are used for patients in vasodilatory shock and noradrenaline remains the first line treatment. Trials have shown noradrenaline superior to dopamine, which causes an increase in dysrhythmias (24.1% vs 12.4%), and preferable to vasopressin as a first line therapy. In this patient, adrenaline was added to provide inotropic support to improve cardiac output. Adrenaline can cause a degree of lactic acidosis and other inotropes, for example dobutamine, could equally well have been chosen. Vasopressin can be used as a second line treatment in vasodilatory shock and although overall it has not been found to improve outcome over noradrenaline support, a posthoc analysis of data derived from the VASST trial has suggested that patients receiving steroid therapy might benefit from vasopressin, with a reduction in mortality from 44.7% to 35.9%. In the same analysis patients without steroid therapy had a worse outcome with addition of vasopressin, with mortality increasing from 21.3% to 33.7%.[6] Although this is not conclusive evidence, it would seem reasonable to ensure that patients have been started on glucocorticoids when commencing vasopressin.

Cardiovascular Monitoring

The balance between fluids, vasopressors and inotropes was guided in this patient by the use of a PICCO monitor. Measurement of cardiac output is widely used to monitor the critically ill patient and can be helpful in guiding management. There is no evidence, however, that cardiac output monitoring is any better than clinical assessment and the use of PICCO in this case was a result of local practice rather than any evidence base. Other methods of guiding management can equally be used. For example fluid responsiveness may be assessed by stroke volume variation and by echocardiography for assessing myo-cardial function. Recent evidence has shown that in the United Kingdom more frequent use of cardiac output monitoring does not translate into improved survival.[7]

Use of Steroids

Addition of hydrocortisone is appropriate in septic patients who need an escalating dose of vasopressor to maintain perfusion pressure despite adequate fluid filling, and was therefore started in our patient. The pathophysiology behind sepsis is complex and not completely understood. There is an increase in proinflammatory and antiinflammatory processes and the holy grail of sepsis research lies in the assumption that this response can be manipu-lated to minimise any organ damage. The cascade of inflammatory mediators, altered gene transcription and molecular processes provide many potential targets for treatment but the effects of interrupting the natural host response cannot easily be predicted. At present the only immunomodulating treatment in common use is glucocorticoid treat-ment. The use of steroids received a renaissance with the publication of Annane's paper in 2002 showing that a combination of mineralocorticoid and glucocorticoid administration improved outcomes in septic patients with 'relative adrenal insufficiency' – that is in those patients who did not achieve an appropriate glucocorticoid response to the short synacthen test. Subsequently the CORTICUS trial did not confirm any benefit from the use of glucocorticoids in septic patients, and this has led to uncertainty about the role of steroids in septic shock.[9]

Nutrition

This patient did not establish full nutrition at any point following his original operation two weeks previously, and was malnourished as a result. Enteral nutrition was not possible postoperatively and parenteral nutrition was therefore started early, as the assumption was made that the patient had less reserve to cope with a further period of starvation.

Patients with sepsis are in a strong catabolic state. The combination of critical illness and immobility leads to rapid muscle loss and providing appropriate nutrition to counter this has been heavily researched. The body has natural mechanisms to deal with illness and it has become apparent that an approach that loads the body with food to offset this does not necessarily help. Early enteral nutrition is accepted as helpful but not all patients can tolerate this in the acute phase of illness. There is some evidence that if full feeding is not possible, low levels of enteral feed can help preserve gut cell structure and so this 'trophic' level of feed should be used if possible. If the enteral route is not possible, parenteral nutrition can be considered. Parenteral nutrition has historically led to worse outcomes, possibly through overfeeding, hyperglycaemia and increased infective risk; however, more recent research is equivocal. Supplemental parenteral nutrition to top up trophic level enteral feeding does not help in the previously well-nourished patient. A period of reduced nutrition of up to a week does not seem to worsen outcome and it would seem reasonable to wait if enteral nutrition is likely to be established within this timeframe in a previously well-nourished patient.[10]

Other Supportive Care

A raft of general measures was introduced to support patients during their stay in the ICU. Supportive care has transformed over recent years to a less aggressive approach than previously. Rather than trying to normalise physiological variables by pushing organ function, the rationale is to rest organs as much as possible during this period of stress while maintaining an environment that allows the patient to survive. Low tidal volume ventilation and the use of renal replacement therapy are examples of this approach, both of which were used successfully in this patient. Other supportive measures are based on best available evidence and include prophylaxis against deep vein thrombosis and stress ulcers, avoiding continuous heavy sedation, and incorporating sedation holds to allow the patient to waken and reducing time spent receiving ventilation. Generally it is best to avoid neuromuscular blockade although 48 hours of paralysis has been used effectively in early ARDS, and this can be considered in patients with poor gas exchange. This patient had good gas exchange and compliance; therefore, neuromuscular blockade was not used.

Follow up studies for patients admitted to intensive care with septic shock have shown that, as in this case, a significant proportion experience a protracted recovery with persistent neuromuscular and musculoskeletal problems. Early and ongoing physiotherapy could potentially help alleviate some of these problems; however, the best approach to minimising these ongoing problems has yet to be elucidated.

Conclusion

The treatment of patients with sepsis has benefitted considerably from a heightened awareness of the disease process and expert implementation of standardised management. Despite this, sepsis remains one of the most common causes of death and improving early diagnosis and treatment of infection currently holds the best chance of further improving outcome.

Key Learning Points

- Sepsis is common and life threatening.
- Early diagnosis and treatment are essential, with delay in antibiotic administration increasing mortality.
- Care bundles aid implementation of best practice and can be adapted as new evidence emerges.
- Recovery from septic shock is protracted and patients may have impaired function for years.

References

1. Rhee C, Gohil S, Klompas M. Regulatory mandates for sepsis care: reasons for caution. N Engl J Med 2014;370(18): 1673–6.

2. Dellinger RP, Levy MM, Rhodes A, et al. Surviving sepsis campaign: international guidelines for management of severe sepsis and septic shock: 2012. Crit Care Med 2013 Feb;41(2):580–637.

3. Van Zanten ARH, Brinkman S, Arbous MS, Abu-Hanna A, Levy MM, de Keizer NF. Guideline Bundles Adherence and Mortality in Severe Sepsis and Septic Shock. Crit Care Med 2014 Aug;42(8): 1890–8.

4. R Ferrer, I Martin-Loeches, G Phillips, et al. Empiric antibiotic treatment reduces mortality in severe sepsis and septic shock from the first hour: results from a guideline-based performance improvement program. Crit Care Med 2014 Apr 8;42(8): 1749–55.

5. Yealy DM, Kellum J A, Huang DT, Barnato AE, Weissfeld L A, Pike F, et al. A randomized trial of protocol-based care for early septic shock. N Engl J Med 2014 May 1;370(18):1683–93.

6. Russell J A, Walley KR, Gordon AC, Cooper DJ, Hébert PC, Singer J, et al. Interaction of vasopressin infusion, corticosteroid treatment, and mortality of septic shock. Crit Care Med 2009 Mar;37 (3):811–18.

7. Ridley S, Harrison DA, Walmsley E, Harvey S, Rowan KM. The Cardiac Output Monitoring EvaluaTion–UK (COMET-UK) study. J Intensive Care Soc 2014;15(1): 12–17.

8. Asfar P, Meziani F, Hamel J-F, et al. High versus low blood-pressure target in patients with septic shock. N Engl J Med 2014 Apr 24;370(17):1583–93.

9. Sprung CL, Annane D, Keh D, et al. Hydocortisone therapy for patients with septic shock. N Engl J Med 2008 Jan 10; 358(2):111–24.

10. Casaer MP, Mesotten D, Hermans G, et al. Early versus late parenteral nutrition in critically ill adults. N Engl J Med 2011 Aug 11;365(6):506–17.

Rhabdomyolysis

Ingi Elsayed and Ajay H Raithatha

Introduction

The epidemiology of acute kidney injury (AKI) remains imprecise. The prevalence of AKI from US data varies between 1.1 and 7.1% of hospital admissions. Data from the UK Intensive Care National Audit and Research Centre (ICNARC) Case Mix Programme (CMP), reported a 6.3% incidence of severe AKI during first 24 hours of admission to ICU, with AKI accounting for 9.3% of all ICU bed-days.[1] It is estimated that about 5% of general ICU patients will require treatment with renal replacement therapy (RRT). Mortality attributable to AKI varies in different reports, from 10% (in uncomplicated AKI) up to 80% in patients with multi-organ failure who also require RRT.

Case Description

A 78 year old male with a past medical history of mild hypertension, hypercholesterolaemia and smoking was admitted to the emergency department, having been found on the floor of his house by a concerned neighbour. The patient was known to live alone and be fully independent with activities of daily living. Of note, medication history revealed he took regular bendrofluazide (2.5 mg), ramipril (5 mg) and atorvastatin (20 mg). His nephew stated he had last seen him three days before. On admission, external examination showed he was cool to touch, and had carpet burn marks and unilateral bruising to his right side. Other findings included hypotension (blood pressure 72/34 mmHg), hypoxia (SpO$_2$ 92% on 15 l/min via a non-rebreathe mask), tachycardia (122 beats per minute) and hypothermia with a core temperature of 34.5 degrees Celsius. Chest auscultation demonstrated right sided bronchial breathing and coarse crepitations. On neurological examination, his Glasgow Coma Score (GCS) was 6/15 (E2 V1 M3), blood glucose was 4.1 mmol/L and there was a right-sided facial droop, in addition to increased right-sided tone with a right-sided extensor plantar reflex.

The patient was intubated and ventilated by the critical care team and was taken for an urgent brain computerised tomography (CT) scan. The imaging showed a left-sided infarction in the territory of the middle cerebral artery (MCA) distribution with presence of the hyperdense MCA sign, but no evidence of haemorrhage or raised intracranial pressure. CT scan of the cervical spine was normal, chest x-ray showed a right basal consolidation and electrocardiogram (ECG) demonstrated atrial fibrillation at a rate of 120–140 bpm. A diagnosis of a left-sided Total Anterior Circulation Infarct (TACI) was made, and the patient was transferred – intubated, ventilated and sedated – to the intensive care unit. Initial arterial blood gas analysis showed pH = 7.28, PaCO2 = 4.8 kPa, PaO2 = 11.5 kPa, HCO3 = 16 mmol/l, BE = −5, Lactate = 2.1 mmol/l and SaO$_2$ = 92%. He remained hypotensive and tachycardic despite receiving 2.5 litres of crystalloid solutions, and was subsequently started on a noradrenaline (NA) infusion. Intravenous antibiotic (piperacillin/tazobactam) was started and sedation was maintained using propofol and alfentanil infusions. The patient was catheterised; however, he only passed 40 mls of dark concentrated urine and subsequently remained oliguric. A urinalysis using bedside orthotolidine dipstick was positive for microscopic haematuria. Later urine microscopy excluded the presence of red blood cells. Blood samples showed evidence of rhabdhomyolysis (RM) with creatine phosphokinase (CK) markedly elevated at 14000 IU/l. Other blood tests included a neutrophil leucocytosis with WCC = 19000 x10^9/l, Hb = 164 g/l, MCV 90 fl, Platelets = 460 x10^9/l. Creatinine was elevated at 440 μmol/l, Urea = 34 mmol/l, Na$^+$ = 139 mmol/l, K$^+$ = 6.2 mmol/l. Baseline creatinine, checked 2 months earlier, was 68 μmol/l, giving him a diagnosis of AKI stage III.

The patient stabilised on invasive ventilation, fluid and vasopressor therapy. He was also given an infusion of 1.4 percent sodium bicarbonate at 50 mls/hr. However, he remained anuric with a worsening base excess and pH: in addition, serum potassium was climbing despite maximal medical management.

Given his anuria and worsening metabolic status despite adequate fluid resuscitation, he was started on RRT. The initial modality was continuous veno-venous hemofiltration (CVVH), provided using a high flux filter with a prescribed filtration dose of 35 ml/kg/hr, prescribed as 70 per cent post-dilution and 30 per cent pre-dilution (a typical prescription for the unit). The circuit was anti coagulated using regional heparinisation.

Additional clinical management was also instituted in line with current recommendations for the treatment of acute ischaemic stroke.[2] The patient subsequently stabilised and improved, and three days later was discharged to the renal unit for ongoing RRT. Three weeks later he no longer needed dialysis and was discharged to the stroke unit for further rehabilitation.

Case Discussion

Pathophysiology

Rhabdomyolysis (RM) is a clinical syndrome characterised by disintegration of skeletal muscles with release of mycoyte contents into the blood stream and urine, subsequently causing electrolyte disturbances and elevation of levels of serum creatine kinase (CK), serum and urinary myoglobin. The clinical presentation varies from asymptomatic, an incidental finding of an elevated CK, to a florid syndrome of severe muscle weakness, myalgia, dark urine and AKI.

The pathogenesis of RM is initiated by unregulated increase in intracellular (myocyte) calcium (Ca). This occurs either through direct sarcolemmic injury or depletion of cellular adenosine triphosphate (ATP), which impairs the function of Ca – regulating pumps (e.g. Na/Ca exchange pump).[3] Unregulated accumulation of intracellular calcium results in unregulated activation of Ca-dependent proteases with subsequent cell lysis and release of cell contents into the bloodstream, including electrolytes (potassium, phosphates), enzymes (CK, LDH, AST and aldolase), uric acid and proteins (myoglobin). Patients with trauma-induced RM suffer further injury through ischaemia-reperfusion and inflammation, caused by infiltrating neutrophils.

Trauma is thought to be the most common of the many causes of RM: the first descriptions followed cases of multiple crush injuries sustained during the London Blitz.[4]

Some of the commonly reported causes of RM are listed in Table 5.1, categorised by mechanism of injury.[5]

AKI is the most serious complication of RM: RM is reported to be the cause of AKI in 7 to 10% of patients in the United States.[5] The incidence of AKI from RM has been reported to be between 13% and 50%, dependent on the definition of AKI.[6] (see Table 5.2 for current AKIN classification system)

Myoglobin is thought to be the main toxin implicated in causing AKI in RM. Following a trigger, intracellular contents including proteins such as myoglobin are released into the bloodstream.[7] The exact mechanism by which RM results in AKI remains unknown; however, experimental data suggests that it is secondary to a combination of renal vasoconstriction, myoglobin-induced toxic tubular injury and formation of intratubular casts.

Table 5.1 Common causes of Rhabdomyolysis

Physical	Hypoxic	Drug induced	Electrolyte/Endocrine	Other
Crush Injury	Vascular thrombosis/ compression	Statins/ Fibrates	Hypokalaemia	Polymyositis
Electrocution	Bariatric/prolonged surgery	Alcohol	Hypothyroidism	Spider bites/ snake venom
Hyper-Hypothermia	sickle cell crisis	Cocaine	Hyperglycaemic / hyperosmolar syndrome	
Burns	carbon monoxide exposure	Heroin	diabetic ketoacidosis	
Malignant Hyperthermia			Adrenal Insufficiency	
Seizures			Hyperaldosteronism	
Extreme exertion				
Neuroleptic malignant syndrome				

Table 5.2 AKIN Classification system (adapted from Mehta RL, Kellum JA, Shah SV, et al. Acute Kidney Injury Network: report of an initiative to improve outcomes in acute kidney injury. *Crit Care* 2007;11:R31)

Stage	Serum creatinine criteria expressed as change from baseline value	Urine output criteria
1	increase in serum creatinine greater than or equal to 150–200% from baseline	<0.5 ml/kg for more than 6 hours
2	increase in serum creatinine greater than or equal to 200%–300% from baseline	< 0.5 ml/kg for more than 12 hours
3	increase in serum creatinine greater than 300% from baseline	< 0.3 ml/kg for 24 hours or anuria for 12 hours

Fluid sequestration in damaged muscles, with subsequent contraction of the intravascular fluid compartment, leads to the activation of renin-angiotensin-aldosterone system (RAAS) resulting in reduction in renal blood flow and renal vasoconstriction (compounded by the reduction in nitric oxide, secondary to the scavenging characteristics of myoglobin.)

Moreover, intracellular antioxidant molecules are overwhelmed with resultant increase in free radicals and reactive oxygen species (ROS).[8] In clinical practice, the AKI associated with rhabdomyloysis results from the contribution of many factors, principally hypovolaemia in combination with effects of other drugs, injuries and metabolic abnormalities on the kidneys.

Diagnosis

Diagnosis is established through history and physical examination, identifying risk factors and possible precipitants of RM. Clinical signs can vary according to cause, with trauma-induced RM being the easiest to identify. Some patients, such as in this case, may be unable to communicate symptoms such as myalgia or muscle tenderness. Simple laboratory investigations can diagnose RM, with elevated serum CK being more specific than other markers of RM. Normal CK is less than 100 IU/l. CK levels of more than five to ten times the upper limit of normal are considered to be clinically relevant, with higher levels correlating with greater degrees of muscle damage. CK levels cannot be used reliably to assess the risk of developing AKI; however, it is generally agreed that a CK greater than 5000 IU/l, warrants close monitoring of kidney functions. Other biochemical features of RM are hyperkalaemia, hyperphosphataemia, low calcium, high LDH and AST. In RM urine testing, using orthotolidine dipstick, is positive for microscopic haematuria whereas microscopy excludes the presence of red blood cells.

Management

Efforts are mainly directed towards prevention of AKI in RM as the treatment of established AKI is mainly supportive. Assessing the risk of developing AKI using levels of CK, myoglobin, LDH, potassium, bicarbonate, albumin or creatinine at presentation have all failed to show that a predictive model or a single marker can reliably predict this risk, given the heterogeneity of causes of RM and the multifactorial AKI in this context.

Therapy should be directed towards attenuating further muscle damage, attempting to prevent AKI and offering organ support, renal replacement therapy (RRT), as indicated.

Attenuating further muscle damage relies on treatment of the cause: removing the, patient from the hazardous or traumatic situation, cessation of known precipitant medications or illicit agents, or treatment of any underlying biochemical or endocrine cause.

Available evidence is weak in support of generally applied preventive measures to avoid AKI in RM.[3,9] Most of the evidence underpinning the commonly available recommendations is either based on animal studies, or on retrospective observational data with small number of patients or case reports or opinions. There are no prospective randomised controlled trials, comparing the impact of type or volume of fluid used, or the effect of alkalinising the urine or addition of mannitol on the incidence of AKI in RM.

Mannitol has been proposed as having a preventive role in AKI; however, experimental animal data has shown that its role is limited mainly to a diuretic effect rather than an antioxidant effect.[10]

The mechanism by which fluid administration prevents AKI in RM is unknown but only early volume expansion has been shown to be effective in preventing AKI. A recently published systematic literature review,[11] examined the available human data to evaluate the evidence-base in relation to widely acceptable recommendations for preventing AKI in RM.[12,13,14]

Early initiation of intravenous fluid therapy has consistently been shown to be associated with a reduced incidence of AKI or reduced need for RRT in patients with RM. This data is from level 4 studies that mainly addressed the question of timing of fluid therapy in relation to trauma.

The volume of fluid needed to prevent AKI is more controversial, with studies (levels 2b and 4) reporting a reduced incidence of AKI in patients receiving higher volumes of fluids in the resuscitation phase. The limitations in these studies are that the exact volumes and types of fluids administered varied, and the criteria used to monitor response or guide volume of fluid therapy also varied. The consistent finding of these studies is that patients whose volume status was corrected earlier had improved outcomes.

Once a patient develops established renal failure, indications for RRT – including persistent hyperkalaemia, significant metabolic acidosis with anuria and possible fluid overload – would necessitate initiating dialysis. There is no role for the use of RRT as a prophylactic measure against the development of AKI in RM, and levels of CK or even myoglobin should not be used to indicate need for dialysis.

Continuous renal replacement therapy is the modality commonly used in patients with AKI on critical care, as opposed to intermittent therapies usually being chosen for patients on renal units. Case reports evaluating myoglobin clearance; have demonstrated better clearance using high permeability membranes,[16,17] but none of these, have reported on the correlation between clearance of myoglobin and survival or renal recovery. A Cochrane review published recently,[18] concluded that whilst CRRT may be beneficial in acute AKI with RM, the poor quality of the involved studies and the absence of data related to clinically relevant outcomes (i.e. mortality or recovery from AKI) limited the ability to recommend CRRT over conventional dialysis (intermittent) in the management of RM induced AKI.

Conclusion

RM is a syndrome caused by a variety of insults and that can have a diverse presentation, with AKI being the most serious consequence. There is currently a paucity of level 1–3 evidence to support using any certain type of fluid, or to support the use of mannitol or sodium bicarbonate infusions to prevent AKI in RM, although some animal and retrospective studies suggest a role for urinary alkalisation. Level 4 human and animal data support starting fluid therapy early. Serial CK monitoring to establish the peak level is prudent, and in patients with markedly raised levels (eg. >15–20,000 IU/l), higher volumes of fluid may be indicated if clinically tolerated. If the patient cannot tolerate this, then earlier renal replacement therapy should be considered.

There is no evidence to suggest routine urinary alkalinisation with sodium bicarbonate and potential risks such as manifestations of hypocalcaemia need to be considered.

In the patient presented, the recommendations based on this review would be to eliminate the cause for RM and to start fluid therapy early, correcting for fluid deficits and ongoing losses. RRT was instituted when indicated, using the modality suitable to the patient's characteristics.

Key Learning Points

- History and physical examination for risk factors and precipitants should indicate those at risk of RM.
- Elevated CK levels greater than five to ten times the upper limit of normal (100 IU/l) are clinically relevant. A CK greater than 5000 IU/l warrants close monitoring of kidney function, although it is not routinely predictive of AKI requiring renal replacement therapy.
- Fluid therapy should be started early, although there is no strong evidence to favour any one type of fluid or to support routine urinary alkalinisation or use of mannitol.
- Additional treatment of RM should be directed towards attenuating further muscle damage, attempting to prevent AKI and offering organ support including renal replacement therapy (RRT), as indicated.

References

1. Kolhe NV, Stevens PE, Crowe AV, Lipkin GW, Harrison DA. Case mix, outcome and activity for patients with severe acute kidney injury during the first 24 hours after admission to an adult, general critical care unit: application of predictive models from a secondary analysis of the ICNARC case mix programme database. *Crit Care* 2008;15(Suppl 1):S2.

2. Raithatha A, Pratt G, Rash A. Developments in the management of acute ischaemic stroke (AIS); implications for critical care. Continuing Education in Anaesthesia, Critical Care & Pain, British Journal of Anaesthesia. *Cont Edu Anaesth Crit Care and Pain*. 2013;13(3):80–86.

3. Giannoglou GD, Chatzizisis YS, Misirli G. The syndrome of rhabdomyolysis: pathophysiology and diagnosis. *Eur J Intern Med* 2007;18:90–100.

4. Beall D, Bywaters EG, Belsey RH, Miles JA. Crush Injury with renal failure. *Br Med J* 1941;1:432–4.

5. Bagley WH, Yang H, Shah KH. Rhabdomyolysis. *Intern Emerg Med* 2007;2:210–18.

6. Melli G, Chaudhry V, Cornblath DR. Rhabdomyolysis: an evaluation of 475 hospitalized patients. *Medicine (Baltimore)* 2005;84:377–85.

7. Singh AP, Junemann A, Muthuraman A, Jaggi AS, Singh N, Grover K, Dhawan R. Animal models of acute renal failure. *Pharmacol Rep* 2012;64:31–44.

8. Boutaud O, Roberts LJ, II. Mechanism-based therapeutic approaches to rhabdomyolysis-induced renal failure. *Free Radic Biol Med*, 2011;51(5):1062–1067.

9. Moore KP, Holt SG, Patel RP, et al. A causative role for redox cycling of myoglobin and its inhibition by alkalinization in the pathogenesis and treatment of rhabdomyolysis-induced renal failure. *J Biol Chem* 1998; 273:31731–7.

10. Zager RA, Foerder C, Bredl C. The influence of mannitol on myoglobinuric acute renal failure: functional, biochemical, and morphological assessments. *J Am Soc Nephrol* 1991;2:848–55.

11. Scharman EJ, Troutman WG. Prevention of Kidney Injury Following Rhabdomyolysis: A Systematic Review. *Ann Pharmacother* 2013;47:90–105

12. Cho YS, Lim H, Kim SH. Comparison of lactated Ringer's solution and 0.9% saline in the treatment of rhabdomyolysis induced by doxylamine intoxication. *Emerg Med J* 2007;24:276–80.

13. Brown CV, Rhee P, Chan L, Evans K, Demetriades D, Velmahos GC. Preventing renal failure in patients with rhabdomyolysis: do bicarbonate and mannitol make a difference? *J Trauma* 2004;56:1191–6.

14. Atef MR, Nadjatfi I, Boroumand B, Rastegar A. Acute renal failure in earthquake victims in Iran: epidemiology and management. *Q J Med* 1994;87:35–40.

15. Zepeda-Orozco D, Ault BH, Jones DP. Factors associated with acute renal failure in children with rhabdomyolysis. *Pediatr Nephrol* 2008;23:2281–4.

16. Naka T, Jones D, Baldwin L, Fealy N, Bates S, Goehl H, Morgera S, Neumayer HH, Bellomo R. Myoglobin clearance by super high-flux hemofiltration in a case of severe rhabdomyolysis: a case report. *Crit Care* 2005;9:R90–R95

17. Sorrentino SA, Kielstein JT, Lukasz A, Sorrentino JN, Gohrbandt B, Haller H, Schmidt BM. High permeability dialysis membrane allows effective removal of myoglobin in acute kidney injury resulting from rhabdomyolysis. *Crit Care Med.* 2011 Jan;39(1):184–6.

18. Zeng X, Zhang L, Wu T, Fu P. Continuous renal replacement therapy (CRRT) for rhabdomyolysis. *Cochrane Database Syst Rev.* 2014 Jun 15;6.

19. Iraj N, Saeed S, Mostafa H, Houshang S, Ali S, Farin RF, et al. Prophylactic fluid therapy in crushed victims of Bam earthquake. *Am J Emerg Med.* 2011 Sep; 29(7):738–42.

Management of Acute Liver Failure

Elizabeth Wilson and Philip Docherty

Introduction

Acute liver failure (ALF) is defined as severe acute liver injury with encephalopathy and impairment of synthetic function (INR >1.5) in a patient without pre-existing cirrhosis or liver disease. A commonly used time frame for definition is failure of less than 26 weeks duration.

This case describes an example of ALF and subsequent management to illustrate the key points for patient management and specialist referral.

Case

A 26-year-old woman presented to her local Emergency Department following a deliberate overdose of paracetamol. Following an argument with her partner and under the influence of alcohol, she took approximately 50 x 500 mg tablets but did not tell anyone until lunchtime the next day when her partner then rang an ambulance. Aside from a mild tachycardia of 110 bpm, her clinical examination was unremarkable.

Initial investigations revealed a paracetamol level of 125 mg/l, raised Alanine transferase (ALT) of 4318 IU/l, a prolonged prothrombin (PT) time of 30 seconds and a creatinine (Cr) of 139 umol/l. Lactate was 11 mmol/l Given these findings she was started on an N-Acetylcysteine (NAC) infusion, resuscitated with crystalloid fluids and following a discussion with the gastroenterology team at the regional transplant centre, arrangements were made to transfer her there. On arrival she was admitted to the intensive care unit where she remained alert and orientated, and despite an initial improvement in heart rate with aggressive fluid resuscitation, was judged to have a significant acute liver injury with an acute kidney injury (AKI) secondary to paracetamol overdose. Repeat bloods 6 hours after the presentation and 22 hours since the overdose showed a lactate of 3 mmol/l, Cr 160 umol/l, ALT 5701 IU/l and hydrogen ions (H+) of 41.5 nmol/l (pH 7.38). The PT had risen to 82 seconds.

Overnight she became progressively drowsy. An earlier psychiatric assessment had indicated that there were no clear contraindications to liver transplantation: specifically no previous suicidal behaviour or longstanding alcohol abuse. Twenty-four hours into her critical care admission, the encephalopathy progressed such that she required intubation and ventilation. Arterial and central venous access was established for haemodynamic monitoring and blood gas sampling. She was oliguric with a measured creatinine of 321 umol/l and PT 106 s. With these parameters and grade 4 encephalopathy (Table 6.1), she met criteria for liver transplantation and was activated as 'super urgent' on the transplant list. Prophylactic antibiotics and anti-fungal agents were started.

Renal replacement therapy (RRT) was started at 30 mls/kg/hr and intra-cranial pressure (ICP) monitored. Insertion of an ICP bolt was preceded with transfusion of blood products,

Table 6.1 Conn Score (Westhaven Classification) for grading hepatic encephalopathy

Grade of encephalopathy	Clinical manifestations
0	no personality or behavioural abnormality detected
1	lack of awareness; shortened attention span, euphoria or anxiety, impaired performance of addition
2	lethargy or apathy; minimal disorientation for time or place; subtle personality change; inappropriate behaviour; impaired performance of subtraction
3	somnolence to semi stupor but responsive to verbal stimuli; confusion; gross disorientation
4	coma (unresponsive to verbal or noxious stimuli)

specifically cryoprecipitate, fresh frozen plasma (FFP) and platelets. The first ICP measurement was 17 mmHg with an adequate cerebral perfusion pressure (CPP) of 60 mmHg. The following day, her mean arterial pressure (MAP) dropped and she was started on a noradrenaline infusion to augment MAP and CPP.

Whilst awaiting a suitable donor, she required several treatments for raised ICP in the form of mannitol and hypertonic saline. Vasopressor and oxygen requirements increased and she developed right-sided infiltrates on the chest x-ray. Antibiotic cover was broadened to treat a presumed pneumonia and a maintenance dextrose infusion started for hypoglycaemia.

On day 5 of her ICU admission a suitable liver became available. She was taken to theatre and had a successful orthoptic liver transplant with 10 litres of intra-operative blood loss requiring cell salvage and almost 30 units of blood products including packed red cells, cryoprecipitate, FFP and platelets. Immunosuppression comprised basimixilab and mycophenolate mofetil (MMF). The ICP bolt was removed on the second post-operative day. Thereafter her post-operative recovery was prolonged due to ongoing respiratory failure. She required a tracheostomy to facilitate weaning from mechanical ventilation and haemofiltration to achieve a negative fluid balance. By day 10 of her ICU admission, she was weaned onto CPAP, coagulation had normalised and as urine output was good, haemofiltration was discontinued. She was successfully decannulated on day 12 and discharged from ICU the following day.

Discussion

The case demonstrates both the severity and breadth of organ dysfunction associated with fulminant hepatic failure. In addition, the timescale reflects the rapid and progressive decline despite optimal therapy. Ultimately liver transplantation may be the only effective therapy in many cases; however, with such a limited resource of suitable organs, great care must be taken to comply with national guidance both in meeting transplant criteria and recipient suitability.

Classification

ALF has been divided into three subgroups; hyperacute, acute and subacute based on time from onset of jaundice to encephalopathy. The case presented here is a typical example of hyperacute liver failure, with paracetamol poisoning being the most common cause in the United Kingdom. The time scales are less than 7 days, 8 to 28 days and 29 days to 8 weeks respectively. This has important ramifications for risk stratification and disease aetiology. Hyperacute cases have a higher mortality from cerebral oedema and kidney injury but show reduced mortality without transplantation. Sub-acute causes typically drug reactions and viral hepatatides have an increased mortality when not transplanted.

Pathophysiology of Paracetamol Toxicity

Normal metabolism of paracetamol yields predominantly non-toxic metabolites, produced by conjugation with sulphate and glucuronide. A small proportion (5%) is oxidised by cytochrome P450 to N-acetyl-p-benzoquinone imine (NAPQI). This highly reactive metabolite is usually detoxified by conjugation with glutathione. In cases of paracetamol overdose excess NAPQI is produced and glutathione stores become rapidly depleted. The liver's ability to compensate is exceeded, resulting in hepatic injury as shown in Figure 6.1. The antidote N-acetylcysteine acts as a precursor for glutathione and also neutralises NAPQI directly.

Setting and Referral

Regardless of the underlying aetiology, the most appropriate setting for a patient with ALF must be considered early in the management strategy. In most cases this often means admission to critical care. Although the cause was known in this case, identifying a cause for the ALF may be problematic and indeed may never be certain. Patients should be discussed with the nearest specialist unit at the earliest opportunity, as in addition to the ability to deliver transplantation, specialist centres have developed expertise in conservative ALF management. Many centres have developed multi-disciplinary teams with associated standardised protocols to achieve optimal care.

Early referral may also facilitate a smoother inter-hospital transfer before the onset of multi-organ failure (MOF). However, care should be taken in transferring even an apparently stable patient with ALF as conscious level and haemodynamics may deteriorate rapidly. Elective ventilation for transfer is often the safest course even if encephalopathy is subtle or travel distance moderate.

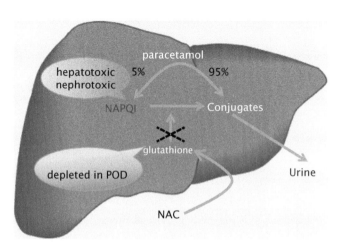

Figure 6.1 Showing metabolism of paracetamol and inability of the liver to cope with excess N-acetyl-p-benzoquinone imine (NAPQI) and glutathione depletion in a paracetamol toxic patient.

Initial Management

A thorough history, examination and standard laboratory blood tests are mandatory and include full blood count, urea and electrolytes), liver function tests, coagulation profile, magnesium, phosphate, paracetamol/salicylate levels and an arterial blood gas (ABG). An ABG will assess metabolic state and lactate. Normal initial values may be falsely reassuring and it may be difficult to assign a raised lactate to liver damage, tissue hypoperfusion or both accurately. When the diagnosis is known as in this case, there is no requirement for a host of specific liver investigations. However some centres' protocols suggest routine testing for hepatitis B and C, Epstein Barr virus, cytalomegalovirus, human immunodeficiency virus and antinuclear and smooth muscle antibodies. Paracetamol levels should be measured and interpreted in the appropriate context of staggered overdoses, patient size and chronic liver disease. N-Acetylcysteine should be started without delay in the case of a suspected toxic dose and subsequently guided by blood levels and liver enzymes.

Priorities by System

As the liver fails, the pathologies relate to failing of a specific functional task of the liver in addition to structural changes, such as development of varices as seen in Figure 6.2.

Cardiovascular

ALF patients are often intravascularly deplete and develop vasoplegia. Delivering timely, appropriate resuscitation may abolish or delay the onset of MOF. The clinical picture is similar to severe sepsis and a combination of initial fluid loading and vasopressor support is often required. The Surviving Sepsis Guidelines[1] is a useful guide to initial cardiovascular management with important caveats. In particular, mixed venous saturations are often elevated, reflecting the hyperdynamic nature of ALF patients.

Fluid resuscitation is usually done with crystalloids initially but may require supplementation with colloid and/or blood products. The vasopressor of choice in fluid-resistant hypotension is usually noradrenaline and may be required in high doses. Lactate, normally an important marker of tissue hypoperfusion, may also reflect direct liver damage. As with

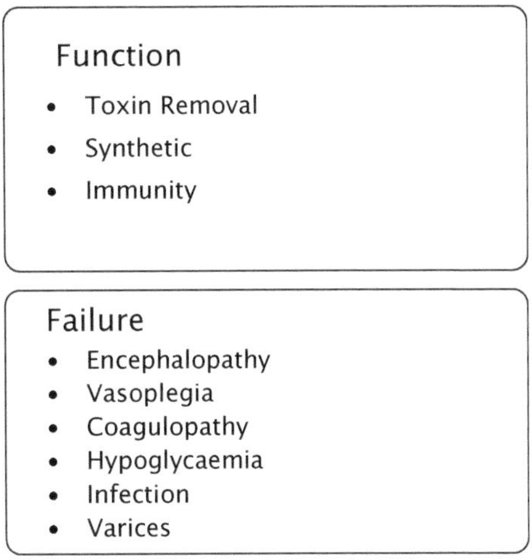

Function
- Toxin Removal
- Synthetic
- Immunity

Failure
- Encephalopathy
- Vasoplegia
- Coagulopathy
- Hypoglycaemia
- Infection
- Varices

Figure 6.2 The failing liver and subsequent clinical manifestations.

this case, an initially elevated lactate may respond to fluid resuscitation and then increase again despite optimal haemodynamic management as the patient's clinical condition deteriorates. Lactate is included in the King's College criteria for liver transplantation [Table 6.1] and has been identified as an important predictor of outcome in critical illness generally and ALF specifically.[2]

Respiratory

The indication for intubation in this case was depressed conscious level, not respiratory distress. Whilst gas exchange may not be impaired initially, patients are at high risk for both infection and development of an acute lung injury (ALI). ALI or acute respiratory distress syndrome (ARDS) may occur in up to 30 per cent of ALF patients with paracetamol toxicity.[3] This is perhaps unsurprising, with the early aggressive fluid resuscitation often given. Subsequent ICP management with deep sedation and muscle paralysis may further predispose to respiratory complications and development of pneumonia.

ARDSnet ventilatory strategies of 6 mls/kg tidal volumes and minimising peak airway pressure is generally accepted management. In ALF, concerns regarding barotrauma may be tempered by prioritising tight PaCO2 control where cerebral oedema and raised ICP are present. Given that our patient required treatment for raised ICP, less than ideal ventilator settings may have been used to maintain normocapnia, thus predisposing to lung injury. Similarly, high positive end expiratory pressure (PEEP) can compromise venous return and MAP further reducing CPP and risking cerebral ischaemia.

With the complex MOF nature of ALF, optimum single organ therapy may require modification from evidence-based protocols to enhance the overall clinical outcome.

Neurological

Encephalopathy has crucial prognostic significance and appears not only in the definition of ALF but also in several of the King's College criteria for liver transplantation (see Table 6.2). These criteria were defined following retrospective analysis of mortality without transplantation.

Management should be aimed at prevention, minimising severity and treating cerebral oedema. Raised intracranial pressure secondary to cerebral oedema is a leading cause of mortality and the development of encephalopathy should raise suspicion.

Insertion of an Intracranial Pressure (ICP) bolt provides qualitative evidence of both ICP and cerebral perfusion pressure but carries significant risk in the presence of deranged

Table 6.2 King's College Hospital transplant criteria for acute liver failure

Paracetamol Overdose	Non-paracetamol overdose
• pH <7.30	• PT >100 seconds
• or ALL of the following . PT >100 seconds . Creatinine >300 umol/l . Grade III/IV encephalopathy	• or THREE of the following . Time from jaundice to encephalopathy >2 days . Non-A, non-B hepatitis, halothane or drug induced liver failure . Age <10 or >40 years . PT >50 seconds . Bilirubin > 300umol/l

coagulation. There is no definitive evidence to guide when, where (intradural or intra-parenchymal) or even if an ICP bolt should be sited. Raised ICP is typically managed with hypertonic fluids, usually mannitol or hypertonic saline.

Renal

This patient had developed an AKI by the time of admission. This is a common finding in ALF generally, but particularly if paracetamol is the aetiology, with an incidence approaching 80 percent.[4] The pathophysiology is similar to septic shock and hepatorenal syndrome with resistant vasoplegia reducing kidney perfusion. There is also some evidence that paracetamol or its metabolites are directly nephrotoxic.[5]

Creatinine is also an important factor when listing patients as super-urgent reflecting the poor prognosis in patients with an associated AKI. RRT is commonly required and can pose several difficulties. In addition to recognised critical illness indications such as acidaemia, fluid overload and hyperkalaemia, there are liver specific indications such as hyperammonaemia. Extending the life of a haemofilter in the context of a complex coagulation picture is also a challenge. Heparin is not recommended and given the very short half-life of prostacyclin (seconds), this represents a safer alternative. Definitive evidence for optimal ultrafiltration rates is uncertain but typically 30 ml/kg/hr exchange is used.

Coagulation

Production of clotting factors is markedly reduced in liver damage. Measurement of prothrombin time (PT) is routine, but whilst it has value in terms of prognostication and transplantation, its significance as an indicator of bleeding risk is less well defined, particularly in ALF. In this setting, pro- and anti-coagulant factors are equally deficient, pre-disposing the patient to the risks of both thrombosis and haemorrhage. Other measurements of clotting such as thromboelastography (TEG) support this view and may give a more accurate view of the overall bleeding risk.[6]

Given the importance of PT with regard to listing for liver transplantation, blood products should only be used when there is active haemorrhage or for complicated invasive procedures. It is NOT routine practice in specialist liver centres to give such products for insertion of arterial lines or central venous lines but if the patient is being transfused, consideration should be given to inserting several lines simultaneously.

Infection

ALF patients are at high risk of developing bacteraemia or fungal sepsis, with rates of 35 per cent and 30 per cent documented respectively.[7] Infection must be actively sought as a proportion of bacteraemias manifest without fever or raised white cell count. Prophylactic antibiotics and anti fungal agents are recommended routinely due to the high prevalence and compromised immune function. There is, however, some evidence that the reduced immune response seen in ALF whilst making recognition of sepsis problematic may confer a mortality benefit.[8]

Transplant

The decision to list a patient as super-urgent for liver transplantation is a key factor in the management of ALF. Unfortunately, meeting King's College Criteria is only the first step. There are several contraindications that may preclude listing including the patient's condition on critical care suggesting surgery would not be of overall benefit, severe co-existent medical disease and specific psychiatric criteria. Once patients meet the criteria, they will be activated nationally as 'super-urgent' and will receive the first appropriate organ. Blood products may then be given to facilitate further invasive monitoring without impacting on listing criteria.

Post-transplant care involves ongoing organ support, immunosuppression and monitoring of coagulation. Patients improve rapidly following transplantation for chronic disease but often those with ALF have a more protracted course. This patient developed pneumonia and required renal replacement therapy, which is not unusual following fulminant hepatic failure. Meticulous attention must be paid to infection control measures and a high index of suspicion maintained for post-operative bleeding. A persistently high lactate and deranged clotting screen are cause for concern. Normally a Doppler ultrasound is performed the day after surgery to assess vascular patency.

Extra-corporeal Techniques

Several new devices have been designed to replace some of the failing functions of the liver. They combine components of dialysis for detoxification and incorporate liver cells into a bio artificial device aimed at replacing some synthetic function. The longest serving device, the molecular absorbent recirculating system (MARS), has been the subject of a clinical trial that showed no survival benefit.[9] Currently such devices are recommended in clinical trial settings only.

Conclusion

ALF can be associated with very rapid and severe multi-organ dysfunction. Timely and optimal critical care management with early involvement of a specialist liver centre is vital, but despite this, liver transplantation can sometimes be the only effective therapy.

Key Learning Points

- ALF may involve rapid onset of MOF. Patients should be discussed early with the nearest referral centre.
- Infection must be actively sought. Both antibiotic and antifungal prophylaxis is recommended.
- Cerebral oedema is a major contributor to mortality and should be suspected particularly in patients with rapidly progressive encephalopathy and paracetamol overdose.
- Blood products should only be given when there is *active bleeding* or once transplant criteria have been met in order to minimise delays in listing patients for transplantation.

References

1. Dellinger RP et al. Surviving Sepsis Campaign guidelines for management of severe sepsis and septic shock. *Crit Care Med.* 2004 Mar;32(3):858–73.

2. Khosravani H, et al. Occurrence and adverse effect on outcome of hyperlactatemia in the critically ill. *Crit Care.* 2009;13(3):R90.

3. Baudouin SV, et al. Acute lung injury in fulminant hepatic failure following paracetamol poisoning. *Thorax.* 1995; 50(4):399–402.

4. Betrosian AP, Agarwal B, Douzinas EE. Acute renal dysfunction in liver diseases. *World J Gastroenterol.* 2007;13(42):5552–9.

5. Eguia L, Materson BJ. Acetaminophen-related acute renal failure without

fulminant liver failure. *Pharmacotherapy.* 1997;17(2):363–70.

6. Stravitz RT, Lisman T, Luketic VA, et al. Minimal effects of acute liver injury/acute liver failure on hemostasis as assessed by thromboelastography. *J Hepatol* 2012;56:129–36.

7. Karvellas CJ, et al. Predictors of bacteraemia and mortality in patients with acute liver failure. *Intensive Care Med.* 2009;35(8): 1390–6.

8. Rolando N, et al. The systemic inflammatory response syndrome in acute liver failure. *Hepatology.* 2000; 32(4 Pt 1):734–9.

9. Saliba F, Camus C, Durand F, et al. Albumin dialysis with a noncell artificial liver support device in patients with acute liver failure: a randomized, controlled trial. *Ann Intern Med* 2013;159: 522–31.

Status Epilepticus

Graeme Nimmo

7

Introduction

Epileptic seizures are a presenting feature of many neurological and systemic disease processes (Box 7.1). They may be generalised (mostly tonic-clonic) or focal. In a proportion of patients the seizure will be an isolated event, affording the time for planned further investigation and treatment by a neurologist with expertise in seizure management. However in 50 percent of patients, their first seizure leads to the condition of status epilepticus (SE). This has been defined as more than 30 minutes of either continuous seizure activity or two or more sequential seizures without full recovery of consciousness between seizures. It is imperative to identify the cause of the seizures to ensure appropriate patient treatment whilst supporting physiology.

There are around 14,000 cases of SE annually in the United Kingdom with an overall mortality approaching 25 percent. The seizures can be categorised as follows:

- Generalised convulsive
- Generalised non-convulsive: absence
- Partial convulsive
- Partial non-convulsive: complex partial

There are many causes of seizure including drug withdrawal, intercurrent illness or metabolic disturbance and progression of disease in those patients with idiopathic epilepsy. Many causes of acute cerebral disturbance such as infection, trauma, cerebrovascular disease and cerebral tumours can also result in seizures, as can acute toxic and metabolic disturbances. (Box 7.1). In some patients with SE no cause is found.

In generalised convulsive (tonic/clonic) SE, the duration of convulsion is important. It is safer to think of between 10 to 20 minutes duration of fitting as a suitable point to aim to start treatment, although clinical research studies use times of up to 30 minutes to define SE. In the heat of the event, the accuracy of timings may also be compromised. The length of time that patients are in uncontrolled SE is important for three reasons:

- Increased risk of cerebral damage
- Increased risk of systemic damage
- Seizures become more resistant to treatment

Two phases of SE are recognised and if seizure activity is not abolished, the patient moves from Phase 1 to Phase 2 of SE.

Phase 1 manifests with recurrent seizures on EEG and tonic-clonic motor effects and associated hypertension, tachycardia and increased cerebral blood flow.

Phase 2 shows periodic epileptiform discharges on EEG and electro-mechanical dissociation. Cerebral perfusion pressure is often compromised due to increased intra-cranial

Box 7.1 Causes of status epilepticus

- Idiopathic
- Traumatic brain injury
- Vascular-intra-cranial haemorrhage; sub-arachnoid haemorrhage; intra-cerebral haemorrhage; sub-dural haemorrhage; extra-dural haemorrhage; cerebral venous and sinus thrombosis
- Stroke
- CNS infection-meningitis; encephalitis; cerebral abscess
- Tumour
- Degenerative CNS diseases-inflammatory; demyelinating
- Toxic-metabolic
- Drugs
- Alcohol
- Hypoxaemia/Hypercapnoea
- Liver failure
- Renal failure
- Hypertensive encephalopathy
- Hypoglycaemia
- Hyperglycaemia (extreme)
- Hyponatraemia
- Hypocalcaemia

pressure in association with systemic hypotension, made more harmful by the loss of autoregulation of cerebral blood flow.

Case Description

A 22 year old female student has been experiencing persistent, dull, bilateral headaches over the last few days, initially responsive to simple analgesia but now worsening. She has had two episodes of abnormal movements of the right upper limb suggestive of focal seizures. Her GP has referred her to the on-call medical team for further assessment with a differential diagnosis of meningitis/encephalitis or a 'space occupying lesion'. She has a past medical history of asthma since aged 12 and her medications are salmeterol two puffs twice daily, salbutamol 2 puffs as required, and the combined oral contraceptive pill.

On arrival in the Medical Admissions Unit, she is assessed by the advanced nurse practitioner (ANP) on duty. Her initial observations are RR 15/min, SpO_2 98 percent on air, pulse 87/min regular and good volume, BP 168/85 mmHg, GCS (E4 V5 M6) = 15, pupils 2 mm and reactive but slightly sluggish and tympanic temperature 37.8°C. Whilst the ANP is taking her history, she collapses with a generalised tonic-clonic seizure. The emergency response team is called and institutes management as follows:

Airway: assessed; attempts to open and maintain it are made difficult by ongoing seizures. High concentration oxygen is administered.

Breathing: assessed and supported with bag-mask-valve apparatus.

Circulation: intravenous (IV) access is secured (taking a sample to measure blood glucose at the bedside and in the lab) and IV 0.9 percent sodium chloride 500 ml is begun.

Disability (and in this case drugs): GCS is assessed as E1, V1, M1, pupils 4 mm equal and unreactive.

Securing the airway is very difficult to achieve, far less optimal, in the seizing patient so abolition of seizures with drugs (D) is a priority whilst establishing monitoring with pulse oximetry, ECG and NIBP and repeated neurological assessment. (Box 7.2 here) Her immediate blood glucose is 5.7 mmol/l so does not require correction with IV glucose. There is no history of alcohol excess or evidence of impaired nutrition so there is no need to add high potency vitamin B and C. (In the United Kingdom this would be IV pabrinex.).

She is treated with IV lorazepam 4 mg (as outlined in Box 7.2) then a further 4 mg, but continues to seize for the next 15 minutes. A phenytoin infusion is started and she is referred to intensive care. In light of the history of headache and the fever, she is given ceftriaxone 2 grams IV and aciclovir 400 mg IV to cover both bacterial and viral CNS infection. It has been confirmed that she has no allergies.

Blood for the following investigations is also sent to help identify the aetiology:

- Blood glucose
- Biochemical profile, Ca^{++}, Mg^{++}, Creatine kinase.
- Arterial blood gas
- Liver enzymes
- Full blood count and coagulation screen

On arrival of the intensive care doctor, she is unconscious (GCS E = 1 V = 1 M = 1) with a partially obstructed airway despite the use of a nasopharyngeal airway, oxygen saturation (SpO_2) of 93 percent on 15 l/min oxygen via a reservoir, pulse rate 127/min in sinus rhythm with BP = 187/95 mmHg. The phenytoin infusion has been started. A decision is made by the ICU doctor to administer anaesthesia to afford airway protection and control of oxygenation and carbon dioxide. Once she is intubated and stabilised (including insertion of a large-bore IV cannula, the rapid administration of another 500 ml 0.9 percent sodium chloride and placement of an arterial line) she is transferred to ICU via the radiology suite where a CT head scan is performed. On arrival in ICU at 22.30 she remains sedated with propofol, paralysed with muscle relaxants and is ventilated. In addition to standard ICU monitoring, she is connected to continuous cerebral electrical activity monitoring and is prescribed further phenytoin 100 mg IV three times daily.

The CT scan is reported as normal with no evidence of ischaemia or infarction, haemorrhage, extra-axial collections, cerebral oedema, tumour or abscess. All bloods (including platelets and clotting) are normal apart from a urea of 7.4 mmol/l and WCC of 14.2×10^9/l.

Box 7.2 Initial anticonvulsive regime for status epilepticus

- Initial treatment with diazepam emulsion (Diazemuls®) or lorazepam.
- Diazepam 2 mg increments up to 10 mg over 5 mins.
- Alternatively lorazepam 4 mg slowly into a large vein.
  - If delay in getting IV access, administer 10–20 mg rectal diazepam
  - Diazepam can be repeated once 15 mins later up to a total of 20 mg and lorazepam can be repeated once 15 mins later up to a total dose of 8 mg.
  - Second line for seizures persisting despite benzodiazepines is phenytoin. Administer 15–20 mg/kg diluted in 0.9 per cent sodium chloride maximum concentration 10 mg/ml i.e. 1 gram in 100 ml. Give slowly or in two divided infusions if the patient is frail, very elderly or there is cardiovascular compromise (acute or chronic).

A lumbar puncture is performed in the left lateral position and the opening pressure is 29 cmH$_2$O. CSF is sent for microscopy, cell count, culture, bacterial and viral PCR, protein and glucose. The muscle relaxant is subsequently discontinued.

On day two, when reviewed, she is still E = 1 Vt M = 1 with sluggish 3 mm pupils, although not apparently fitting. She has received alfentanil 2 mg/hour and propofol 250 mg/hour (25 ml 1 per cent) overnight. The propofol is stopped and the alfentanil infusion rate is halved. Three hours later her GCS, has not changed. Results from CSF examination are returned:

No cells or organisms on microscopy

Glucose 4.6 mmol/l with concurrent plasma glucose 5.9 mmol/l

Protein 524 mg/l (reference range 200–400 mg/l)

An EEG is performed and shows she is still in SE (non-convulsive). Serum phenytoin concentration (corrected with respect to albumin level) is 15.6 mg/l (therapeutic range 10 to 20). Propofol is re-instituted at 27 ml/hour (she is 68 kg: maximum dose 4 mg/kg/hr) and the seizure activity is virtually abolished. A loading dose of 10 mg midazolam is given and a midazolam infusion is started at 14 mg/hr (0.2 mg/kg/hr). Sodium valproate is added in consultation with the neurology consultant who recommends arranging a CT venogram or an MRI scan to diagnose a possible cerebral venous sinus thrombosis. The CT venogram confirms cerebral venous sinus thrombosis and systemic heparinisation is begun as treatment following discussion with neurology and interventional neuro-radiology specialists. On sedation hold the following day, she is E = 3 Vt M = 6 with 2 mm symmetrical and reactive pupils. EEG shows no evidence of seizure activity. Ventilation is weaned over the next twenty-four hours. A repeat CT scan is performed looking for brain swelling or haemorrhage and this shows a small area of infarction related to the thrombosis but no other worrying changes. She is extubated uneventfully and is E4 V4 M6 with good power in all four limbs. She is transferred to Neuro HDU the following day.

Case Discussion Including a Summary of the Evidence Base

The definition of SE is currently under review, and debated, but a shorter length of seizure activity is now accepted as discussed in the introduction.

SE has multiple causes as listed in Box 7.1, and a wide range of physiological derangements and complications which are detailed in Box 7.3.

This patient had an underlying structural reason for her seizure activity necessitating the combination of seizure management and treatment of the cause.

Seizure Management

In a randomised controlled trial[1] of lorazepam vs diazepam vs placebo, using a five-minute threshold in 205 patients, SE was terminated by lorazepam in 43% and by diazepam in 21%. Respiratory complications were similar in the lorazepam and diazepam groups (11% vs 10%) but higher in the placebo group (23%), presumably due to continuing seizure activity.

In a double blind trial with a ten minute threshold for SE, 1705 patients were screened and 570 studied.[2] Success was defined as abolition of all clinical and EEG seizure activity at 20 minutes, for up until 1 hour. Four IV regimes were studied:

Box 7.3 Complications of SE

- Airway obstruction; apnoea; hypoxia; hypercapnoea
- Massive catecholamine release, tachycardia, arrhythmias, labile BP
- Raised cerebral O_2 consumption and cerebral blood flow (CBF)
- Loss of cerebral autoregulation
- Hypotension and reduced CBF
- Hyperpyrexia, hyperglycaemia
- Systemic and cerebral hypoxia
- Neurogenic pulmonary oedema
- Rhabdomyolysis, acute renal failure, hyperkalaemia
- Lactic acidosis
- Hepatic necrosis
- Disseminated intravascular coagulation

Diazepam plus phenytoin; lorazepam; phenobarbitone;, phenytoin alone.

Success rates were diazepam/phenytoin 56%; lorazepam 65%; phenobarbitone 58%; phenytoin alone 44%. Mortality in generalised convulsive SE was 27%.

SIGN guideline 70[3] synthesises the evidence into a treatment protocol which is very similar to that in Box 7.1

In patients who continue to have seizures despite this, specialist input is vital and an example treatment protocol for SE is appended. See Appendix.

Cerebral Venous and Sinus Thrombosis

Cerebral venous and sinus thrombosis (CVST) is rare, accounting for less than 1 per cent of all strokes. The exact incidence in adults is unknown. The peak incidence in adults is in the third decade, and oral contraceptives are a significant risk factor. The diagnosis is frequently missed or delayed because of the varied presentations and the often, indolent onset. Headache is the most frequent symptom of CVST and occurs in almost 90 percent of all cases. The headache may be very similar to the headache experienced by patients with subarachnoid haemorrhage. Forty percent of all patients with CVST will suffer seizures. Focal neurological signs (including focal seizures) are the most common finding in CVST. Of all clinical signs reported in CVST, coma at admission is the most consistent and strongest predictor of a poor outcome. Saposnik and colleagues have reviewed this condition comprehensively, including presentation, investigation and treatment.[4]

Patients with CVST without contraindications for anticoagulation should be treated either with body weight-adjusted subcutaneous low molecular weight heparin or with dose-adjusted intravenous unfractionated heparin, but this should always be done in consultation with specialists as noted above.

Conclusion

Prompt control of seizures in SE is the immediate goal of therapy, whilst searching for a cause. SE continues to have a high mortality which might be improved by earlier specialist involvement of expert teams: neurology, neuro-radiology and neuro-intensive care.[5] This is worthy of future research.

Key Learning Points

- SE (like left ventricular failure or sub-arachnoid haemorrhage) is not a definitive diagnosis but a syndrome for which the cause must be sought.
- Control of airway, breathing and circulation may not be possible until motor features of seizures are abolished
- Following initial treatment of SE, and abolition of motor seizure activity, lack of improvement in conscious level often indicates sub-convulsive seizure activity. Access to full EEG recording, with specialist interpretation, is mandatory.
- In a patient with a normal CT brain scan but with a high opening pressure at LP (+/- raised CSF protein), cerebral venous and sinus thrombosis should be sought and, if present, treated.

References

1. Alldredge BK, Gelb AM, Isaacs SM, et al. A comparison of lorazepam, diazepam, and placebo for the treatment of out-of-hospital status epilepticus. *N Engl J Med.* 2001 Aug 30;345(9):631–7.

2. Treiman DM, Meyers PD, Walton NY, et al. A comparison of four treatments for generalized convulsive status epilepticus. Veterans Affairs Status Epilepticus Cooperative Study Group.*N Engl J Med.* 1998 Sep 17;339(12):792–8.

3. Diagnosis and management of epilepsy in adults. Guideline No 70 April 2003, Updated October 2005. Currently under review.

4. Saposnik G, Barinagarrementeria F, Brown RD Jr, et al. for American Heart Association Stroke Council and the Council on Epidemiology and Prevention. Diagnosis and management of cerebral venous thrombosis: a statement for healthcare professionals from the American Heart Association/American Stroke Association. *Stroke.* 2011 Apr;42(4):1158–92.

5   Wijdicks EFM. *The clinical practice of critical care neurology.* Oxford University Press 2003. Excellent primer in neuro-intensive care.

Appendix: Critical Care Guideline for the Treatment of Status Epilepticus

SE is defined as more than 30 minutes of:

Continuous seizure activity or;

Two or more sequential seizures without full recovery of consciousness between seizures

Management of SE is conveniently described by a stepwise approach. Critical Care is usually involved from stage 2 or 3 onwards or where intubation and ventilation are required.

Stage 1

0–30 mins.
Early SE.
Treat with benzodiazepines, diazepam (or lorazepam).

Stage 2

30–120 mins.
Established SE.
Treat with IV anti-epileptic drugs eg. phenytoin.

Stage 3

>120 mins.
Refractory SE.
Treat with general anaesthesia, e.g. propofol and intubation,
ventilation and
propofol +/- midazolam by continuous infusion.

Stage 4

>24 hrs.
Super refractory SE.

Complex specialist treatment requiring neurologist/ neurophysiology and EEG input. Drug therapies include the above plus sodium valproate, barbiturates and ketamine.

Investigation

History and examination.
Identify and treat the underlying causes of seizures.
Blood glucose: identify and treat hypoglycaemia.
Imaging: CT, MRI, EEG. CSF examination, metabolic screen, anti-receptor antibody assay, NMDA

Drug Treatment Guidelines

The general stepwise addition of drug treatment is outlined below.

Stage 1

Early SE 0–30 mins.
Initial treatment with **diazepam** emulsion (Diazemuls®).

2 mg increments IV initially up to 10 mg over 5 mins.
Alternative is IV lorazepam 4 mg slow IV into a large vein.
Repeat diazepam once 15 mins, later up to total 20 mg if required.
Repeat lorazepam once 15 mins later up to a total of 8 mg, if required. [1]

Stage 2

30–120 mins.
Established SE.

Load with **phenytoin** and start maintenance dose.

Loading dose 20 mg/kg (see appendix 2 for dosing in obesity).

Caution in frail and elderly as it may cause significant hypotension.
Consider loading in two divided doses.

Maintenance dose 100 mg 8 hourly IV. Check level morning following loading to check adequate loaded.

Stage 3

>120 mins.
Refractory SE.
Induce general anaesthesia. Intubate and ventilate with general supportive ICU care. Use drugs as follows in a stepwise fashion.

Propofol

Initial bolus to induce anaesthesia. Maintenance infusion of up to 4 mg/kg/hr.[4,5]

Midazolam

Loading dose bolus: 0.1–0.2 mg/kg.
Maintenance infusion 0.05–0.4 mg/kg/hr. If breakthrough SE give a further bolus and increase the infusion every 3–4 hours by 0.05–0.1 mg/kg/hr.[4,5,6]

Sodium Valproate

Loading dose of 30 mg/kg, i.e. 2100 mg if 70 kg. If patient is obese, use ideal body weight.
Maintenance infusion of 2400 mg over 24 hours. Ammonia levels should be performed for patients started on valproate approximately two days after starting valproate.

Stage 4

>24 hrs.
Super refractory SE. SE that has continued despite general anaesthesia. This requires complex specialist treatment

involving a collaborative approach with neurology and neurophysiology, EEG input and continuous EEG monitoring. By this stage the seizures are often nonconvulsive.

Phenobarbitone

Loading dose of 10 mg/kg IV up to a maximum of 1000 mg.
Maintenance dose of 120 mg once daily IV.[2,3]

Thiopentone

Using a 25 mg/ml solution for a 70 kg adult infuse approximately:
40 ml/hr for 1 hour
24 ml/hr for 2 hours
12 to 20 ml/hr thereafter.[14]

Ketamine

There is evidence on the use of ketamine; it is mostly based on isolated case reports. From the information available:
Loading dose of 50 mg.
Maintenance infusion of 1–5 mg/kg/hr.[7,8,9,10,11,12]
It is recommended that increased intracranial pressure should be excluded before ketamine is administered. There are few published data on the theoretical risk of neurotoxic effects when the drug is used for prolonged periods and its safety in prolonged use is largely untested.

Other Treatments

Inhalational anaesthetic agents.
Magnesium infusion.
Hypothermia.
Ketogenic diet.
For auto-immune encephalitis: high dose steroids, immunoglobulin and plasma exchange, in consultation with neurologist specialist/ epileptologists.

References

1. Lothian Adult Medical Emergencies Handbook.

2. British National Formulary 64, September 2012.

3. Personal communication Dr Matthew Walker. UCL.

4. Liegrel S, Bedos JP, Azoulay E. Managing Critically Ill Patients with Status Epleticus. Annual Update in Intensive Care and Emergency Medicine 2010. Edited by J.L. Vincent.

5. Brophy GM, Bell R, Claassen J, Alldredge B, Bleck TP et al. Guidelines for the evaluation and management of status epilepticus. *Neurocrit Care* 2012 Aug;17 (1):3–23.

6. Shorvon S. The management of status epilepticus. *J Neurol Neurosurg Psychiatry* 2001;70 (suppl II):ii22–ii27.

7. Kramer AH. Early ketamine to treat refractory status epilepticus. *Neurocrit Care* (2012);16:299–305.

8. Shorvon S, Ferlisi M. The treatment of super-refractory status epilepticus. *Brain.* 2011;134(10):2802–18.

9. Chen JWY, Wasterlain CG. Status epilepticus:pathophysiology and management in adults. *Lancet Neurol* 2006;5:246–56.

10. Sheth RD, Gidal BE. *Refractory status epilepticus: response to ketamine.* Neurology. Dec 1998;51:1765.

11. Nathan BR, Smith TL, Bleck TP. The use of ketamine in the treatment of refractory status epilepticus. *Neurology* April 2002;58: (Suppl 3). A197.

12. Synowiec AS, Singh DS, Yenugadhati V, Valeriano JP, Schramke CJ et al. Ketamine use in the treatment of refractory status epilepticus. Epilepsy Research 2013; in press.

13. Ubogu EE, Sagar SM, Lerner AJ, Maddux BN, Suarez J et al., Ketamine for refractory status epilepticus: a possible ketamine-induced neurotoxicity. *Epilepsy Behav* 2003; 4:70–5. LUHD Critical Care monograph for administration of thiopentone.

Acute Ischaemic Stroke

Samir Matloob and Martin Smith

Introduction

Stroke is a collection of clinical syndromes that are the most common cause of mortality and long-term disability worldwide. Acute ischaemic stroke (AIS) accounts for 85 percent of all stroke cases and haemorrhage for the remainder. There have been significant advances in the management of AIS over the last two decades following the introduction of four interventions that are supported by class I evidence: care on a stroke unit, intravenous tissue plasminogen activator (tPA) within 4.5 hours, aspirin within 48 hours and decompressive craniectomy for supratentorial malignant hemispheric infarction.[1] Approximately 15% to 20% of patients require admission to an intensive care unit (ICU) and this chapter highlights important aspects of the critical care management of AIS.

Case Description

A 55-year-old man developed sudden onset left-sided weakness and facial droop. Following confirmation of potential stroke by the attending paramedics, he was transferred directly to the local hyperacute stroke unit (HASU). On admission to hospital, his Glasgow Coma Score (GCS) was 15 (Eyes = 4, Verbal = 5, Motor = 6) but he had a dense left hemiparesis and left facial droop. Blood pressure was 205/110 mmHg and blood glucose was within normal limits. Past medical history included hypertension and coronary artery disease for which a drug-eluting coronary stent had been inserted three months previously. Medication included ramipril, bisoprolol, atorvastatin, aspirin and ticragrelor. An urgent non-contrast cranial computerised tomography (CT) scan confirmed early signs of right middle cerebral artery (MCA) infarction, thrombus in the M1 segment of the MCA and no evidence of haemorrhage (Figure 8.1). The patient received intravenous thrombolysis with alteplase 85 minutes after symptom onset and was then transferred to the acute stroke ward for observation and further management. A repeat CT scan at 24 hours showed extensive areas of infarction in the right MCA territory, causing only slight mass effect (Figure 8.2a). Although his neurological status was unchanged at this stage, the patient was transferred to the neurocritical care unit (NCCU) for close monitoring in view of the CT findings. Twelve hours later his GCS fell to 13 (E3, V4, M6) and a repeat scan showed worsening mass effect (Figure 8.2b). An urgent decompressive hemicraniectomy was undertaken after multi-disciplinary review and patient consent.

The patient was sedated and ventilated post-operatively and his intracranial pressure (ICP) monitored. A postoperative CT scan (at 24 hours) showed a good decompression with no complications. Sedation was reduced but the patient had a generalised seizure so was resedated and started on levetiracetam 500 mg bd. On the following day an

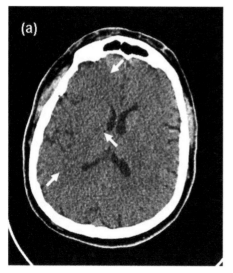
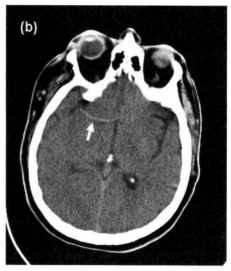

Figure 8.1 Admission cranial computerised tomography scans. (a) Early hypodensity is evident in the right middle cerebral artery (MCA) territory (arrows) consistent with hyperacute ischaemic stroke. There is mild mass effect of the ipsilateral ventricle but no midline shift and no signs of haemorrhage. (b) The hyperdense right MCA is suggestive of acute thrombus (arrow).

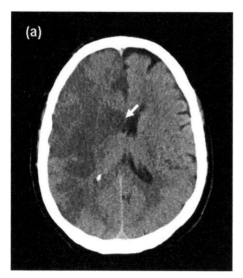
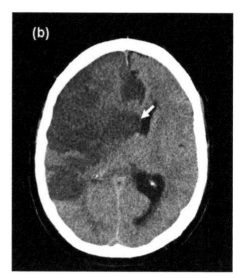

Figure 8.2 Cranial computerised tomography scans. (a) Extensive right hemispheric subacute infarction is seen within the right middle cerebral artery territory, causing mass effect compressing the ipsilateral lateral ventricle (arrow). (b) Twelve hours later there is markedly worse mass effect with midline shift towards the left (arrow).

electroencephalogram (EEG) showed no epileptiform activity. Hypertension was initially treated with a labetolol infusion and subsequently the patient's usual antihypertensive agents were reintroduced. Blood glucose was maintained between 7 to 11 mmol/L with intravenous insulin, and an episode of chest sepsis treated with piperacillin/tazobactam.

Aspirin was re-introduced two days after craniectomy following multi-disciplinary discussion among cardiology, neurosurgery, stroke and critical care teams. Clopidogrel was subsequently added two weeks after stroke onset. The patient was extubated seven days after admission to the NCCU and subsequently discharged back to the stroke unit six days later. His dense left hemiparesis persisted but he was otherwise neurologically normal.

Discussion

An understanding of the underlying pathophysiology of AIS is crucial to the delivery of effective and timely treatment. Key to this is the concept of a central area of tissue ischaemia surrounded by a hypoperfused but potentially salvageable penumbral zone. Blood flow to the ischaemic core is too low to maintain electrophysiological activity and cellular integrity whereas the surrounding penumbra has potential for complete functional recovery if blood flow is restored in a timely manner and to a sufficient degree. Beyond the urgent need for tissue reperfusion, there are further intracranial and systemic sequelae of AIS that must be identified and treated in a timely manner.

Stroke Care Pathways

Pre-hospital stroke scales facilitate identification of potential stroke by patients and first-responders, allowing direct transfer to a HASU so that treatment can be expedited if the diagnosis is confirmed. In the United Kingdom, the Cincinnati Pre-hospital Stroke Scale, also known as the Face Arm Speech Test (FAST), is widely used (Table 8.1). Immediate assessment and stabilisation after arrival at the HASU and urgent neuroimaging facilitates timely thrombolysis in eligible patients.

Indications for ICU Admission

While it is known that management by a multidisciplinary team in an acute stroke unit improves outcome after AIS, there is little evidence guiding management in the ICU. Indications for ICU admission include intracranial complications such as infarct extension, haemorrhagic transformation and malignant stroke syndromes, and management of non-neurological complications.[2] Monitoring and optimisation of systemic physiology, including blood pressure, glucose and temperature control, are key components of the ICU management of AIS (Table 8.2).

In determining the suitability for ICU admission, the potential reversibility of any neurological deterioration and likely outcome should be considered, taking into account the patient's pre-morbid state and wishes (if possible to ascertain). Overly pessimistic

Table 8.1 Face Arm Speech Test (FAST) pre-hospital stroke scale

	Yes	No
Facial droop?		
Arm drift?		
Speech abnormal?		
Positive screen if response to any question is positive		

Table 8.2 Management of systemic physiological variables after acute ischaemic stroke

Oxygenation and ventilation	• Routine administration of oxygen is not recommended • Administer supplemental oxygen only if SpO_2 <95% • Intubation and mechanical ventilation may be required in patients with decreased conscious level, severe bulbar palsy and risk factors for intracranial hypertension
Blood pressure	• Routine blood pressure lowering not recommended • Cautious BP lowering in patients not receiving thrombolysis if BP > 220/120 mmHg • Lower BP to less than 185/110 mmHg before thrombolysis and maintain for 24 hours afterwards • Treat significant hypotension (systolic BP < 90 mmHg) with volume expansion and vasopressors
Glucose	• Maintain blood glucose between 7–11 mmol/l (with iv insulin as required) • Treat hypoglycaemia (blood glucose < 2.8 mmol/l) with 10% dextrose
Temperature	• Symptomatic treatment with paracetamol if temperature >37.5°C • Exclude or treat infective cause of pyrexia

prognostication should be avoided in the early days as many patients can have a good recovery if complications are prevented or treated.

There is little evidence to support routine neuromonitoring after AIS, although intracranial pressure (ICP) is often measured in patients with large space-occupying infarction and oedema. However, measured ICP can be normal despite large ischaemic tissue volumes, and reliance on clinical and radiological findings (rather than on ICP alone) is appropriate in most cases. In the postoperative period, ICP monitoring can be useful in identifying intracranial complications early.

Thrombolysis

Thrombolysis with intravenous tissue plasminogen activator (tPA) is an evidence-based intervention for patients less than 80 years of age presenting within 4.5 hours of stroke onset, although earlier thrombolysis is always of greater benefit.[3] The number needed to treat to achieve one functionally independent patient increases from 4.5 to 15 when tPA is delayed from 90 minutes to 4.5 hours after stroke onset, emphasising the need to minimize 'stroke-to-needle' time. Interventional procedures such as intra-arterial thrombolysis, mechanical embolectomy and angioplasty/stenting are options in some patients who are ineligible for, or fail to respond to, intravenous tPA and may extend the treatment window to 6–8 hours.

Haemorrhage is the most significant complication of thrombolytic therapy although haemorrhagic transformation of infarcted tissue can also occur in non-thrombolysed patients. Post-thrombolysis haemorrhage is reported in up to 6 per cent of patients and its risk is increased by hypertension immediately prior to treatment, older age, hyperglycaemia, pre-existing diabetes and larger infarct volume. A cranial CT scan should be performed routinely at 24 hours to assess for haemorrhagic complications.

Airway and Respiratory Management

Dysphagia is common after AIS and increases the risk of aspiration pneumonia. All patients should undergo a swallow assessment soon after admission, and remain nil by mouth until an adequate swallow has been confirmed.

Hypoxaemia is common after AIS (Box 8.1) but routine oxygen supplementation does not improve outcome and can in fact be detrimental. The National Institute for Health and Care Excellence recommends that oxygen should be administered only if SpO_2 falls below 95 percent[4].

Endotracheal intubation and mechanical ventilation should be considered in patients with decreasing conscious level, severe bulbar palsy and pathology that might lead to intracranial hypertension. The need for intubation should be assessed on an individual basis depending on likely outcome and patient and family preferences. Studies report high mortality (60% to 80%) amongst ventilated stroke patients, although 50 to 60% of survivors (including up to 25% of those older than 65 years) have reasonable long-term functional outcome.[5] It is likely that the introduction of more aggressive management strategies has greatly improved outcome in patients who require mechanical ventilation.

Between 15% and 35% of AIS patients managed in the ICU require a tracheostomy and this is most likely in those with severe dysphagia and bulbar palsies or after prolonged periods of mechanical ventilation. Tracheostomy should be considered after one week of mechanical ventilation if a reasonable outcome is predicted.

Blood Pressure Management

Approximately 80 percent of patients are hypertensive at presentation (systolic BP greater than 140 mmHg), but blood pressure decreases spontaneously in most over the subsequent hours and days. Hypertension is likely related to chronic hypertension, raised ICP, or stress or neuroendocrine responses. There is a U-shaped relationship between blood pressure and outcome after AIS, with both high and low pressure being associated with adverse outcome. Hypertension can contribute to worsening brain injury by exacerbating cerebral oedema and increasing the risk of haemorrhagic transformation, whereas low blood pressure can compromise cerebral perfusion and potentially increase infarct volume. Despite this, studies of blood pressure interventions have failed to show outcome benefit.[6] Current guidance recommends that cautious blood pressure lowering (less than 15% in 24 hours) should be considered in those not receiving thrombolysis only when blood pressure is greater than 220/120 mmHg.[7] In patients undergoing thrombolysis, blood pressure should be less than 185/110 mmHg before commencing treatment and for 24 hours afterwards.[4] Labetalol is a

---

Box 8.1 Common causes of hypoxaemia following stroke

- Pulmonary aspiration
- Pneumonia
- Pulmonary embolus
- Acute lung injury/Acute respiratory distress syndrome
- Central respiratory depression/arrhythmias
- Obstructive sleep apnoea
- Respiratory muscle weakness

reasonable first-line agent in such circumstances. If longer term anti-hypertensive treatment is required, angiotensin-converting-enzyme inhibitors or angiotensin-receptor blockers are the preferred agents.

Hypotension, defined by the individual's pre-morbid blood pressure or when systolic pressure is less than 90 mmHg, should be treated with fluid resuscitation in the first instance. Vasoactive agents such as norepinephrine are indicated in those unresponsive to volume replacement.

There are no data to guide blood pressure management after decompressive craniectomy in stroke patients but, as ICP is reduced after surgery, a lower arterial pressure is required to maintain adequate cerebral perfusion. Blood pressure targets should take into account the original stroke as well as the need to minimise the risks of postoperative bleeding and brain swelling. Systolic blood pressure between 120 and 160 mmHg is a reasonable target in most patients.

Decompressive Craniectomy

Pooled analysis of data from three European randomised controlled trials confirm that decompressive hemicraniectomy performed within 48 hours of symptom onset reduces mortality from 78% to 29% and significantly improves favourable outcomes in patients with malignant MCA infarction, aged between 18 and 60 years.[8] The benefits of surgery are impressive, with a number needed to treat of two for survival, and four for survival with mild-to-moderate disability. More recently, the DESTINY II trial evaluated the benefit of hemicraniectomy in patients aged over 60 years. Surgery again conferred a large mortality benefit (mortality rate 33% compared to 70% in controls) but, in this age group, at the cost of more survivors with poor neurological function. The potential risks (of survival with severe disability) as well as benefits of hemicraniectomy should therefore be discussed with the patient or family members before proceeding to surgery, in those over 60 years of age. Hemicraniectomy should be offered early to all patients under age 60 with large MCA infarctions who previously had good functional status.

Decompressive craniectomy is most effective when performed early and certainly before a significant deterioration in neurological status. Patients with a reduction in conscious level (a fall in GCS of one or more points) should be referred for surgical intervention within 24 hours and decompressed within 48 hours of the neurological change.

Glycaemic Control

Hyperglycaemia occurs in more than 40 percent of patients after AIS and is associated with a range of deleterious effects including larger infarct volume, higher risk of post-thrombolysis haemorrhage and higher rates of infection, particularly pneumonia.[9] Persistence of hyperglycaemia beyond the first four hours is strongly associated with worse outcome. Randomised controlled trials have been inconclusive in terms of outcome benefits of tight glycaemic control with intensive insulin therapy (IIT) after AIS, but all have shown that that IIT is associated with a high rate of hypoglycaemia which is a particular concern in brain-injured patients.[10] The optimal blood glucose target after AIS is uncertain although moderate level control, aiming to maintain serum glucose between 7.0 to 11.0 mmol/L whilst avoiding large swings in glucose levels, is usually recommended.[4]

Antiplatelet Agents

Administration of aspirin within 48 hours of AIS is associated with overall benefit and it should be routinely administered at a dose of 300 mg daily, decreasing to 75 mg after two weeks.[4] In patients who have received thrombolysis, aspirin should be delayed for 24 hours as co-administration with tPA increases the rate of intracerebral haemorrhage without improving outcome. There is some evidence that dual antiplatelet therapy administered within 72 hours of stroke onset might bring additional benefits in terms of reduced stroke recurrence, and it does not appear to be associated with an increased risk of major bleeding. This is an important consideration in patients taking dual antiplatelet agents for another indication (e.g. drug eluting coronary stent) and suggests that dual therapy can be safely re-introduced early in some patients. However, relative contraindications to dual antiplatelet therapy, such as haemorrhagic transformation or cranial neurosurgery, mean that decisions should be made on a case-by-case basis after multi-disciplinary consultation.

Infection

AIS is associated with a period of relative immunosuppression resulting in hospital-acquired infections in 30 to 45 percent of patients. Pneumonia occurs in 6 percent of AIS patients overall but is most common in those who are mechanically ventilated. It is associated with the highest mortality of all non-neurological stroke complications. Independent risk factors for the development of pneumonia include mechanical ventilation, dysphagia, dysarthria and age greater than 65 years.

Up to 50 percent of patients develop fever after AIS and this is independently associated with poor outcome. Symptomatic treatment with paracetamol is advocated after exclusion or treatment of an infective cause.

Seizures

Early seizures (within 1–2 weeks) occur in approximately 3 to 8 percent of patients after AIS and are most commonly associated with cortical infarction. Although controlled seizures do not adversely affect outcome up to 25 percent of patients who develop seizures progress to status epilepticus and this is associated with higher rates of mortality. Seizures should always be treated aggressively but there is insufficient evidence to support the routine use of prophylactic anticonvulsants for primary or secondary seizure prevention, and some evidence that phenytoin might be detrimental.[2] Whether newer anticonvulsants such as levetiracetam are more effective or safer is yet to be confirmed. EEG monitoring should be undertaken in all patients with unexplained and/or persistently altered consciousness to exclude seizures as the cause of the altered neurological state.

Conclusion

AIS is a common and often devastating condition. Its management is complex and requires a multi-disciplinary team approach. Redesign of stroke services has allowed rapid access to investigation and intervention which has resulted in improved outcomes for patients. Increasing numbers of stroke patients are being admitted to the ICU for management of intracranial and systemic complications, and physiological optimisation. ICU management focuses on airway and ventilation management, haemodynamic and fluid optimisation, glycaemic, fever and seizure control, and surgical interventions for malignant MCA infarction.

Key Learning Points

- Acute ischaemic stroke is a medical emergency and early diagnosis, stabilisation and intervention are associated with improved outcomes.
- The management of acute ischaemic stroke is complex and requires a multidisciplinary team approach.
- Increasing numbers of stroke patients are being admitted to the ICU where management is focussed on the prevention and treatment of intracranial and systemic complications.
- Optimisation of systemic physiology is a key component of the ICU management of AIS and includes airway and ventilation management, haemodynamic and fluid optimisation, glycaemic and temperature control and control of seizures.
- Decompressive craniectomy is life-saving in patients with malignant MCA infarction.

References

1. Donnan GA, Fisher M, Macleod M, Davis SM. Stroke. *Lancet* 2008;371:1612–23.

2. Kirkman MA, Citerio G, Smith M. The intensive care management of acute ischemic stroke: an overview. *Intensive Care Med* 2014;40:640–53.

3. Lees KR, Bluhmki E, von KR, et al. Time to treatment with intravenous alteplase and outcome in stroke: an updated pooled analysis of ECASS, ATLANTIS, NINDS, and EPITHET trials. *Lancet* 2010;375:1695–1703.

4. National Institute for Health and Care Excellence (2008). Diagnosis and initial management of acute stroke and transient ischaemic attack. www.nice.org.uk/guidance/cg68/resources/guidance-stroke-pdf. (accessed 20 August 2014)

5. Foerch C, Kessler KR, Steckel DA, et al. Survival and quality of life outcome after mechanical ventilation in elderly stroke patients. *J Neurol Neurosurg Psychiatry* 2004;75:988–93.

6. Geeganage C, Bath PM. Interventions for deliberately altering blood pressure in acute stroke. *Cochrane Database Syst Rev* 2008; CD000039.

7. Jauch EC, Saver JL, Adams HP, et al. Guidelines for the early management of patients with acute ischemic stroke: a guideline for healthcare professionals from the American Heart Association/American Stroke Association. *Stroke* 2013;44: 870–947.

8. Vahedi K, Hofmeijer J, Juettler E, et al. Early decompressive surgery in malignant infarction of the middle cerebral artery: a pooled analysis of three randomised controlled trials. *Lancet Neurol* 2007; 6:215–22.

9. Luitse MJ, Biessels GJ, Rutten GE, Kappelle LJ. Diabetes, hyperglycaemia, and acute ischaemic stroke. *Lancet Neurol* 2012; 11:26171.

10. Bellolio MF, Gilmore RM, Ganti L. Insulin for glycaemic control in acute ischaemic stroke. *Cochrane Database Syst Rev* 2014: CD005346.

Chapter 9

Subarachnoid Haemorrhage

Alex Trotman and Peter Andrews

Introduction

Aneurysmal subarachnoid haemorrhage (aSAH) accounts for only 5 percent of strokes, with the UK incidence being around nine cases per 100,000 of the population.[1] The incidence of aSAH rises with age, peaking between the ages of 40 and 60 years. Despite advances in its diagnosis and management, outcomes after aSAH remain poor, with estimated mortality over 50 percent, and significant morbidity for a large number of survivors.[1] Despite a wide range of clinical presentations, multidisciplinary management in a surgical neurosciences centre is required for all cases. Aneurysm treatment modalities have evolved over time, and scientific evaluation of these has led to guideline development and changes in practice. Likewise, we now have evidence to support management strategies for the life-threatening complications that may develop following aSAH.[1,2] We discuss these interventions whilst looking at a patient's journey following presentation with aSAH.

Case Presentation

A 58-year-old female was brought to the accident and emergency department by ambulance complaining of a sudden onset of severe headache. She vomited in the ambulance and in the emergency department she complained of nausea and photophobia. Her past medical history included hypertension controlled with an ACE inhibitor, and mild COPD secondary to a 40-year history of smoking. On initial examination she had a GCS of 15 and no focal neurology was demonstrated. There were no other abnormalities found on examination. After she was in the emergency department for one hour, her conscious level deteriorated suddenly, and her GCS decreased to 8/15 (Eyes = 1, Verbal = 2 Motor = 5). At this point, anaesthetic staff attended to perform rapid sequence intubation and transferred the patient for non-contrast CT imaging of her head.

As intracranial pathology was suspected, a cranial CT scan was performed to establish a diagnosis. This showed a moderate subarachnoid blood load ('star sign' distribution) with some intraventricular blood, but no signs of hydrocephalus. She was then transferred to ICU for further management.

On ICU she was sedated to allow invasive mechanical ventilation and monitoring. Ventilator settings were optimised to provide adequate oxygenation and maintenance of $PaCO_2$, within the lower end of the normal range without excessive inspiratory pressures. A urinary catheter was inserted to monitor accurate fluid balance.

Due to initial inadequate sedation on ICU, her blood pressure was 180/95 mmHg. A systolic blood pressure limit of 160 mmHg was set as a threshold to start antihypertensive treatment, with the aim of reducing the risk of further aneurysm rupture (rebleeding).

Specific therapy for aSAH was started in the form of enteral nimodipine 60mg, given every 4 hours, to reduce delayed cerebral ischaemia.[2] A nasogastric tube was inserted to allow enteral administration of the nimodipine therapy.

Subsequent imaging showed an anterior communicating artery aneurysm, which was amenable to endovascular coiling. This procedure was carried out 24 hours after admission to ICU. Following the procedure, she returned to ICU under general anaesthetic for ongoing management. Over the following days, repeated neurological assessment was made using daily sedation holds to monitor and detect any complications. As the aneurysm was now secured, control of blood pressure to a higher target pressure was achieved, as the previous risk of rebleeding from the unsecured aneurysm was no longer present. Although there is no evidence-based data to suggest an optimal limit, we believe a systolic blood pressure of 180 mmHg is a reasonable upper limit for intervention once an aneurysm has been secured.

During her admission to ICU, our patient developed clinical and radiological signs of lower respiratory tract infection, which was treated with antibiotics. She also required treatment of moderate hyponatraemia and serial assessments for delayed cerebral ischaemia using bedside Doppler imaging. Her GCS was assessed with regular sedation holds, and this improved to Eyes = 3 Verbal = T Motor = 6 over the days following aneurysm coiling. Her respiratory support was weaned but unfortunately she failed a trial of extubation on day 11 of her admission. Following reintubation a percutaneous tracheostomy was performed and she successfully weaned from respiratory support and was discharged to the neurosurgical high dependency ward for further rehabilitation.

Discussion

Epidemiology and Presentation

In the majority of cases, SAH occurs due to rupture of an intracranial aneurysm, but can also be due to other cerebrovascular diseases, such as vasculitis or blood vessel malformations. These pre-existing conditions can lead to spontaneous bleeding, but SAH may also occur in a healthy individual following trauma. Factors that increase the risk of SAH include hypertension, smoking, atherosclerosis and cocaine and alcohol abuse. There is a familial preponderance due to certain inherited conditions associated with intracranial aneurysms, for example autosomal-dominant polycystic kidney disease and connective tissue disorders.[1]

The most common sites of aneurysm formation are at bifurcations of the major blood vessels around the Circle of Willis, shown in Figure 9.1.

Although not present in this case, other typical symptoms of aSAH include neck stiffness and focal neurology. In severe cases, cardiac arrest may occur. The symptoms of sudden onset 'thunder-clap' headache, nausea, vomiting, photophobia and a fall in conscious level seen in this case were highly suggestive of aSAH.

As there is a wide variation in presentation, from a neurologically intact patient with headache to a comatose patient with signs of raised ICP, attempts have been made to create a severity grading system that reflects the different clinical presentations. The World Federation of Neurological Surgeons (WFNS) grading scale is recommended, which is shown in Table 9.1 below. Prognosis decreases with increasing grade, as shown by the outcome figures. As implied by the WFNS grading scale, the neurological condition of the patient is the most important determining factor for patient outcome following aSAH.

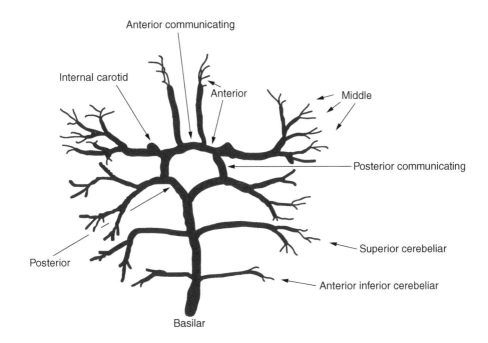

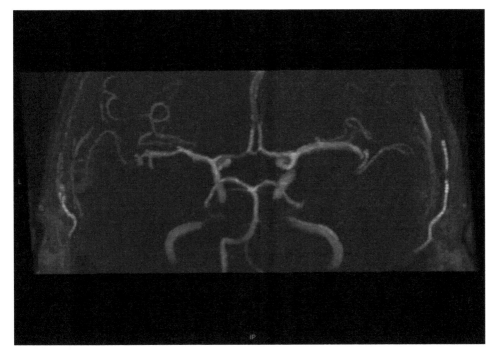

Figure 9.1 a) Circle of Willis b) MR angiogram showing Circle of Willis.

Table 9.1 The World Federation of Neurological Surgeons grading scale

WFNS grade	Criteria	Patients with poor outcome
I	GCS 15	14.8%
II	GCS 13–14 No focal deficits	29.4%
III	GCS 13–14 Focal deficits present	52.6%
IV	GCS 7–12	58.3%
V	GCS 3–6	92.7%

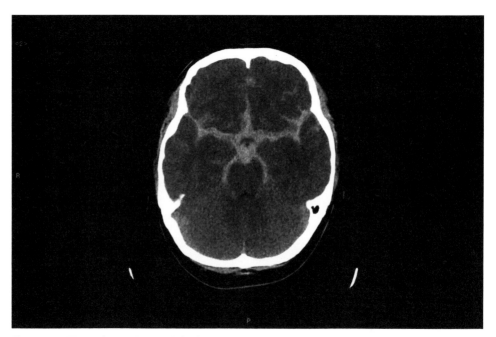

Figure 9.2 CT scan showing 'star sign' distribution.

Other factors that are most closely linked to outcome are patient age and the volume of extravasated blood visible on cranial imaging.[1]

Diagnosis

In the early stages following an aneurysm rupture, CT scanning is a sensitive method of detecting subarachnoid blood, but this early high sensitivity diminishes over time due to resorption and redistribution of blood. After five days only 85 per cent of cases will demonstrate subarachnoid blood on CT imaging, and after two weeks this falls to 30 per cent of cases. Magnetic resonance imaging (MRI) is comparable with CT imaging in the acute phase following aSAH, then becomes superior to CT over the ensuing days as sensitivity of the latter decreases.[1] If CT or MRI scans fail to demonstrate subarachnoid blood, a lumbar puncture (LP) should be performed 6 and 12 hours following the suspected bleed. Laboratory testing of cerebrospinal fluid (CSF) using a spectrophotometer can positively diagnose SAH due to the time-dependent degradation of subarachnoid blood, causing elevated bilirubin levels. Net bilirubin absorbance (NBA) greater than 0.007 absorbance units (AU) and net oxyhaemoglobin absorbance (NOA) greater than 0.02 AU is consistent with SAH. Serum bilirubin and CSF total protein levels may be required to allow interpretation of spectrophotometry that does not fulfil the above criteria.[3] As our patient had a positive CT diagnosis, LP was not indicated.

In order to determine the precise location of the aneurysm and to plan for securing the aneurysm, CT angiography (CTA) or magnetic resonance angiography (MRA) can be performed. For the detection of small aneurysms, MRA demonstrates a higher sensitivity than CTA, but digital subtraction angiography (DSA) is the most sensitive method available at present.[1] Due to expected improvements in CTA and MRA technology in the future, the use of DSA is anticipated to decrease, and will be reserved for cases when no bleeding source is found on CTA or MRA.

Management

Our patient had a grade IV aSAH requiring intubation and mechanical ventilation and admission to ICU. Patients with better grades (I to III) may be monitored with regular GCS assessment in a neurosurgical HDU (Better Critical Care, Level II). For all cases, neurosurgeons and neuroradiologists will assess the imaging and choose the most appropriate time and method for securing the aneurysm.

Clipping Versus Coiling

Options for definitive management of aSAH are either endovascular Guglielmi detachable coil (GDC) embolisation, or neurosurgical clipping of the aneurysm. Regardless of the technique chosen, until the aneurysm is secured there is a risk of further bleeding from the aneurysm causing clinical deterioration, and ultimately a much worse prognosis. Estimates for risk of early recurrent SAH range from 4 percent to 15 percent over the first 24 hours after the initial haemorrhage. The risk then falls to 1 percent to 2 percent per day over the next few weeks. For conservatively managed aneurysms, around half will have a further episode of aneurysmal rupture within six months. Approximately one third of this conservatively managed group who survive the initial haemorrhage will die as a consequence of secondary bleeding. After the initial six-month period, the risk posed by an unsecured aneurysm decreases to 3 percent over the following ten years, but a recurrent bleed has a very high mortality of over 60 percent.[1] These figures show that early definitive management for suitable patients will reduce morbidity and mortality from secondary haemorrhage, but the timing of when to secure an aneurysm will vary depending upon the clinical condition of the patient, and discussion amongst the multidisciplinary team. Management is also influenced by the potential complications that can arise, and these will be discussed later. However, it is our view that early securing of aneurysms improves outcomes.

Until the early 1990s neurosurgical clipping was used to secure cerebral aneurysms. Since 1995, and following development of the GDC, endovascular coiling has become widely used to secure both unruptured and ruptured aneurysms. A GDC is a platinum detachable coil that can be placed under radiological guidance to occlude blood flow into the aneurysm sac and prevent further rupture (shown in Figure 9.3). The International Subarachnoid Aneurysm Trial (ISAT) was undertaken to investigate safety and efficacy of endovascular treatment compared to surgical clipping. It was a multicentre clinical trial

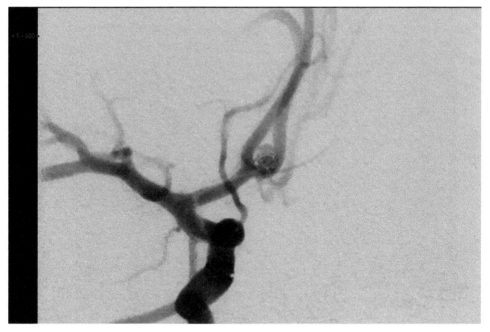

Figure 9.3 GDC placement under radiological guidance.

with patients randomised to either endovascular treatment with GDC or neurosurgical craniotomy and clipping. The findings showed a significant improvement in independent survival in the endovascular treatment group, but an increased risk of early rebleeding post-procedure after endovascular techniques. A limitation of the trial was that recruited patients tended to have a good clinical grade with small anterior circulation aneurysms, and patients with poor clinical grade and posterior circulation and middle cerebral aneurysms were under-represented. Also, unfavourable aneurysm anatomy can rule out endovascular management, and these patients are more likely to be referred for surgical intervention.[4,5,6]

In general, ISAT has shown that for aneurysms that can be managed with either technique, endovascular coiling is significantly more likely to result in survival without disability to one year post SAH, when compared to neurosurgical clipping. The decision to perform clipping or coiling will also depend on patient factors, such as age, comorbidity and presence of intracranial haemorrhage, plus procedural factors, such as logistics and availability of staffing and services.[6]

There are some prophylactic measures carried out for all SAH patients aimed at reducing the risk from complications. Repeated assessment and monitoring is required to identify the complications that are discussed below. Once an aneurysm is secured, the risk of rebleeding is greatly reduced, and systolic blood pressure control can be somewhat relaxed (up to 200 mmHg). Targets should provide a balance between adequate cerebral perfusion and prevention of DCI, and avoidance of the general risks associated with acute hypertension. This will require consideration of individual patient factors such as pre-morbid disease state and previous blood pressure.[2]

The use of pharmacological agents for thromboprophylaxis is contraindicated before securing the aneurysm, but the combined use of graduated compression stockings and pneumatic calf compression devices is recommended. Once the aneurysm is secured, low molecular weight heparin should be started at the discretion of the clinical team.[2]

Complications

Delayed Ischaemic Deficit (DCI)

Around one third of patients will develop new focal neurological deficit or a drop of two or more points of their GCS. Patients are most at risk of this between 4 to 10 days after the initial bleed. This can be reversible, but may progress to cause cerebral infarction, which has high morbidity and mortality rates. DCI often occurs with associated arterial vessel narrowing (aka vasospasm) which can be seen radiologically. Serial angiography is considered the gold standard for visualising this, but transcranial Doppler studies can be performed at the bedside, and are a quick, non-invasive method of detecting raised cerebral artery blood velocity, and avoids the need for moving the patient around the hospital. However, there is uncertainty regarding the exact pathogenesis of DCI, as patients may have neurological deterioration without radiographic evidence of vessel narrowing.[7,8]

A Cochrane review found a relative risk of 0.81 for death or dependence in patients treated with calcium antagonists. Although statistically significant, the findings depend heavily on a single large trial. Regardless of this, guidelines recommend the use of nimo-dipine in all patients with aSAH. Ideally this should be given enterally, as intravenous preparations have not shown benefit.[9]

Rebleeding

Modulation of coagulation using antifibrinolytic drugs has produced evidence of a reduced risk of bleeding from SAH. A Cochrane review of nine randomised trials showed that despite the reduction in risk, there was no influence on outcome. Recombinant factor VIIa has also been tested in small numbers of patients, however despite efficacy in reducing rebleeding, reports of arterial and venous thrombus formation mean it cannot be recommended for this use.[1] At present, there is no medical treatment that will improve patient outcome by a reduction in rebleeding.

Hydrocephalus

Hydrocephalus occurs in around 20 percent of patients with SAH and is usually diagnosed by a reduction in GCS and cranial CT imaging.[1] The cause of hydrocephalus following SAH is obstruction of the normal flow of CSF by blood from the aneurysm rupture. The risk of acute hydrocephalus following SAH rises with increasing amounts of intraventricular haemorrhage. Treatment of acute hydrocephalus is commonly a ventricular drain, but this presents added risks of infection and rebleeding. Chronic hydrocephalus will require consideration of ventriculo-peritoneal or ventriculo-atrial shunt insertion.

Hyperglycaemia & Hyperthermia

Both occur frequently after aSAH, and are independently associated with poor outcome. Pyrexia is often present without infection, and is thought to be an inflammatory response to subarachnoid blood. Evidence for an improved outcome after correcting hyperglycaemia is lacking, although it may reduce infection rates. Similarly, there is limited evidence to suggest that control of temperature is beneficial, and a single randomised trial of mild induced hypothermia during aneurysm surgery showed no benefit. Despite the evidence gap, treatment of blood glucose greater than 10 mmol/L and normothermia are recommended.[1]

Seizures

Seizures may occur following SAH, but evidence on their impact on outcome is lacking. If there are clinically apparent seizures, or EEG evidence of seizure activity in a comatose patient, anticonvulsants should be started. There is no evidence for the use of anti-convulsants prophylactically.[1]

Neurogenic Pulmonary Oedema (NPE)

NPE is a term used to describe hypoxaemic respiratory failure with associated pulmonary oedema following an acute brain injury. Other causes of pulmonary oedema that may be cardiac in origin must be ruled out. Estimates of the incidence of NPE following aSAH are around 2 percent, but prevalence may be much higher in fatal aSAH.[10] There is debate surrounding the pathogenesis of NPE, with two proposed mechanisms. Acute brain injury following aSAH can lead to a massively increased sympathetic activity, leading to acute myocardial dysfunction and pulmonary venous constriction, giving a hydrostatic aetiology of NPE. Another potential mechanism is due to increased permeability of pulmonary vasculature, possibly caused by cytokines released from injured brain tissue.[10] Diagnosis may be aided by echocardiogram, and pulmonary artery occlusion pressures. Therapeutic interventions for NPE – such as fluid restriction, diuretics, and lung protective ventilation – are often detrimental to the management of aSAH. This is reflected by a high incidence of poor outcomes in this patient group. Therefore any treatment should target well-defined goals to avoid worsening outcomes.

Hyponatraemia

Serum sodium levels less than 135 mmol/l are seen in approximately 30 to 40 percent of patients in the acute phase after aSAH.[10] There is a wide differential diagnosis for hyponatraemia, but syndrome of inappropriate antidiuretic hormone (SIADH) and cerebral salt wasting (CSW) syndrome are both common following aSAH. Diagnosis requires assessment of volaemic status, serum and urine osmolalities. If hyponatraemia is severe (less than 120 mmol/L) treatment will require hypertonic saline. If less severe, treatment is targeted at the underlying aetiology. For SIADH this requires restriction of free water, and for CSW syndrome intravascular volume and total body sodium restoration is required.

Summary

Presentation of aSAH varies due to a spectrum of intracranial insult following the aneurysm rupture. Grading systems help predict morbidity and mortality, in addition to improving multidisciplinary communication and management decisions. Once this is diagnosed, we believe early intervention will improve outcome, and radiological coiling should be considered in all appropriate cases. Monitoring of the patient before and after coiling is required to allow early detection of complications and targeted interventions, with the hope of improving outcome.

Key Learning Points

- Grading of severity at initial presentation is the best predictor of morbidity and mortality
- All patients should be managed in a neurosurgical centre by multidisciplinary teams
- Interventions to reduce risk of rebleeding and other complications are crucial to improving outcome

- Regular enteral nimodipine should be started as soon possible
- Coiling of ruptured aneurysms improves outcome compared with surgical clipping
- Close monitoring and vigilance are required to identify complications early an initiate appropriate treatment

References

1. Steiner T et al. European stroke organisation guidelines for management of intracranial aneurysms and subarachnoid haemorrhage. *Cerebrovascular Dis* 2013;35:93–112.

2. Stevens RD et al. Intensive care of aneurysmal subarachnoid haemorrhage: an international survey. *Intensive Care Med* 2009;35:1556–66.

3. Cruickshank A et al. Revised national guidelines for analysis of cerebrospinal fluid for bilirubin in suspected subarachnoid haemorrhage. *Ann Clin Biochem* 2008;45:238–44.

4. Bairstow P et al. Comparison of cost and outcome of endovascular and neurosurgical procedures in the treatment of ruptured intracranial aneurysms. *Australasian Radiology* 2002;46:249–51.

5. Scott RB et al. Improved cognitive outcomes with endovascular coiling of ruptured intracranial aneurysms. *Stroke* 2010;41:1743–7.

6. Molyneux A et al. (International Subarachnoid Aneurysm Trial [ISAT] Collaborative Group) International Subarachnoid Aneurysm Trial (ISAT) of neurosurgical clipping versus endovascular coiling in 2143 patients with ruptured intracranial aneurysms: a randomised trial. *Lancet* 2002;360:1267–74.

7. Etminan N et al. Effect of pharmaceutical treatment on vasospasm, delayed cerebral ischaemia, and clinical outcome in patients with aneurysmal subarachnoid hemorrhage: a systematic review and meta-analysis. *Journal of Cerebral Blood Flow & Metabolism* 2011;31:1443–51.

8. Vergouwen MDI et al. Definition of delayed cerebral ischaemia after aneurysmal subarachnoid hemorrhage as an outcome event in clinical trials and observational studies. *Stroke* 2010;41:2391–5.

9. Dorhout Mees S et al. Calcium antagonists for aneurysmal subarachnoid haemorrhage. *Cochrane database of systematic reviews* 2007, Issue 3. Art. No: CD000277

10. Stevens RD, Nyquist PA. The systemic implications of aneurysmal subarachnoid haemorrhage. *Journal of the Neurological Sciences* 2007;261:143–56.

Chapter 1

Management of Traumatic Brain Injury

Matthew Wiles

Introduction

Trauma is the leading cause of death in people aged 15 to 44 and traumatic brain injury (TBI) is responsible for the majority of these deaths. The incidence of TBI in Europe is 150 to 300 per 100,000 populations per year, which is equivalent to more than 750,000 new TBI cases each year. The long-term neurological sequelae of TBI in terms of disability is associated with significant financial implications, both in ongoing healthcare provision for survivors and the loss of their ability to work. It is estimated that over six million people in Europe are living with some level of disability secondary to TBI.

The management of TBI is becoming more complex due to changing patient demographics. TBI was once predominantly a disease of young men, but although TBI remains more common in men (3:1 male to female ratio), the mean age of a patient has increased significantly over the past 30 years and is now around 45 years. This has resulted in a greater number of comorbid medical problems that must be considered when managing brain injury. This increase in patient age is reflected in the mechanism of injury with the most common cause of TBI now being falls (50 percent); road traffic collisions (30 percent) and assaults (10%) are some way behind. To further complicate their management, around 40% of patients with TBI will have an associated major extracranial injury and a similar number will be intoxicated on admission to hospital.

The optimal early management of TBI, with the prevention of secondary brain injury, is crucial in determining outcome. The six-month mortality of TBI in the UK is approximately 25 percent; of the survivors only 25 percent will make a good recovery, with 25 percent having a moderate disability and 50 percent remaining severely disabled. It is, therefore, vital that brain protective strategies are employed meticulously throughout the patient's critical care stay.

Case Description

A 45 year old male motorcyclist was involved in a high-speed road traffic collision (motor-cycle versus car) on his way to work. At the scene his GCS was 13 (Eyes = 3 Motor = 5 Verbal = 5) with no other injuries identified. He was rapidly transferred to the local Major Trauma Centre where his primary survey revealed no obvious injuries to chest, abdomen or pelvis but by this stage his GCS had fallen to 7 (E1 M4 V2). He was anaesthetised, his trachea intubated and he was transferred for a trauma CT scan (head to sacrum). He was stable throughout this time from both a cardiovascular and pulmonary perspective. The CT brain revealed a large subdural haematoma with evidence of significant mass effect, as demonstrated by midline shift and uncal herniation. There were no other injuries identified in the thorax, abdomen or pelvis. He was immediately transferred to theatre for a craniotomy where the neurosurgical team evacuated the haematoma. Before replacing the bone flap was replaced, an intracranial pressure (ICP) monitor was inserted. He has now returned to the ICU for 48 hours of 'brain-protection' before a decision will be made about attempting to reduce sedation and awaken him.

This chapter will subsequently discuss how an isolated head injury should be optimally managed on critical care, with a particular focus on how to address increases in ICP during that time.

Discussion

Type of Brain Injury

The nature and location of the brain injury can give a guide as to the severity of the insult and the likelihood of increases in ICP. The types of TBI encountered in patients admitted to critical care can broadly be classified as follows:

Subdural haematoma: this most commonly occurs as a result of blunt trauma and is usually a venous bleed secondary to tearing of bridging cortical veins. This is the most common type of brain injury and is often associated with trauma to the underlying brain parenchyma.

Extradural haematoma: this is usually secondary to damage to the middle meningeal artery and requires urgent neurosurgical decompression. It is associated with a better prognosis than other types of injury.

Cerebral Contusion: this is caused by direct parenchymal damage and may be associated with intraparenchymal haemorrhage. These injuries tend to have associated cerebral oedema and may increase in size over a period of 24 to 72 hours.

Traumatic Subarachnoid Haemorrhage: this is caused by damage to small arteries within the subarachnoid space. Complications are similar to those seen following aneurysmal rupture and include hydrocephalus and delayed cerebral ischaemia (DCI; previously called vasospasm).

Diffuse Axonal Injury: this is caused by acceleration/deceleration forces causing axonal disruption. The CT appearance classically shows deep-seated, small punctuate haemorrhages, which may be widespread. This injury is strongly suggestive of a severe, irreversible brain injury.

Physiological Basis for Management Strategies

The early management priorities of a patient with TBI admitted to critical care are based upon prevention of secondary brain injury. The most common strategies used to achieve this are by the maintenance of an optimal cerebral perfusion pressure (CPP) and minimisation of increases in ICP, whereby CPP equals MAP minus ICP (or MAP minus CVP if CVP is greater than ICP). The basis for this strategy is the Monroe–Kellie doctrine, which is a simplified model of the pressure–volume relationships of the contents of the craniospinal space. The model assumes that the craniospinal space is a non-compliant box and consists of four volumes: brain tissue, intravascular blood, cerebrospinal fluid (CSF) and other (potential) space-occupying lesions, such as haematoma or oedematous tissue. An increase in the volume of one component (for example, a subdural haematoma) will increase the pressure within the box, and, therefore, the ICP. This pressure increase will initially be compensated for by a shift in another component (usually displacement of CSF in the spinal cord), but once this buffering capacity is exhausted, the ICP will increase exponentially, with a subsequent decrease in CPP and the risk of cerebral hypoxia as oxygen delivery falls.

Management of Intracranial Pressure

As per the Monroe–Kellie doctrine, in order to reduce ICP, it is necessary to reduce the volume of one of the four components of the craniospinal space.

1. Reduction in CSF volume: this can be achieved by either removal (via external ventricular drain) or diversion (via ventricular shunt) of cranial CSF.
2. Reduction in brain/potential space-occupying lesion: these are surgical treatments and involve either the removal of haematomas or, in extreme cases, brain tissues (frontal lobotomy).
3. Reduction in cerebral blood volume (CBV): this forms the basis of the majority of TBI management on critical care, although in fact most interventions are actually targeted at reductions in cerebral blood flow (CBF), which is controlled by the variations in cerebral arteriolar diameter.

   a. Carbon Dioxide Control

   An increase in $PaCO_2$ leads to a reduction in CSF pH and induces cerebral vasodilation. The relationship between $PaCO_2$ and CBF is fairly linear across normal clinical values, with an elevation in $PaCO_2$ of 1 kPa increasing CBF by 20 to 30 per cent over a period of only a few minutes. The effect is transient, as the changes in CSF pH normalise over 6 to 12 hours and CBF returns to baseline. Marked hyperventilation should be avoided as at low $PaCO_2$ levels (less than 2.5 kPa) there may actually be reflex vasodilation due to cerebral hypoxia caused by excessive vasoconstriction.

   b. Cerebral Oxygenation

   A reduction in cerebral arterial oxygen content results in cerebral vasodilation and an increase in CBF. This inverse relationship is relatively linear and occurs regardless of the underlying cause of the reduction in oxygen content (e.g. hypoxia, anaemia).

   c. Blood Pressure

   Due to autoregulation, CBF remains constant for a CPP of 50 to 150 mmHg although in patients with long-standing hypertension, the curve is shifted to the right, making them more likely to be able to maintain CBF should the MAP fall. In TBI, the autoregulatory process may be impaired and CBF may become pressure-dependant with changes in CBF directly mirroring alterations in MAP. Accurate blood pressure management is vital and the arterial line transducer should be placed at the tragus of the ear in order to accurately measure brain MAP and therefore reflect CPP.

   d. Cerebral Metabolic Rate for Oxygen ($CMRO_2$)

   The brain is metabolically highly active, accounting for 20 percent of both the body's cardiac output and oxygen consumption, with a close correlation between CBF and $CMRO_2$. In TBI the aim is to minimise $CMRO_2$ by decreasing cortical activity through sedation, control of seizures and temperature regulation with avoidance of pyrexia; there is a 7 percent increase in CBF for each 1°C rise in body temperature.

e. Avoidance of Venous Obstruction

This primarily consists of avoiding any factors that will impede cerebral venous drainage, such as tight endotracheal tube ties and rigid cervical collars in conjunction with the application of 10 to 15° of head-up tilt. The use of PEEP of up to 15 cm H_2O in patients with TBI has been shown not to increase ICP; open-lung ventilatory strategies are recommended in TBI, as atelectasis and pulmonary infection have the potential to impair oxygenation and carbon dioxide removal, which are far more significant factors in terms of ICP control.

Within neurosurgical centres, these physiological effects will be targeted according to protocolised care, an example of which is shown in Figure 10.1. The Brain Trauma Foundation (BTF) guidelines form the basis of many of the treatment targets, although other groups have also published therapeutic goals (Table 10.1), with no overall consensus. A large part of the care bundles used in TBI are identical to those used for other ITU conditions, with infection control, nutritional support and ventilator care bundles being of similar importance.

BTF, Brain Trauma Foundation; EBIC, European Brain Injury Consortium; AAGBI, Association of Anaesthetists of Great Britain and Ireland, SpO_2, arterial oxygen saturation; PaO_2, partial pressure of oxygen in arterial blood; $PaCO_2$, partial pressure of carbon dioxide in arterial blood; SBP, systolic arterial blood pressure; MAP, mean arterial blood pressure; ICP, intracranial pressure; CPP, cerebral perfusion pressure.

Many aspects of TBI management remain controversial, with differing opinions and contrasting study results cited found throughout the published literature. Some of these will be discussed more fully below.

Areas of Controversy

Hypotensive Resuscitation

Although permissive hypotension is increasingly used in the management of the unstable trauma patient, its use is contraindicated in moderate to severe TBI, as hypotension (SBP less than 90 mmHg) is associated with a significant increase in mortality. The optimal way to restore systemic blood pressure is yet to be determined, but a combination of crystalloid and colloid solutions and vasopressor therapy (e.g., noradrenaline infusion) is most commonly used. Dextrose containing solutions and albumin should be avoided, as these are associated with increases in cerebral oedema and ICP.

'Rosner' vs. 'Lund' Strategies

Cerebral perfusion pressure protocols (first described by Rosner in 1995)[1] focus on the maintenance of an adequate CPP by a combination of inducing a high-normal MAP and control of ICP; this is the most commonly used strategy for TBI management in ICUs in the United Kingdom. The Lund Principle (named after the Swedish hospital where it was developed) is an alternative strategy that aims to decrease cerebral oedema by decreasing $CMRO_2$ and CPP.[2] This is primarily achieved with normalisation of plasma osmotic pressure with transfusions of albumin and packed red blood cells and a reduction in capillary hydrostatic pressure with the use of alpha- and beta-blockers. The use of barbiturate coma, osmotherapy, CSF drainage and head-up tilt are avoided. Although proponents of both strategies claim excellent results, there are no trials that directly compare the two.

Intracranial Pressure/Cerebral Perfusion Pressure Management Strategy

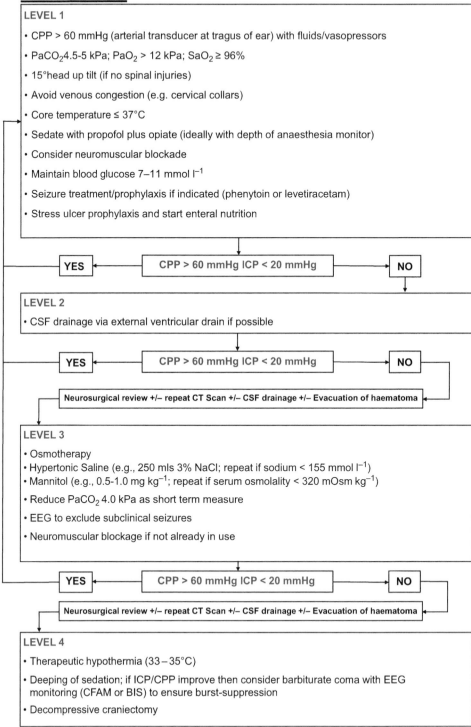

LEVEL 1

- CPP > 60 mmHg (arterial transducer at tragus of ear) with fluids/vasopressors
- $PaCO_2$ 4.5-5 kPa; PaO_2 > 12 kPa; SaO_2 ≥ 96%
- 15°head up tilt (if no spinal injuries)
- Avoid venous congestion (e.g. cervical collars)
- Core temperature ≤ 37°C
- Sedate with propofol plus opiate (ideally with depth of anaesthesia monitor)
- Consider neuromuscular blockade
- Maintain blood glucose 7–11 mmol l^{-1}
- Seizure treatment/prophylaxis if indicated (phenytoin or levetiracetam)
- Stress ulcer prophylaxis and start enteral nutrition

YES ← CPP > 60 mmHg ICP < 20 mmHg → NO

LEVEL 2

- CSF drainage via external ventricular drain if possible

YES ← CPP > 60 mmHg ICP < 20 mmHg → NO

Neurosurgical review +/– repeat CT Scan +/– CSF drainage +/– Evacuation of haematoma

LEVEL 3

- Osmotherapy
- Hypertonic Saline (e.g., 250 mls 3% NaCl; repeat if sodium < 155 mmol l^{-1})
- Mannitol (e.g., 0.5-1.0 mg kg^{-1}; repeat if serum osmolality < 320 mOsm kg^{-1})
- Reduce $PaCO_2$ 4.0 kPa as short term measure
- EEG to exclude subclinical seizures
- Neuromuscular blockage if not already in use

YES ← CPP > 60 mmHg ICP < 20 mmHg → NO

Neurosurgical review +/– repeat CT Scan +/– CSF drainage +/– Evacuation of haematoma

LEVEL 4

- Therapeutic hypothermia (33 – 35°C)
- Deeping of sedation; if ICP/CPP improve then consider barbiturate coma with EEG monitoring (CFAM or BIS) to ensure burst-suppression
- Decompressive craniectomy

Figure 10.1 Intracranial pressure algorithm.

Table 10.1 Therapeutic targets in the management of traumatic brain injury

Parameter	BTF (2007)	EBIC (1997)	AAGBI (2006)
Respiratory	AVOID $SpO_2 < 90\%$ $PaO_2 < 8$ kPa $PaCO_2 < 3.3$ kPa	TARGET $SpO_2 > 95\%$ $PaO_2 > 10$ kPa $PaCO_2$ 4.0–4.5 kPa	TARGET $PaO_2 > 13$ kPa $PaCO_2$ 4.5–5.0 kPa
Cardiovascular	AVOID SBP < 90 mmHg	TARGET MAP > 90 mmHg	TARGET MAP > 80 mmHg
Neurological	TARGET ICP $\leq$ 20 mmHg CPP 50 to 70 mmHg	TARGET ICP < 20 to 25 mmHg CPP > 60 to 70 mmHg	Not stated

Transfusion Triggers

Anaemia occurs in around 50 per cent of patients with TBI, but the optimum haemoglobin concentration for these patients is yet to be determined. Anaemia may decrease cerebral oxygen delivery but this needs to be balanced against the undesirable effects of transfusion of red blood cells. In the absence of definitive evidence, there is a general consensus that the restrictive transfusion trigger used in general ICU (70 g l^{-1}) is not applicable in TBI and that a higher trigger of 90 g l^{-1} should be used. A trial is currently underway examining whether erythropoietin is of value in moderate/severe TBI.[3]

ICP and Multimodal Monitoring

Intracranial pressure monitoring has been the bedrock of TBI management for many years, despite uncertainties over the indications for its use and the lack of evidence of outcome benefit. The use of ICP as a value treated in isolation is likely to be of little value, but when used as part of an overall management strategy appears to be associated with better outcomes. Intraventricular pressure monitors are the gold standard, but parenchymal bolts (which are more prone to calibration drift) are more commonly used in the United Kingdom. There is a drive to improve the way in which the injured brain is monitored, thereby allowing an individualised target for CPP and ICP to be determined. Brain tissue oxygenation (PbtO$_2$) guided therapy shows the most promise, with some studies suggesting improved functional outcomes with its use. Other modalities such as cerebral microdialysis to measure lactate: pyruvate ratios, transcranial Doppler ultrasound and jugular bulb venous oxygen saturation measurement which are all used in some centres, despite the lack of evidence from RCTs supporting their use.

Prophylaxis for Venous Thromboembolism

Venous thromboembolic events are common following TBI, especially in the context of polytrauma, where rates of DVT are in excess of 20 per cent. Mechanical preventative measures such as graduated compression stocking and intermittent pneumatic compression should be used unless contraindicated. The use of low-molecular weight heparin (LMWH) as prophylaxis remains controversial, due to the potential for worsening of intracranial bleeding. However, this risk appears minimal 48 to 72 hours post-injury and LMWH therapy should be considered at this point.

Hypothermia

Following TBI many cellular pathophysiological processes are initiated that lead to neuronal damage. Many of these are temperature dependant, which led to the investigation of therapeutic hypothermia as a treatment for TBI and the management of raised ICP. At present, however, there are no high-quality studies that have demonstrated any improvement in mortality or neurological outcome with induced hypothermia, and there may be a greater incidence of pneumonia and a reduction in CPP with its use.[4] At the present time, therefore, therapeutic hypothermia for the routine management of TBI cannot be recommended.

Barbiturate Coma

Barbituates are used in the management of refractory intracranial hypertension as they reduce CBF, $CMRO_2$ and ICP, although at the cost of hypotension (and reduction in CPP) and immunosuppression. Doses are titrated using EEG monitoring (either cerebral function analysing monitor [CFAM] or the bispectral index [BIS]) aiming for burst suppression. Although barbituates reduce ICP, there are no data demonstrating that their use is associated with improvements in mortality or neurological outcome.

Decompressive Craniectomy

Like barbituates, decompressive craniectomy is an effective treatment for the management of refractory intracranial hypertension, but has also not been shown to reduce mortality or unfavourable neurological outcomes.[5] Concerns remain that the use of decompressive craniectomy may result in poor quality survival in TBI patients; that is, the salvage of highly-disabled individuals who would have otherwise died.

Glycaemic Control

Hyperglycaemia is common in patients with TBI and is associated with a worse neurological outcome. However, the higher rates of hypoglycaemia seen with the use of intensive insulin therapy regimens used in general critical care patients, may be similarly detrimental from a neurological perspective. A meta-analysis demonstrated that intensive-insulin therapy in patients with TBI was not associated with improvements in mortality or neurological outcome, although infection rates were decreased.[6] As such, the current recommendation for glucose control in patients with TBI is within a range of 6 to 10 mmol/l.

Osmotherapy

Osmotic agents, usually mannitol or hypertonic saline, are common used in the management of raised ICP despite uncertainties regarding the correct dose and a lack of evidence of long-term benefit. Both agents will acutely decrease ICP by similar amounts, although neither treatment has been shown to improve mortality or neurological outcome. Mannitol decreases ICP in two ways: first, by inducing a reduction in blood viscosity which leads to an increase in cerebral blood oxygen delivery and subsequent cerebral vasoconstriction and second by causing osmotic shift of fluid from brain extracellular fluid to plasma (if the blood-brain barrier is intact). A typical dose of mannitol is 0.25 to 1 mg kg^{-1} (targeted to keep serum osmolality less than 320 mOsm kg^{-1}), with a therapeutic effect of 1 to 4 hours. Hypertonic saline exerts its effect on ICP in a similar osmotic manner to that of mannitol. Doses depend upon the formulation used, with concentrations varying from 1.7 to 29.2 per cent, and may be given as intermittent boluses (aiming for serum sodium less than 155 mmol/l) or as a continuous infusion.

Seizure Prophylaxis

Prophylaxis for post-traumatic seizures is recommended for the first seven days following injury in those at high-risk for seizures (GCS less than 10, depressed skull fracture, intracranial bleeding, cerebral contusion, penetrating TBI or seizures within 24 hours of injury). Phenytoin has been the traditional agent used although levetiracetam is increasingly being utilised due to its superior side-effect profile of less cardiovascular instability.

Other Pharmacological Interventions

Magnesium is thought to attenuate the cellular damage caused by trauma-induced ischaemia. However, a meta-analysis by the Cochrane group was unable to demonstrate that the administration of magnesium improved either neurological outcome or mortality in TBI. Similarly, the Medical Research Council CRASH study of over 10,000 patients showed that the administration of corticosteroids in TBI was associated with a greater risk of death and disability.[7] The beneficial effects of progesterone in animal models of TBI have not been seen in human studies, with two large RCTs showing no improvements in neurological outcome or mortality with the administration of either very early, or later progesterone therapy.[8]

Timing of Tracheostomy

Patients who suffer acute brain injury are more likely to undergo a tracheostomy compared to other ICU patients. Although the results of the TracMan trial suggested no overall benefit in terms of mortality or length of critical care stay with early tracheostomy (within four days) compared to late tracheostomy (more than ten days), it is important to remember that this study excluded chronic neurological conditions and patients with acute intracranial pathologies made up less than 4 per cent of the cohort.[9] There is a paucity of high-quality, prospective trials specifically examining the timing of tracheostomy in patients with severe TBI, although recent data have suggested that early tracheostomy (less than 7 days post-injury) in patients with severe TBI (GCS less than or equal to 8) may be associated with better neurological outcomes and a reduced length of stay.

Prognositication

Outcome prediction in TBI is extremely difficult due to the heterogeneous nature of both the brain injury and the patient population. In an attempt to correct this variability, various outcome prediction models have been developed, the most widely used being the IMPACT model (International Mission for Prognosis and Analysis of Clinical Trials in traumatic brain injury). However, no model can predict the outcome for an individual patient and most commonly used in clinical trials to ensure cohorts are comparable. The major predictors of poor outcome remain age greater than 46 years, reduced GCS motor score and absence of pupillary reactivity. The most promising prognostic biomarker is S100-β, which is a subunit of a calcium binding protein that is primarily found in Schwann and glial cells, the concentration of which is positively associated with both mortality and neurological outcomes in the short, medium and long-term. There are uncertainties regarding the time of measurement and precise concentration of S100-β that is associated with worse outcomes, but this measure may help further refine prognostic models.

Conclusion

Despite the extensive investigation of numerous therapeutic targets and pharmacological agents, no single intervention has been shown to improve mortality or neurological outcomes following TBI. The improvements in mortality that have been seen over the past decades are largely due to the implementation of several packages of care, which includes the use of ICP monitoring in addition to the care bundles already widely used in general ICU, such as those for ventilator and infection control care. However, due to the heterogeneous nature of TBI, both in terms of the injury itself and the patient population, the onus is on intensivists to try to individualise the care they provide rather than routine application of generic protocol with no consideration of patient specific factors. Advances in cerebral monitoring technology beyond simple ICP measurement may make this most challenging aspect of TBI management somewhat easier in the future.

Key Learning Points

- The five key pillars of TBI management are the maintenance of 'normal', namely normoxia, normocarbia, normotension, normothermia and normoglycaemia.
- Hypotension must be avoided at all costs in TBI; a single episode of SBP less than 90 mmHg leads to a doubling in mortality.
- Permissive hypotension has no place in the management of the polytrauma patient with a head injury.
- The arterial line transducer should be placed at the tragus of the ear in order to accurately reflect CPP.
- End-tidal carbon dioxide does not reliably correlate with $PaCO_2$. If in doubt, do a blood gas.
- Intracranial pressure values are a measurement, not a therapy, and should be interpreted in the context of the global clinical picture.
- Do not forget the value of general intensive care interventions such as nutrition, venous thromboembolism prophylaxis, infection-control bundles and gastric protection.

References

1. Rosner MJ, Rosner SD, Johnson AH. Cerebral perfusion pressure: management protocol and clinical results. *Journal of Neurosurgery* 1995;83:949–62.

2. Grände PO. The "Lund Concept" for the treatment of severe head trauma: physiological principles and clinical application. *Intensive Care Medicine* 2006;32:1475–84.

3. Nichol A, French C, Little L et al. Erythropoietin in traumatic brain injury: study protocol for a randomised controlled trial. *Trials* 2015;16:39 doi: 10.1186/s13063-014–0528-6.

4. Georgiou AP, Manara AR. Role of therapeutic hypothermia in improving outcome after traumatic brain injury: a systematic review. *British Journal of Anaesthesia* 2013;110:357–67.

5. Cooper DJ, Rosenfeld JV, Murray L, et al. Decompressive craniectomy in diffuse traumatic brain injury. *New England Journal of Medicine* 2011;364:1493–502.

6. Zafar SN, Iqbal A, Mauricio FF, Kamatkar S, de Moya MA. Intensive insulin therapy in brain injury: a meta-analysis. *Journal of Neurotrauma* 2011;28:1307–17.

7. Edwards P, Arango M, Balica L et al. Final results of MRC CRASH, a randomised placebo-controlled trial of intravenous corticosteroid in adults with head injury-outcomes at 6 months. *Lancet* 2005;365:1957–9.

8. Skolnick BE, Maas AI, Narayan RK et al. A clinical trial of progesterone for severe traumatic brain injury. *New England Journal of Medicine* 2014;371:2467–76.

9. Young D, Harrison DA, Cuthbertson BH et al. Effect of early vs late tracheostomy placement on survival in patients receiving mechanical ventilation: the TracMan randomized trial. *Journal of the American Medical Association.* 2013;309:2121–9.

Variceal Haemorrhage

Gregor McNeill

Introduction

Variceal haemorrhage is a medical emergency that can challenge the intensive care clinician on several fronts as initial resuscitation and management is often difficult. Airway compromise, circulatory collapse and the need for definitive haemorrhage control may need to be addressed simultaneously. Transfer of this patient group may also pose particular issues. Once on the ICU, careful attention must be paid to a variety of organ systems to ensure the best outcome is achieved.

Case Description

A 54-year-old man was found collapsed at home by a neighbour who alerted the emergency services. On arrival in the Emergency Department (ED), he was noted to be drowsy with signs of airway compromise. He had vomited altered blood during the transfer to hospital. The attending emergency staff noted that he was clammy, pale and looked very unwell. A radial pulse was not palpable but brachial and femoral pulses were present. His initial pulse rate was recorded as 140/minute and blood pressure was unrecordable. An initial venous blood gas revealed a pH 6.8, bicarbonate of 6.7 mmol/l, lactate of 19 mmol/l, haemoglobin (Hb) level at 32 g/l, Base Excess at -26 mmol/l, pO2 of 3.04 kPa and pCO2 at 4.55 kPa. The patient's Glasgow Coma Score (GCS) was 12. His abdomen was soft with a previous midline laparotomy scar. There was no immediate history of any previous medical problems. A focussed ultrasound examination performed by the ED staff did not reveal any abnormality. During this initial assessment the patient proceeded to develop cardiorespiratory arrest and required 3 cycles of cardio pulmonary resuscitation (CPR) before restoration of circulation was achieved. He was intubated and ventilated at this time. The hospital Major Haemorrhage protocol was initiated and the patient was administered 4 units of O negative blood. An urgent Computed Tomography (CT) scan of chest, abdomen and pelvis and CT Aortogram were performed. This revealed an irregular looking liver consistent with liver cirrhosis and some peri-hepatic free fluid. No definite bleeding source was identified. There were no other significant findings.

Following six units of blood and two units fresh frozen plasma, haemodynamic parameters stabilised with pulse rate of 123/minute and BP 115/70. An arterial line was placed and a further blood gas analysis revealed pH of 7.13, pCO2 4.86 kPa, pO2 28.3 kPa, bicarbonate of 12.3 mmol/l, BE -17.1 mmol/l, haemoglobin of 72 g/l and a lactate of 12.1 mmol/l. Corroborative history from family members confirmed heavy alcohol use over many years and the midline laparotomy scar related to a knife injury some years before. A focussed clinical examination confirmed signs of chronic liver disease. Baseline blood tests taken before his cardiac arrest revealed Hb 31 g/l, white blood count (WBC) 22.7 10^9/l, Platelet count of 366 10^9/l, Prothrombin Time (PT) 17 s, Activated Partial Thromboplastin Time (APTT) of 35 s, Thrombin Time (TT) 24 s, Fibrinogen 1.9 g/l, sodium 133 mmol/l, potassium 4.6 mmol/l, urea 8.3 mmol/l, creatinine 76umol/l, alanine aminotransferase (ALT) 19 u/l, total bilirubin 18 umol/l, total alkaline phosphatase 92 u/l and albumin of 24 g/l. The patient was reviewed by the on-call surgical team who felt, given the signs of chronic liver disease, that the next step should be upper GI tract endoscopy. The patient was transferred to the emergency theatre for the procedure.

Endoscopy revealed stigmata of recent bleeding within the oesophagus.

Three large varices (at the 11, 1 and 4 o'clock positions) with red signs showing recent bleed were seen. There were also gastric varices at the fundus of stomach but no blood in the stomach. Five bands were applied to the three oesophageal varices.

Following endoscopy the patient was transferred to the intensive care unit for on-going care. He was started on terlipressin 2 milligrams 4 hourly, regular intravenous ranitidine, intravenous antibiotics and lactulose therapy. Over the next 12 hours he stabilised: coagulopathy improved, he remained free of signs of further bleeding and did not require any on-going cardiovascular support. He was therefore extubated and plans were made to transfer to ward-based care.

However on day five following admission, the patient had an episode of vomiting fresh blood and passing melaena. Haemoglobin level was noted to drop from 95 g/l to 70 g/l. He was transferred to the emergency theatre again where another gastroscopy was performed under general anaesthesia. There was a large volume of fresh blood seen in the oesophagus and stomach.

Three further varices were seen at the 2, 6 and 11 o'clock positions and additional bands were applied but the fresh bleeding continued.

A Sengstaken–Blakemore tube was therefore inserted by the endoscopist and the patient was transferred to the Interventional Radiology Department where a transjugular intrahepatic portosystemic shunt (TIPS) was placed. Prior to the TIPS procedure, the hepatology and intensive care teams agreed that if the procedure failed to achieve haemorrhage control then the patient should be palliated.

Initial porto-systemic pressure gradient was noted to be 22 mm Hg and this dropped to 11 mm Hg post TIPS. Following the procedure the patient returned to the ICU, and as he remained haemodynamically stable, the Sengstaken–Blakemore tube was removed. He was successfully extubated 24 hours later, and there were no signs of on-going hepatic encephalopathy. Following ward transfer, the patient was successfully transferred home one week later.

Discussion

Variceal haemorrhage remains a lethal complication of chronic liver disease. Oesophageal and gastric varices develop as a consequence of portal hypertension. The most common cause is cirrhotic liver disease although rarer causes such as portal or splenic vein thrombosis should also be considered. In patients with cirrhotic liver disease presenting with GI haemorrhage, 70 percent will have a variceal source. Although recent years have seen significant advancements in therapeutic strategies,[1] variceal haemorrhage is a condition that still carries a significant risk of mortality.[2] The risk of death appears to be related the significance of the underlying liver disease as defined by the Childs-Pugh grading of chronic liver disease (Table 11.1 and 11.2).

Table 11.1 Assigning a Child-Pugh score

Parameter	Score		
	1	2	3
Ascites	none	Mild	moderate or severe
Encephalopathy	none	1–2	3–4
Bilirubin (micromol/L)	<35	35–50	>50
Albumin (g/L)	>35	25–35	<28
INR	<1.7	1.8–2.3	>2.3

Table 11.2 Classification of Child Pugh score with grade

Child Pugh Grade	Child Pugh Score
A	5–6
B	7–9
C	10–15
Adapted from [11]	

The diagnosis should be considered in any patient presenting with evidence of hypovolaemic shock or GI bleeding. As in the above case, there may not always be a confirmed history of either variceal haemorrhage or liver disease. Evidence of stigmata of liver disease such as icterus, spider naevi or ascites should prompt the intensivist to consider the possibility of a variceal cause.

Initial Resuscitation

Resuscitation of patients with variceal haemorrhage should follow a standard 'ABCDE' approach. While the initial management focus is often circulatory support, careful consideration should be made to airway assessment. Endotracheal intubation may be required for airway protection if there is torrential upper GI haemorrhage particularly if there is coexisting encephalopathy. Endotracheal intubation may also be indicated if prolonged endoscopic therapy or insertion of a Sengstaken–Blakemore tube (or similar) is likely to be required. Given the risks of worsening cardiovascular instability in an under resuscitated patient, the timing of induction of anaesthesia should be carefully considered.

The main focus of the initial resuscitation is likely to be around circulatory support. The priority should be peripheral wide bore intravenous access. An urgent cross-match should be sent. Fluid resuscitation should be principally with blood and group specific or O negative blood may be required depending on the acuity of presentation. Arterial line placement may aid monitoring of the cardiovascular response to resuscitation. Caution should be advised to avoid over-resuscitation as this theoretically risks raising portal pressure and could lead to further bleeding.

Coagulopathy should be corrected and clinicians should be aware of their local major haemorrhage protocols that may best facilitate timely, rapid issue of blood products when haemorrhage is severe. Patients may be coagulopathic due to both overwhelming haemorrhage as well as pre-existing decompensated chronic liver disease. Fresh frozen plasma should be given if the prothrombin time is prolonged and cryoprecipitate if the fibrinogen level is low. Platelet transfusion should also be considered if thrombocytopenia is present. Vitamin K should be administered routinely in case of coexisting vitamin K deficiency.

Medical Therapy

Antibiotics

Variceal haemorrhage is associated with bacterial infection. After blood cultures have been obtained, broad spectrum antimicrobials should be commenced. There is evidence that use of antimicrobials in variceal haemorrhage may be associated with both a reduction in rebleeding as well as overall mortality.[3] The benefit is possibly greatest in those with more advanced liver disease.

Therapy to Reduce Portal Pressure

Terlipressin, a synthetic analogue of vasopressin, is effective at reducing portal pressure (2 milligrams 4 hourly reducing to 1 milligram 4 hourly once haemorrhage control is achieved). It causes both splanchnic and peripheral vasoconstriction. It differs from vasopressin in that it has a longer half-life and a better side effect profile with less risk of cardiac and peripheral ischaemia. It should be continued for up to 72 hours to reduce the risk of rebleeding. A meta-analysis has found a statistically significant reduction in mortality with terlipressin when compared to placebo.[4]

Administration of the somatostatin analogue octreotide has been used as an additional therapy to reduce portal pressure; however a recent Cochrane review found no significant effect on either mortality or transfusion requirements.[5]

Although beta blockers such as propranolol have been shown to reduce the risk of bleeding from oesophageal varices, they do not have a role in the acute management of variceal haemorrhage. They should, however, be considered once the patient has been stabilised.

Endoscopic Therapy

Endoscopic therapy has both a diagnostic and therapeutic role in the management of variceal haemorrhage. It should therefore be performed as soon as the patient has been resuscitated and appropriately stabilised. The setting for any endoscopic therapy should be carefully considered by both the endoscopist and the intensive care team. The need for access to endoscopic interventions must be balanced by the need for the intensive care team to provide on-going resuscitation and close monitoring. Often an emergency theatre setting may be more appropriate than an endoscopic suite.

Endoscopy allows accurate diagnosis of the location of variceal haemorrhage and also allows the exclusion of another source of haemorrhage.

Therapeutic options for oesophageal varices include both sclerotherapy and band ligation. Recent meta-analysis suggests band ligation is the intervention of choice.

Although both sclerotherapy and band ligation are both successful in causing cessation of bleeding in around 90 percent of cases, rates of rebleeding are lower when band ligation is used.[6] Gastric varices can be more challenging to treat and band ligation appears less effective: injection with N-butyl-2-cyanoacrylate tissue glue may be effective.[7] If bleeding is torrential, endoscopic therapy may not be feasible, and in this circumstance, temporising measures such as direct tamponade may be required prior to definitive haemorrhage control using Transjugular Intrahepatic Portosystemic Shunt (TIPS) as in this case.

Balloon Tamponade

When other methods have proved ineffective and as an emergency temporising measure prior to definitive therapy, variceal bleeding can be controlled by applying direct pressure to the bleeding point using a balloon. The most widely used is the Sengstaken–Blakemore tube. This encompasses an oesophageal balloon, a gastric balloon and a gastric suction port. A modified version of the Sengstaken–Blakemore tube, termed the Minnesota tube with an additional oesophageal suction port, is also available. The patient should be intubated prior to insertion. The balloons should also be checked before insertion. The tube should be passed to 50 to 60 cm. If passage of the tube proves difficult, a successful position may be achieved by endoscopy-assisted placement. Once placed, the gastric balloon should be inflated with either 250 mls of water or oral contrast medium, and traction should be applied to the tube until resistance is felt, indicating the gastric balloon abutting the gastro-oesophageal junction. The tube should then be secured while maintaining traction either by affixing it securely to the side of the mouth with sticking plaster or by using a pulley system attached to a 250 to 500 g weight (such as a 500 ml bag of fluid). A chest x-ray should performed to confirm position. In general only the gastric balloon should be inflated. The oesophageal balloon should not be routinely inflated as this can lead to additional serious complications such as oesophageal necrosis and perforation. The tube should be left in situ for 24 to 48 hours, with the gastric balloon deflated every 12 hours to check for signs of rebleeding.

Transjugular Intrahepatic Portosystemic Shunt

TIPS should be considered in the 10 to 20 per cent of patients in whom endoscopic and vasoactive therapy fails to control bleeding or in patients who experience further bleeding during the acute admission. More recent evidence suggests that TIPS may also have a role as a first line therapy in reducing rebleed as well as mortality in those at high risk of treatment failure.[1] TIPS has largely superseded surgical shunt techniques which carry a higher morbidity and mortality.[8]

TIPS is a radiologically guided procedure that involves placement of a shunt between the hepatic vein and an intrahepatic branch of the portal vein. The aim of the procedure is to reduce the portovenous pressure to less than 12 mmHg as in this case. It is suggested that this will achieve haemostasis in over 90 per cent of cases. Complications of TIPS includes worsening of porto-systemic encephalopathy. Although it is clearly effective at controlling haemorrhage, the demonstrable risk of increasing morbidity means the exact timing of TIPS remains controversial.[9]

On-going Intensive Care Support

Once patients have received definitive haemorrhage control, they are likely to require on-going ICU care. Management strategies will focus on observation for rebleeding and ongoing organ support. Hepatic encephalopathy should be treated aggressively, particularly in those who have undergone TIPS. Lactulose 30 mls 8 hourly should be started, and thiamine and multivitamin replacement should be considered.

As with any patients presenting to the ICU with acute or chronic liver failure, careful consideration should be given to the benefits of multi-organ support. Recent analysis suggests that the main determent of outcome is number of failing organs rather than the specific severity of liver disease.[10] In addition, those presenting with bleeding may represent a subgroup with lower mortality when compared to other presentations of decompensation.

Conclusion

Patients presenting with variceal haemorrhage continue to represent a group with high morbidity and mortality. Optimal outcome requires effective early resuscitation and close liaison with the specialty hepatology team to ensure timely and effective treatment.

Key Learning Points

- Careful consideration should be given to early intubation for airway protection and to facilitate oesophageal therapy.
- Emergency endoscopic therapy should be performed in an area adequately equipped to provide on-going resuscitation.
- Terlipressin is the vasoactive treatment of choice.
- Balloon tamponade is a temporising measure and should be considered as a bridge to definitive therapy.
- TIPS is increasingly used as a definitive method of haemorrhage control.

References

1. Garcia-Pagan JC, Caca K, Bureau C et al. Early use of TIPS in patients with cirrhosis and variceal bleeding. *N Engl J Med.* 2010;362:2370–9.

2. Krige JE, Kotze UK, Bornman PC et al. Variceal recurrence, rebleeding, and survival after endoscopic injection sclerotherapy in 287 alcoholic cirrhotic patients with bleeding esophageal varices. *Ann Surg* 2006;244:764–70.

3. Chavez-Tapia NC, Barrientos-Gutierrez T, Tellez-Avila F et al. Meta-analysis: antibiotic prophylaxis for cirrhotic patients with upper gastrointestinal bleeding - an updated Cochrane review. *Aliment Pharmacol Ther.* 2011;34: 509–18.

4. Ioannou G, Doust J, Rockey D C. *Terlipressin for acute esophageal variceal hemorrhage.* Cochrane Database Syst Rev. 2003.

5. Gotzsche PC. *Somatostatin or octeotide for acute bleeding oesophageal varices.* Cochrane Database Syst Rev. 2000.

6. Laine L, Cook D. Endoscopic ligation compared with sclerotherapy for treatment of esophageal variceal bleeding. *A meta-analysis. Ann Intern Med.* 1995;123:280–7.

7. Lo GH, Lai KH, Cheng JS et al. A prospective, randomized trial of butyl cyanoacrylate injection versus band

ligation in the management of bleeding gastric varices. *Hepatology* 2001;33:1060–4.

8. Rikkers LF, Jin G. Emergency shunt. Role in the present management of variceal bleeding. *Arch Surg.* 1995;130:472–7.

9. de Franchis R. Revising consensus in portal hypertension: report of the Baveno V consensus workshop on methodology of diagnosis and therapy in portal hypertension. *J Hepatol.* 2010;53:762–8.

10. Moreau R, Jalan R, Gines P et al. Acute-on-chronic liver failure is a distinct syndrome that develops in patients with acute decompensation of cirrhosis. *Gastroenterology.* 2013;144: 1426–37.

11. Pugh RN, Murray-Lyon IM, Dawson JL, Pietroni MC, Williams R. Transection of the oesophagus for bleeding oesophageal varices. *The British Journal of Surgery* 1973; 60(8):646–9.

12 Surgical Management of Pancreatitis

Qaiser Jalal and Ahmed Al-Mukhtar

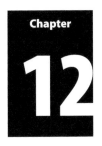

Introduction

Pancreatitis is a common cause of admission to a surgical ward, with an incidence in the United Kingdom of 22.4 people per 100,000 that appears to be rising.[1] Pancreatitis commonly presents as severe abdominal pain radiating to the back with a raised serum amylase and lipase levels greater than three times normal and radiological findings of pancreatitis on CT, MRI or ultrasound.

Early diagnosis and resuscitation are of paramount importance in the initial management and prevention of subsequent complications. Appropriately timed investigations and interventions are also required to deal with the consequences of severe pancreatitis as this case illustrates.

Case Description

A 59-year-old gentleman presented to his local hospital with a short history of abdominal pain and vomiting on a background history of hypertension and depression. His BMI was 40. He was diagnosed as suffering from gallstone–induced severe pancreatitis with severe systemic inflammatory response syndrome (SIRS) that necessitated admission to intensive care, ventilation and NJ feeding for nutrition. By the second week of his ICU admission, his clinical condition had not improved and a CT scan was performed which showed diffuse inflammation and fluid around the pancreas but no evidence of necrosis or abscess formation (Figure 12.1).

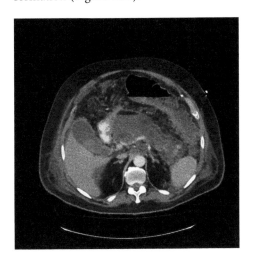

Figure 12.1 Diffuse pancreatitis.

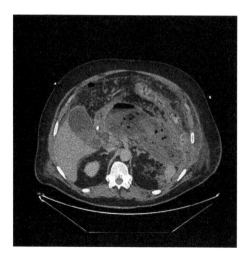

Figure 12.2 Infected pancreatic necrosis.

As a result, he was started on broad spectrum antibiotics and antifungal therapy as empirically he was deemed to have an ongoing need for inotropic support suggestive of inadequately treated infection. His condition failed to improve and he remained ventilator dependant with increasing inotropic support but maintaining good renal and hepatic function. A tracheostomy was performed in the third week of admission in anticipation of prolonged ventilation and weaning. A repeat CT, done because of failure to progress on the sixth week post admission, now showed signs of necrosis which prompted discussion with and transfer of the patient to a tertiary care hepatobiliary (HPB) unit.

A further CT performed at the tertiary centre showed the presence of gas in the retroperitoneum in addition to the pancreatic necrosis suggesting infected necrosis, which was treated with CT guided percutaneous drainage.

After this he required continuing inotropic support and developed raised intra-abdominal pressure and deteriorating renal function. A repeat CT scan showed what was thought to be semisolid necrosis that was not amenable to percutaneous drainage. The accuracy of determining whether the necrosis is liquid or solid using CT scanning is reasonable and there was the therapeutic option of replacing the existing drain with a larger bore drain, but following discussion with radiology, it was thought that this would not be of benefit in achieving drainage in this case.

The patient was therefore taken to theatre and minimal invasive retroperitoneal necrosectomy was performed and repeated a further four times over the next four weeks with good results.

Following this intervention, the patient was gradually weaned off ventilation and drain output decreased. Enteral feed was gradually introduced with diabetic team input due to the patient developing diabetes.

The patient's care was stepped down to the surgical ward as nutrition and mobility improved and he was able to be returned to the referring hospital for his recovery phase with a drain in situ (Figure 12.3) and a plan to do an elective cholecystectomy once his condition was stabilised and he was out of the catabolic phase of his illness.

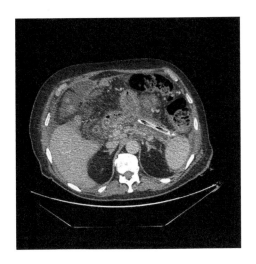

Figure 12.3 Drain in situ with good results.

Discussion

Assessment of Severity

Common causes of pancreatitis are listed below:

Causes of Pancreatitis

Gall stones
Alcohol
ERCP induced
Hyperlipidemia
Hypercalcemia
Drugs (corticosteroids, azathioprine, valporic acid)
Viral
Ampullary tumour
Pancreatic divisum
Trauma
Genetic
Autoimmune
Idiopathic

Once the diagnosis of pancreatitis is made the next step is prompt and adequate resuscitation maintaining end organ perfusion, analgesia and nutrition as in this case.

Approximately 80 percent of patients who present with acute pancreatitis will make an uneventful recovery and risk stratification plays a part in the management and early evaluation of severity in an attempt to allow the clinician to predict the patient's clinical course, estimate prognosis, and help determine the need for early intensive care involvement or admission. Several scoring systems are used, none of which is particularly accurate and there is evidence to suggest that stratification is best done using an Early Warning Scoring system (EWS); a high EWS at presentation predicts a more severe attack (2) Other common scoring systems are based on criteria developed by Imrie in Glasgow (Table 12.1) who described features in a population of patients with gallstone pancreatitis and the Ranson criteria (Table 12.2) developed from an American population of alcohol induced pancreatitis. The Apache II scoring system can also be used.

If the modified Glasgow score is greater than or equal to 3, severe pancreatitis is likely and intensive care input is needed. A score less than 3 suggests severe pancreatitis is unlikely.

Table 12.1(a) Modified Glasgow scoring

Parameter	Value
Arterial Po2	<60 mmHg
Serum albumin	<32 g/l
Serum Ca	<2 mmol/l
WBC	15,000/mm^3
AST	>200 IU/l
LDH	>600 IU/
Glucose	>10 mmol/l
Serum urea	>16 mmol/l

Table 12.1(b) Modified Glasgow Score and mortality

Modified Glasgow Score	Mortality %
0–2	2
3–4	15
5–6	40
7–8	100

Table 12.2(a) Ranson's score on admission

Parameter	Value
Age	>55
WBC	16000/mm^3
Glucose	>200 mg/l
LDH	>350 IU/L
AST	>250 IU/L

Table 12.2(b) Ranson's score within 48 hours of admission

Parameter	Value
Drop in Hematocrit	>10%
Serum Ca	<8 mg/dl
Base deficit	>4 mEq/l
Increase in serum urea from admission	>5 mg/dl
Fluid requirements within 48 hours	>6 l
Arterial Pao2	<60 mmHg

Team Working in Pancreatitis

Pancreatitis can prove life-threatening and at times, as in this case, has longer term debilitating effects on patients that require a cohesive team work involving surgeons, intensivists, radiologists, dieticians, microbiology and nursing staff.

Aggressive management would ideally be focussed on breaking the cascading events of pancreatitis but there are no specific interventions to do this at present. Hence, current care is supportive, aimed at early recovery and rehabilitation. Eighty percent of patients presenting with pancreatitis settle with simple measures and symptomatic treatment and 20 percent end up having severe pancreatitis with organ dysfunction or failure. Patients with end organ dysfunction need intensive support and management co-ordinated by intensive care specialists.[3] The majority will still recover without further complications but worsening organ dysfunction is associated with increasing mortality.[4] Mortality associated with mild pancreatitis is as low as 1 percent and severe pancreatitis is associated with long ICU stay and increased mortality.[6] UK data suggests that patients with severe acute pancreatitis admitted to intensive care have unit and hospital mortality of 32 percent and 42 percent respectively.[7]

Patients with severe pancreatitis can have systemic and local complications, including pleural effusion, ARDS, ileus, gastric ulceration, renal failure and cardiovascular compromise. Local complications include acute fluid collection leading to gastric outlet obstruction, pseudocyst, abscess, necrosis, pseudoaneurysm of the splenic artery and fistulation into an adjacent hollow viscus.

Imaging in Pancreatitis

All patients presenting with pancreatitis should have an ultrasound of their biliary system within 24 hours of admission[5] to look for gallstones as there may be an indication for early ERCP if the patient is sufficiently jaundiced. (Many patients with pancreatitis will have a mildly elevated bilirubin.) Repeated and careful clinical examination is of paramount importance in deciding on the type and timing of imaging and any interventions.

Cross-sectional imaging in the first two weeks of an acute attack of pancreatitis is generally unhelpful unless the primary reason for the scan is diagnostic doubt, for instance to exclude another cause such as a perforated viscus or to confirm the diagnosis of pancreatitis when the biochemical tests are equivocal. The main reason for this is that no major therapeutic options are available that will change the course of the disease in the first two weeks. There are also issues about the accuracy of the scans in terms of defining the type of necrosis and there is some suggestion that the contrast agent may make the pancreatitis itself worse.

In this case, the decision to perform the CT scan was made on the basis that the patient was still unwell at the end of two weeks and at that stage evidence of pancreatic necrosis with or without liquefaction and infection should be sought.

Surgery in Pancreatitis

Minimally invasive necrosectomy is performed by dissection of a drain track to the source of the necrosis. There is no convincing evidence that the outcomes from this minimally invasive approach are better than from open surgery which is carried out with an anterior approach and a major laparotomy. This may well reflect disease severity and either approach can be associated with significant complications.

The rationale for cholecystectomy when a patient has recovered sufficiently is to reduce the risk of a recurrent attack of acute pancreatitis if the trigger is thought to be gall stone related.

Conclusion

The majority of patients presenting with pancreatitis recover uneventfully without critical care support but a significant minority develop organ dysfunction requiring management by both surgeons and intensivists.

Initial CT scans may not show evidence of necrosis which becomes evident at a later stage illustrating the need for reassessment and an open minded approach to management. Infected necrosis which does not respond to antibiotics should be considered for treatment by percutaneous drainage, especially if there is no evidence of the presence of a solid component of the necrosis which is not amenable to percutaneous intervention.

Minimally invasive pancreatic necrosectomy can produce good results but does require repeated visits to theatre. The clinical course of pancreatitis can be unpredictable and multidisciplinary input is the key to good outcomes. The case described above is a good example of the progression of pancreatitis with appropriate timely interventions giving desired results.

Key Learning Points

- Early identification and management of organ failure and aggressive resuscitation to optimise tissue perfusion is important in cases of severe pancreatitis.
- Stratification of severity and the early involvement of the critical care team offer the best chance of a favourable outcome.
- Patients with severe pancreatitis should be managed by a multidisciplinary team with an interest in pancreaticobiliary disease. Patients with complications of severe pancreatitis should be discussed by a specialised unit with access to specialised interventions including percutaneous drainage, ERCP and minimal invasive; necrosectomy and having the expertise to do an open necrosectomy if required.
- Cholecystectomy in cases of mild gallstone-induced pancreatitis should be performed within 2 weeks of discharge. In cases of severe pancreatitis, surgery should be performed once the patient has recovered.

References

1. Roberts SE, Williams JG et al. Incidence and case fatality for acute pancreatitis in England: geographical variation, social deprivation, alcohol consumption and aetiology: a record linkage study. *Alimentary Pharmacology and Therapeutics* 2008;28(7):931–41.

2. Garcea G, Gouda M, et al. Predictors of severity and survival in acute pancreatitis: validation of the efficacy of early warning scores. *Pancreas* Oct 2008;37(3):e54–61.

3. Neoptolemos JP, Raraty, M et al. Acute pancreatitis: the substantial human and financial costs. *Gut* 1998;42(6): 886–91.

4. Butter A, Imrie CW, Carter CR et al. Dynamic nature of early organ dysfunction determines outcomes in acute pancreatitis. *Br J Surg* 2002;89(3):298–302.

5. UK guidelines for management of acute pancreatitis. Gut 2005;54(suppl.3):iii1–9.

6. Uhl W, WarshawA, Imrie C et al. IAP guidelines for the surgical management of acute pancreatitis. *Pancreatology* 2002; 2(6):565–73.

7. Harrison DA, D'Amico G, Singer M. Case mix, outcome, and activity for admissions to UK critical care units with severe acute pancreatitis: a secondary analysis of the ICNARC case mix programme database. *Critical Care* 2007;11(1) article S1.

13 Intra-abdominal Hypertension and Abdominal Compartment Syndrome

Helen Ellis and Stephen Webber

Introduction

The potentially harmful effects of high intra-abdominal pressure (IAP) were first recognised over one hundred years ago, but it was not until the 1980s that pressures were measured in clinical practice. Several case reports subsequently appeared in the medical literature describing abdominal compartment syndrome (ACS) and the resolution of renal function following surgical decompression. Over the past ten years, there has been a resurgence of interest on this topic, with the World Society of the Abdominal Compartment Syndrome (WSACS) being founded in 2004. Definitions (Figure 13.1) and guidelines were published by 2007, then revised in 2013[1] to aid the diagnosis and management of intra-abdominal hypertension (IAH) and ACS.

An epidemiological study in 2004 suggested the prevalence of intra-abdominal hypertension in critically ill patients was as high as 50.5 percent, with 8.2 percent of these having ACS.[2] Particular patient groups appear to be at increased risk, including trauma patients, those with severe acute pancreatitis and those having undergone large volume crystalloid fluid resuscitation prior to ICU admission.[3]

IAH and ACS are not interchangeable concepts. ACS is the syndrome of organ dysfunction that occurs as a result of intra-abdominal hypertension. The pathophysiology of ACS is that of any other compartment syndrome. Increasing pressures within a relatively fixed compartment not only compromise arterial perfusion of the viscera, but also venous drainage. This results in visceral oedema, which further increases compartment pressure. Integrity of the gut mucosal barrier is compromised, allowing bacterial translocation and increasing the risk of sepsis. Ischaemia and necrosis of vital organs will occur, resulting in multi-organ failure and a high mortality, even with surgical decompression.[4]

Definitions

IAH: a sustained or repeated pathological elevation in IAP ≥ 12mmHg

ACS: a sustained IAP > 20mmHg that is associated with new organ dysfunction/failure

IAP is graded as follows:
- Grade I, IAP 12 – 15mmHg
- Grade II, IAP 16 – 20mmHg
- Grade III, IAP 21 – 25mmHg
- Grade IV, IAP > 25mmHg

Figure 13.1 World Society of the Abdominal Compartment Syndrome (WSACS) definitions of intra-abdominal hypertension and abdominal compartment syndrome.

Case Description

A 66-year-old man presented to the Emergency Department with a five-hour history of severe abdominal pain. Past medical history included hypertension, type II diabetes mellitus and a body mass index (BMI) of 52.

Clinical examination revealed tachycardia, hypotension and a pulsatile abdominal mass. A contrast enhanced Contrast Tomography (CT) scan of the abdomen confirmed a 7.9 cm ruptured abdominal aortic aneurysm and the patient was transferred rapidly to the Operating Department. Open repair of the aneurysm was performed with an infra-renal cross clamp time of 110 minutes. A large retroperitoneal haematoma was noted, and the patient underwent a massive transfusion in addition to receiving 6 litres of crystalloid intravenously.

Post-operatively the patient was kept ventilated and sedated and was transferred to the intensive care unit (ICU). On initial assessment, the airway was secured with an appropriately placed endotracheal tube, ventilation was maintained with an inspiratory pressure of 22 cmH$_2$O and 5 cmH$_2$O of positive end expiratory pressure (PEEP), and oxygen saturations were 94 per cent. Heart rate was 112 bpm and blood pressure 92/55 mmHg on a noradrenaline infusion running at 0.45 mcg/kg/min. There was a nasogastric tube in situ and a urinary catheter with 45 ml of urine in the collecting chamber. The abdominal wound appeared dry and both feet were cool and mottled.

An arterial blood gas (ABG) performed with a FiO$_2$ of 0.60 revealed the following results: pH 7.19, PaO$_2$ 9.05 kPa, PaCO$_2$ 4.9 kPa, HCO$_3^-$ 19 mmol/l, BE -6.8 mEq/l, lactate 8.5 mmol/l and haemoglobin 69 g/l. The patient underwent respiratory recruitment and PEEP was increased to 12 cmH$_2$O.

Over the course of the first post-operative night, a further 500 ml of crystalloid and two units of packed red cells were administered. Coagulation results demonstrated the need for further cryoprecipitate and fresh frozen plasma, and urea and creatinine rose to 9.8 mmol/ and 223 μmol/ respectively.

Despite further fluid administration, urine output remained less than 20 ml/hr. IAP monitoring was instituted via the urinary catheter with an initial pressure of 18 mmHg. Cardiac output monitoring was begun which revealed a cardiac index of 2.3 l/min/m^2, a systemic vascular resistance index (SVRI) of 1230 dynes/s/cm^5/m^2 with a stroke volume variation of 8 per cent. The noradrenaline was increased to maintain a mean arterial pressure (MAP) of 75 mmHg and inspiratory pressure on the ventilator was increased to 28 cmH$_2$O to maintain tidal volumes of 6 ml/kg predicted body weight.

Four hourly IAP measurements were requested, and continuous veno–veno haemofiltration (CVVH) was commenced given a serum potassium of 7.1 mmol/l and ongoing oliguria. Nasogastric aspirates were high so enteral feed was not commenced and prokinetics were started. IAPs remained relatively stable for the remainder of that day, and the vascular team was updated.

On the second post-operative day, the nursing staff noted a rise in IAP to 23 mmHg. Sedation was deepened and an infusion of a neuromuscular blocking drug commenced. Despite this, IAP continued to rise and reached 28 mmHg on the third post-operative day. Cardiorespiratory parameters deteriorated with a fall in cardiac index and tidal volumes, whilst repeat ABGs demonstrated progressive hypercarbia and a climbing lactate. The surgeons were consulted and the decision was made to take the patient to the operating theatre for a decompressive laparotomy.

The patient returned from theatre with a Bogota bag™ covering the open abdominal wound and IAP measurements remained within acceptable limits. The operative findings noted that the bowel looked generally oedematous and a large amount of old retro-peritoneal haematoma had been evacuated. Respiratory compliance improved and inspiratory pressures were reduced to 24 cmH$_2$O. Reapplication of cardiac output monitoring showed a cardiac index of 2.8 l/min/m^2, a systemic vascular resistance index (SVRI) of 2200 dynes/s/cm^5/m^2 and a MAP of 92 mmHg, which permitted rapid weaning of vasopressor support. Given this, the ICU team decided to pursue a negative fluid balance using CVVH.

On post-operative day four, the surgical team exchanged the Bogota bag for a vacuum assisted closure (VAC®) device and began negative pressure wound therapy in the ICU.

Over the next few days, the patient's oxygen requirements reduced and a negative fluid balance of over three litres was achieved. Enteral feed was successfully titrated up to meet full nutritional requirements with low nasogastric aspirates.

On post-operative day nine, the patient returned to theatre for a successful primary abdominal closure. The following day the patient was extubated onto non-invasive ventilation.

Over subsequent days, the patient began to pass good volumes of urine, CVVH was stopped and creatinine and urea plateaued. The patient was moved to the High Dependency Unit on post-operative day 13 and discharged from Critical Care on day 16.

Case Discussion

IAH has been defined as a sustained or repeated pathological elevation in IAP greater than or equal to 12 mmHg[1] although adverse effects have been noted with pressures as low as 10 mmHg. 'Normal' IAPs in critically ill ventilated patients are expected to range between 5 mmHg and 7 mmHg, varying with respiration. The WSACS further subdivides IAH into grades I to IV on the basis of the IAP measurement (Figure 13.1). ACS is defined as a sustained rise in IAP greater than 20 mmHg that is associated with new organ dysfunction or failure.

Both IAH and ACS can be described as being primary or secondary in nature depending on whether the condition causing raised IAP originates from the abdomino-pelvic region or not. Abdominal trauma or acute haemorrhage would be considered a primary cause, whereas burns or sepsis a secondary cause. The condition can also be described as recurrent if it redevelops following treatment, and chronic if the onset occurs over a more prolonged period of time.

Both medical and surgical critically ill patients are vulnerable to developing IAH and ACS. Particular groups at risk are those having sustained abdominal trauma, burns to over 30 percent body surface area, patients undergoing liver transplantation, those with acute severe pancreatitis and those having undergone large volume crystalloid resuscitation.[3] Risk factors for IAH and ACS can be subdivided as follows:

- Decreased abdominal wall compliance: e.g., prone positioning, major trauma, major burns, abdominal surgery.
- Increased intra-luminal contents: e.g., gastroparesis, ileus, colonic obstruction.
- Increased intra-abdominal contents: e.g., pancreatitis, blood, pus, tumour, ascites, carbon dioxide insufflation.
- Capillary leak: e.g., acidosis, hypothermia, massive transfusion or fluid resuscitation, critical illness.

- Miscellaneous factors: e.g., sepsis, coagulopathy, head-up position, mechanical ventilation, obesity, PEEP greater than 10 cmH_2O, peritonitis, pneumonia, shock.

Presentation of IAH/ACS in non-ventilated patients is less common, but conscious patients may complain of shortness of breath, abdominal pain, bloating, weakness or dizziness. In patients with grade III and IV IAH, there may be evidence of the sequelae of ACS such as oligo-anuria, high ventilatory requirements or cardiovascular instability. Although the vast majority of patients will have a tight, distended abdomen, diagnosis on clinical grounds alone lacks sensitivity and specificity.[5]

Although imaging may help determine the aetiology and guide management, the IAP should be measured to make a diagnosis of intra-abdominal hypertension. The WSACS recommend monitoring of IAPs in a protocolised manner using the trans-bladder technique (Figure 13.2) when any known risk factor for IAH is present. Direct measurement of compartment pressures is possible, but carries an increased risk compared to the indirect trans-bladder method. Measurement of IAP via trans-urethral bladder catheters has been shown to have good correlation with direct intra-peritoneal pressure monitoring.[6] It should be noted however that regional variations in IAP may be present.

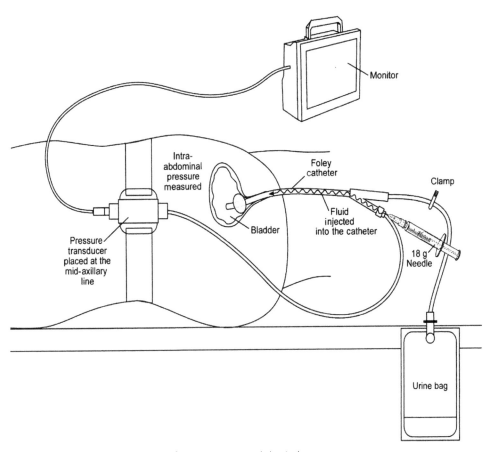

Figure 13.2 Trans-bladder technique for measuring intra-abdominal pressure.

To obtain a measurement, the patient is positioned supine, the bladder emptied and the urinary catheter clamped distally. A transducer set is attached to the bladder catheter via a three-way port, and zeroed in the mid-axillary line. No more than 25 ml of normal saline is instilled into the bladder as larger volumes than this risk precipitating detrusor spasm, falsely elevating pressure readings. A single pressure measurement is taken, then the three-way port is closed and the urinary catheter unclamped. Whilst continuous pressure measurement is possible, it is impractical and generally unnecessary. Most ICUs perform measurements four to six hourly in at-risk patients.

A sustained pathological rise in IAP does not just impact organs within the abdominal cavity, but has multi-system effects.[7]

High IAP reduces venous return to the heart from the inferior vena cava, reducing preload and hence cardiac output. It will also effectively increase afterload, increasing myocardial work and decreasing cardiac output further. Obstruction to venous return can cause venous stasis, increasing the risk of thromboembolic events in this already high-risk population. Cephalad movement of the diaphragm can cause decreased myocardial compliance and distortion of the great vessels. A compensatory tachycardia may occur, placing further stress on the myocardium.

Diaphragmatic splinting will reduce functional residual capacity, residual volume and total lung capacity. Pulmonary atelectasis will result in significant respiratory shunt and ventilation-perfusion mismatch. The high ventilatory pressures that may be required due to reduced respiratory compliance can cause barotrauma. Hypoxic pulmonary vasoconstriction may occur over time, placing additional stress on the right heart.

The renal system is most often referred to when discussing the complications of IAH and ACS. Not only does compromise occur to renal arterial and venous blood flow, but also to the renal outflow tract. High pressures are transmitted back to the glomeruli, reducing the filtration gradient and compromising renal function further. The fall in cardiac output also activates the renin-angiotensin-aldosterone system, causing further renal vasoconstriction. This manifests itself as oligo-anuria that may fail to correct with increased perfusion pressure, and often does not resolve until decompression is undertaken.

The impedance to venous drainage of the bowel itself causes oedema and further worsens IAP. High pressure can directly compromise the arterial blood supply to the gut, resulting in bowel ischaemia and infarction. Hypo-perfusion of the gut wall has been shown in animal studies to increase risk of bacterial translocation, putting the patient at risk of sepsis. The ischaemia and resultant metabolic acidosis is compounded by reduced hepatic clearance of lactate.

High IAPs have also been demonstrated to contribute to raised intra-cranial pressure, thereby compromising cerebral perfusion. Coupled with the reduction in cardiac output and the hypercarbia caused by respiratory embarrassment, this can have profoundly negative effects for the brain-injured patient.

The concept of abdominal perfusion pressure (APP) can be thought of being analogous to cerebral perfusion pressure:

$$APP = MAP - IAP$$

As such, targeting higher mean arterial pressures whilst simultaneously attempting to reduce IAP may optimise abdominal perfusion pressure. However there is currently no robust evidence available to recommend a target APP.

In patients known to be at high risk of developing IAH/ACS, consideration should be given to prophylactic measures. These may include supine positioning, limiting the volume of crystalloid resuscitation, delaying the administration of enteral nutrition and even leaving the abdomen open after damage-control surgery in severe abdominal trauma.

The WSACS has developed a management algorithm for IAH/ACS (Figure 13.3).

If an obvious precipitating cause has been identified such as intra-abdominal haemorrhage, clearly that should be addressed as a priority. Other extra luminal space-occupying lesions contributing to high IAP such as collections of pus or ascites should be reviewed for intervention. The WSACS recommends attempts at percutaneous drainage of intra-peritoneal fluid if present before progressing to operative intervention.

Measures to increase abdominal wall compliance such as analgesia, sedation and trials of neuromuscular blocking drugs can be used. Consideration should be given to the optimum patient position balancing the risk of increasing IAP with sitting up beyond 20 degrees, against the potential risks of the supine position. The volume of intra-luminal contents can be reduced by nasogastric and flatus tubes, or prokinetics if ileus is thought to be a contributing factor. Avoidance of the administration of large volume crystalloid infusions after initial resuscitation has been completed is recommended, and consideration should be given to achieving a negative fluid balance.

In overt cases of abdominal compartment syndrome, surgical decompression is the only recognised treatment. It is performed via a midline incision into the intra-abdominal cavity. The abdomen is then usually maintained with a form of temporary closure to prevent desiccation and evisceration. This may be done with patches, meshes or silo techniques such as the application of a Bogota bag™. Bogota bags have the added benefit of being transparent and non-adherent. Whichever method is used, it must be loosely applied to prevent the recurrence of IAH/ACS. There are currently no randomised controlled trials in support of decompressive laparotomy, and no guidance available on optimal timing of this intervention.

Temporary closure can be combined with negative pressure wound therapy (NPWT), also known as VAC® therapy.[8] This allows removal of infected material as well as measurement of fluid loss. A foam sponge covers the abdominal contents, whilst the entire wound is enclosed with an adhesive dressing and attached to a suction system. The system also helps counteract the lateral retraction of the fascia by the abdominal wall muscles, making primary closure of the abdomen more feasible.

Potential complications of the open abdomen include fluid and protein loss, lateral fascial retraction, ventral herniae and fistulae formation. Extubation and enteral feeding are not contra-indicated, and depend on other patient factors.

Attempts at early fascial closure are recommended. The longer the abdomen is left open, the lower the chances of achieving primary closure and the higher the likelihood of developing fistulae. If primary closure is not possible, functional closure with mesh or skin-only closure can be performed. Grafting or leaving the wound to heal via secondary intention may be necessary if the skin itself cannot be closed.

Development of intra-abdominal hypertension has a significant impact on critically ill patients. It increases length of stay, ventilated days, severity of organ failure and has an independent association with mortality.[9] ACS results in tissue hypo-perfusion, multi organ failure and has a mortality of between 40 percent and 100 percent.

INTRA-ABDOMINAL HYPERTENSION (IAH) / ABDOMINAL COMPARTMENT SYNDROME (ACS) MANAGEMENT ALGORITHM

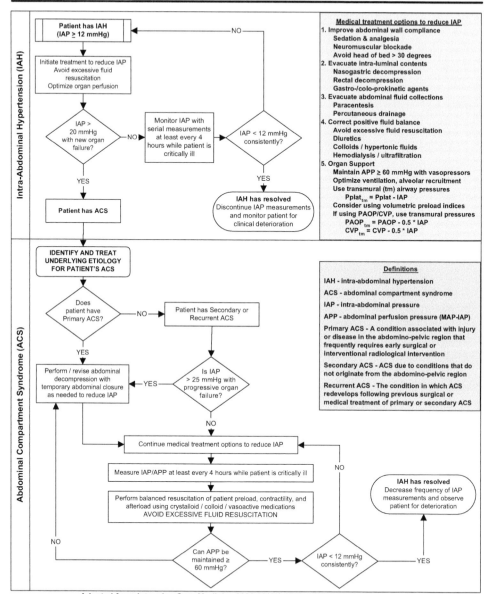

World Society of the Abdominal Compartment Syndrome (WSACS)
ZNA Stuivenberg, Lange Beeldekensstraat 267, B-2060 Antwerpen 6, Belgium
Tel: +32 3 2177092 Fax: +32 3 2177279 e-mail: info@wsacs.org
Website: www.wsacs.org

Figure 13.3 World Society of the Abdominal Compartment Syndrome (WSACS) algorithm for managing intra-abdominal hypertension and abdominal compartment syndrome.

Conclusion

This patient was at high risk of IAH given the presenting condition and the large volume crystalloid resuscitation received. The development of ACS, diagnosed via trans-bladder pressure measurements, led to a multi-system deterioration. The situation was temporised with medical management pending definitive surgical decompression and subsequent staged abdominal closure.

Key Learning Points

- Intra-abdominal hypertension is a relatively common occurrence in the critically ill, and occurs in both surgical and medical patients.
- Intra-abdominal hypertension is defined as a sustained or repeated pathological elevation in IAP greater than or equal to 12 mmHg, and graded I to IV by the WSACS.
- Abdominal compartment syndrome is defined as a sustained rise in IAP greater than 20 mmHg that is associated with new organ dysfunction or failure.
- Patients with any risk factors for developing IAH/ACS should have IAP measured four to six hourly on admission to critical care.
- Consideration should be given to preventative measures in certain high-risk patient groups, for example temporary abdominal closure after damage control surgery in the polytrauma patient.
- Guidelines for the management of IAH have been developed by the WSACS. Measures should be aimed at maximising organ perfusion, increasing abdominal wall compliance and decreasing the volume of intra-abdominal contents.
- The only recommended treatment for ACS is decompressive laparotomy, although there are no randomised control trials to support this approach.
- Vigilance for potential complications whilst managing the open abdomen is necessary and plans should be made for early or same stay closure.
- The incidence of organ dysfunction and mortality remains high in ACS, even if treated with decompressive laparotomy.

References

1. Kirkpatrick AW, Roberts DJ, De Waele J et al. Intra-abdominalhypertension and the abdominal compartment syndrome: updated consensus definitions and clinical practice guidelines from the World Society of the Abdominal Compartment Syndrome. *Intensive Care Med* 2013; 39:1190–1206.

2. Malbrain ML, Chiumello D, Pelosi P et al. Prevalence of intra-abdominal hypertension in critically ill patients: a multicenter epidemiological study. *Intensive Care Med* 2004;30:822–9.

3. Holodinsky JK, Roberts DJ, Ball CG et al. Risk factors for intra-abdominal hypertension and abdominal compartment syndrome among adult intensive care unit patients: a systematic review and meta-analysis. *Crit Care* 2013;17:R249.

4. Cheatham, ML, Safcsak K. Is the evolving management of intra-abdominal hypertension and abdominal compartment syndrome improving survival? *Crit Care Med* 2010;38:402–7.

5. Sugrue M, Bauman A, Jones F et al. Clinical examination is an inaccurate predictor of intra-abdominal pressure. *World J Surg* 2002;26:1428–31.

6. Iberti TJ, Lieber CE, Benjamin E. Determination of intra-abdominal pressure using a transurethral bladder catheter:

clinical validation of the technique. *Anesthesiology* 1989;70:47–50.

7. Hunter LD, Damani Z. Intra-abdominal hypertension and the abdominal compartment syndrome. *Anaesthesia* 2004;59:899–907.

8. National Institute for Health and Care Excellence (2013). *Negative pressure wound therapy for the open abdomen. NICE interventional procedure guidance 467.* London: National Institute for Health and Care Excellence.

9. Vidal MG, Weisser JR, Gonzalez F et al. Incidence and clinical effects of intra-abdominal hypertension in critically ill patients. *Crit Care Med* 2008;36:1823–31.

Management of the Ventilated Asthmatic Patient

Jochen Seidel

Introduction

Asthma is a common disease across all age groups with up to 5.4 million patients in United Kingdom receiving treatment for the condition. This patient group generated 65,000 hospital admissions with a primary diagnosis of asthma in 2011–12. Mortality from asthma is generally on the decline over the past three decades; however the extremes of age (0 to 9 years and over 75 years) are excluded from this trend and their mortality figures are broadly static.[1] In an American study of ~30,000 asthma related hospital admissions, 10 percent of patients required admission to critical care and 20 percent of critical care patients required intubation and ventilation. Mortality for invasively ventilated asthmatics in modern health care systems is generally around 5 percent.[2]

There is a paucity of clinical trial data specific to asthma patients requiring invasive ventilation and guidelines for management of this subset of patients are equally scarce. However, due to the distinct pathophysiology of near fatal asthma, some principles of care (mostly relating to ventilation technique) have been developed and should be adhered to.

Clinical Scenario

A 43-year-old known heroin abuser was referred to critical care from the emergency department with a four-day history of worsening shortness of breath, wheeze and discoloured sputum. He was a known asthmatic with five hospital admissions in the last six months, but had never been admitted to critical care before. On this admission, he had already been treated with nebulised salbutamol (repeatedly) and ipratropium, 200 mg of hydrocortisone intravenously, an aminophylline infusion (without a loading dose) and a bolus of 8mmol magnesium, but had not responded to treatment after two hours. On examination, he was in obvious respiratory distress with a silent chest. He was only able to speak in two word sentences and his respiratory rate was 14 breaths / minute. Cardiovascular observations revealed a heart rate of 140 beats / minute (sinus tachycardia) with a blood pressure of 145 / 80 mmHg. He was awake and orientated; no signs of confusion or obvious intoxication were found. Arterial blood gas analysis showed a worsening pattern of type II respiratory failure with elevated $PaCO_2$ and respiratory acidosis. He denied having injected any excessive amounts of heroin or using other illicit substances unfamiliar to him.

Further Clinical Course

Due to concerns about rapidly worsening fatigue, the patient was sedated and intubated with a modified rapid sequence induction, using ketamine and suxamethonium. Initial hand ventilation revealed a significantly 'stiff chest' and paralysis with a non-depolarising neuromuscular blocker was required to facilitate ventilation. Mechanical ventilation was continued with a pressure controlled mode, using a frequency of 11 breaths / minute and an inspiratory: expiratory (I:E) ratio of 1: 3.5. Inflation pressure was set at 26 cm H_2O, PEEP at 4 cm H_2O, delivering tidal volumes around 450 ml. In addition to propofol and alfentanil, an infusion of ketamine was started at 0.5 mg/kg/hr and the aminophylline was continued. No further paralysis was needed to achieve acceptable ventilation parameters at this stage and over the next 12 hours, the elevated $PaCO_2$ returned to near normal values. However, on attempted weaning of sedation, the patient developed severe bronchospasm again and required further paralysis. Nursing interventions such as turning to prevent pressure sores had to be suspended at times, as it provoked further attacks of bronchospasm, so that ventilation could only be achieved with additional paralysis with neuromuscular blockers. Salbutamol nebulisation was changed to an intravenous infusion and further magnesium boluses (2 x 8 mmol) were given in the first 48 hours of care. Steroids were used for seven days, intravenously for the first 48 hours, then via the enteral route. Sputum cultures were positive for pseudomonas aeruginosa and antibiotics were adjusted accordingly. The patient slowly improved and it was possible to reduce and stop the intravenous bronchodilator therapy (ketamine and salbutamol) over the next three days. He was extubated on day six, but suffered from agitation and symptoms of heroin withdrawal. Ongoing sedation with enteral clonidine and intermittent periods of continuous positive airway pressure via a hood device were required. On day 11 he was discharged from intensive care, continued to improve on the ward and left hospital 16 days after admission.

Discussion

A number of points should be considered in managing the ventilated asthmatic patient.

Identification of the Asthmatic at High Risk of Requiring Invasive Ventilation

The report of the Royal College of Physicians 'Why asthma kills' and the British Thoracic Society (BTS) guidelines clearly identify patient and disease characteristics, which act as red flags to the potential for attacks of life threatening asthma.[1,3] Some of these risk factors are listed below.

Box 14.1   Disease characteristics of the high risk patient

Disease characteristics of high risk patients:

- Not on inhaled steroids,
- Excessive use of bronchodilators (>2 canisters / month)
- Long acting beta-agonist as monotherapy
- Recent need for GP home visit
- Never seen by specialist
- Required recent emergency treatment / admission
- Accelerating frequency of attacks ± ED visits
- Previous critical care admission ± ventilation

> **Box 14.2** Psycho-social characteristics of patients at high risk
>
> Psycho-social characteristics of patients at high risk:
>
> - Current smoker
> - Obesity
> - Low socio-economic status
> - Heroin abuse (smoking)
> - Presence of significant psychological or psychiatric co-morbidity

Even in the absence of any of the above factors, suffering from lifelong asthma alone may increase the risk of a severe attack. Patients exhibiting wheezing in the first year of life and with symptoms that persist through to adult life have the most severe baseline limitations of airflow.[4] The assumption is that this group suffers from congenital and acquired deficits in airway function, making them the most likely subjects to develop non-fully reversible airway obstruction. This may also explain why there is a clinically important co-existence of irreversible airflow obstruction (chronic obstructive pulmonary disease, COPD-phenotype) in some patients, whose primary disease is characterised by reversible airflow obstruction (asthma phenotype).[5] Unsurprisingly, this group of patients have an increased risk of mortality from their respiratory disease.

Pathophysiology of Asthma

Acute asthma is characterised by three main pathophysiological features:

1. Bronchospasm, secondary to smooth muscle contraction
2. Airway inflammation with mucosal oedema formation
3. Mucus production ± retention

All of these features lead to narrowing of the airways and significant airflow reduction, mostly on expiration. Due to mucus plugging, some peripheral airways may even be completely excluded from gas exchange, ultimately leading to areas of collapse / consolidation. Dynamic hyperinflation contributes to unfavourable respiratory mechanics and impaired working conditions for the diaphragm, but poses a real threat to the invasively ventilated patient (see Figure 14.1). Hypoxia develops and is always a feature of life-threatening asthma. Coughing attacks triggered by mucus may precipitate further bronchospasm or even apnoea episodes. Work of breathing increases significantly as airways become narrower and the length of the asthma attack continues. As exhaustion develops, arterial $PaCO_2$ levels normalise from their initially low values and ultimately rise in the near fatal stage of exhaustion. Blood lactate levels may also be elevated at this stage.

Given the pathophysiology of asthma, key elements of emergency treatment therefore must include:

- Oxygen, as hypoxia is always a feature of near fatal asthma
- Bronchodilators, e.g., nebulised β_2-agonists and anticholinergics
- Steroids

Established Treatment Strategies

Invasive ventilation is an established and life-saving treatment for asthma. The decision to intubate, however, is not always easy or obvious, other than for patients in extremis or in

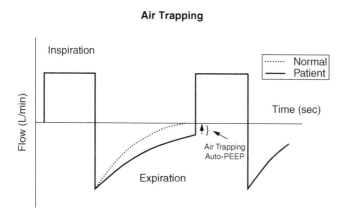

Air Trapping

Figure 14.1 Flow / Time diagram for a patient with incomplete exhalation and potential for DHI.

respiratory arrest. The possibility of a significant increase in bronchospasm after intubation is very real and the cardiovascular side-effects of induction in a (likely) fluid depleted patient can be highly unpredictable. The intubation process, however, is no different than for any other patient who requires emergency intubation. An endotracheal tube of at least 8.0 mm in diameter should be selected for an adult patient to facilitate removal of secretions and decrease inspiratory airway resistance. In any case, the decision to intubate and the peri-intubation management of the patient requires experience and skill and needs to be undertaken by senior personnel rather than novices.

Ketamine (1–2 mg/kg iv) is a good choice of induction agent, as it has clear broncho-dilatory properties and preserves cardiovascular status better than most other anaesthetic induction agents. As most asthmatics will need invasive ventilation for a number of days, troublesome emergence phenomena from a single dose of ketamine should not pose a problem. While most anaesthetists may be more familiar with thiopentone, it has the potential to induce laryngo- and bronchospasm.

Preoxygenation may well be difficult in a patient with a silent chest, who can be very anxious or even agitated. The use of a textbook rapid sequence induction with suxamethonium and a deliberate period of apnoea may therefore not be ideal. Depending on the risk of aspiration, a modified induction with a large dose of rocuronium 0.6 mg/kg iv (with less histamine release), followed by cricoid pressure and ventilation may avoid worsening hypoxia and provide the same intubation conditions as the use of suxamethonium.

The main goals of ventilation are oxygenation, reduction of the work of breathing, avoidance of dynamic hyperinflation (DHI) and slow reduction in $PaCO_2$ levels. Existing DHI can be worsened dramatically by mechanical ventilation and there may be a case for manual ventilation of the asthmatic patient at very low frequency after intubation to allow complete expiration. The respiratory rate on the ventilator should be set low (10 to12 / minute) and I:E ratio needs to be long e.g. 1:3 to 1:4. Figure 14.1 illustrates the scenario of persisting expiratory flow, generating intrinsic PEEP and DHI. External PEEP should be set no higher than measured intrinsic PEEP (ideally less than or equal to 80 percent) and some authors argue that PEEP provides no benefit at all.[6]

Hypercarbia will be a feature of the post-intubation period and there is no need to correct this aggressively. As bronchoconstriction and mucosal oedema settle over time, hypercarbia will improve gradually.

There is no data to favour pressure- controlled or volume- controlled modes of ventilation for this group of patients. Compliance may vary significantly over short periods of time (due to mucus plugs, new onset of bronchoconstriction, etc.), making close monitoring of pressures and tidal volumes paramount. Lung protective ventilation strategies (plateau pressure less than 30 cm H_2O, limited tidal volumes) equally apply to asthmatics and a decelerating flow pattern during inspiration may help to avoid DHI. Good humidification of the ventilator circuit is very important as mucus production is increased and it may be difficult to remove. Repeated aggressive suctioning can be detrimental, however, as it may provoke coughing and further episodes of bronchospasm. Neuromuscular blockade is often necessary in the beginning of the ventilation period, but it should be used as bolus therapy rather than as an infusion. The necessary use of steroids combined with neuromuscular blockers (NMBs) puts patients at higher risk of critical illness myopathy. While atracurium has the benefit of being eliminated irrespective of renal and hepatic function, it does cause clinically relevant histamine release frequent enough to cause concern about its use in this patient group. A steroid- based NMB or cisatracurium may provide a more favourable profile.

Bronchodilators and their delivery: Inhaled beta-agonists are considered standard therapy for near fatal asthma. While there is very good evidence to support their role in non-ventilated patients, there is a paucity of evidence to support their use in ventilated patients. A Cochrane review in 2011 failed to identify any suitably rigorously conducted studies to support their use in ventilated asthma patients.[7] The authors, however, did clearly state that they support the ongoing use of this practice 'because ancillary evidence suggests that beta2-agonist treatment in intubated patients may be beneficial'. The technical aspects of delivery of beta-agonists by nebulisation or via pressurised metered-dose inhalers (pMDI) have been reviewed.[8] Box 14.3 lists the main variables affecting drug delivery for pMDIs and jet nebulisers.

Steroids are a cornerstone of asthma therapy. The patient with an acute asthma attack requires systemic steroids, rather than inhaled steroids alone. BTS guidelines suggest that there is no difference in the effect of enteral steroids compared to intravenous delivery if enteral absorption is effective. Prednisolone 40 to 50 mg once daily for at least 4 to 5 days (or 4 x 100 mg hydrocortisone intravenously) is adequate and higher doses offer no treatment advantage. As the onset of any effects from therapeutic steroids is not immediate (usually 6 to 12 hours from administration) they should be given as early as possible on presentation to hospital. Tapering of steroids is not necessary in a steroid naive patient and they can be

---

Box 14.3 Factors affecting drug delivery in nebulisers and pMDI-devices

Variables affecting both devices:

- Gas temperature and degree of humidification
- Positioning of device in circuit (distance to endotracheal tube)
- Density of gas in circuit

Variables affecting each device separately:

pMDI	Nebuliser
• Appropriate priming of device	• Type of device (jet, ultrasonic, mesh)
• Synchronisation of delivery with inspiration	• Mode of nebulisation (continuous, intermittent)
• Interval of puff delivery (>15s)	• Drug volume in nebulisation chamber
• Use of a spacer chamber	• Flow-rate of driving gas
	• Composition of driving gas

stopped abruptly. There is little evidence to support the use of inhaled steroids in addition to systemic steroid therapy.

Non-established Treatment Strategies

In addition to above described established treatment strategies, a variety of pharmacological therapies have been tried, usually outside any guidelines or even outside licenses for these drugs. As with many other aspects of critical care, good evidence is often difficult to obtain for these patients.

Aminophylline: There is no trial evidence to support use of aminophylline in near fatal asthma or for the ventilated asthmatic. The risk of arrhythmias in patients with electrolyte shifts (from beta-agonist therapy), hypercarbia and high endogenous levels of catecholamines is high and they may prove difficult to control. Continuous infusions of aminophylline may contribute significantly to fluid loading of the asthmatic patient, unless administered in concentrated solutions via central access. There is, however, plenty of anecdotal evidence of aminophylline therapy being useful as an adjunct to established best practice. If aminophylline is used, tight monitoring of electrolytes and diuresis must be exercised, in order to limit its side-effects. The loading and maintenance doses used for other indications (COPD) are unchanged in asthma. Plasma levels should be monitored regularly.

Magnesium: Magnesium is an established treatment for severe asthma as a single intravenous bolus of 1.2 to 2 g (4.8 to 8 mmol). Its role for asthmatics requiring invasive ventilation, however, is very poorly defined. Due to its action as a relaxant of smooth muscle, it acts as a bronchodilator, but it also has anti-inflammatory actions and has actions relating to mast cells and histamine release. Again, it has been used successfully (including as a continuous infusion) in ventilated patients refractory to standard therapy, but this practice is currently not supported by evidence from trials.

Ketamine: This is a dissociative anaesthetic agent and exerts its bronchodilator effects by blockade of smooth muscle calcium channels. There is limited trial data available, but a number of case report the safety and effectiveness of a ketamine-infusion (0.3–1 mg/kg/hr) in ventilated asthmatics unresponsive to other treatment strategies.[9] One randomised study found no benefit from the addition of ketamine, but this study only examined patients not in need of mechanical ventilation. The frequency of unpleasant dreams and hallucinations with ketamine make its use more difficult, even when patients are heavily sedated.

Anaesthetic volatile agents: Inhaled anaesthetic agents such as isoflurane and sevoflurane are bronchodilators and have been successfully used in ventilated asthmatics. Their delivery into the ventilator circuit on an intensive care unit may prove technically challenging (due to management of waste gases), but specialised delivery devices (e.g. Anaconda™) exist. Hypotension is a likely and significant side-effect, but the use of an anaesthetic agent should allow a substantial reduction of other intravenous sedatives.

Intravenous beta-agonists: There is no evidence that intravenous beta-agonists are superior to nebulised therapy in non-ventilated patients in the emergency department. The situation in ventilated patients is less clearly understood. The potential side-effects of intravenous salbutamol or even adrenaline are quite significant (cardiovascular system instability, lactic acidosis, alterations in blood sugar level, electrolyte disturbances etc.) and may prove too difficult to control in exchange for very little benefit in additional bronchodilatation.

The role of Non-invasive Ventilation

Non-invasive ventilation (NIV) is established as first line support for patients with severe exacerbations of COPD. Its role in asthma is much more controversial and its use should be limited to an intensive care setting with immediate access to invasive ventilation. Systemic review has shown no benefit in mortality or avoidance of invasive ventilation for asthma patients.[10] A variety of respiratory parameters were improved by NIV, but these were secondary outcomes of the studies included. As a general comment, it should be noted that all the studies only included patients with moderate to severe asthma, rather than life-threatening or near-fatal asthma.

Discharge from Critical Care and Follow-up

Weaning from mechanical ventilation should be performed in a standard way and the asthma patient may well require NIV-support post extubation, especially if lung consolidation develops during invasive ventilation. Discharge from critical care should only be performed during daytime hours to a respiratory ward after a comprehensive handover including frequency of beta-agonists and ongoing antibiotic therapy. Specialist respiratory care while in hospital and timely outpatient follow-up (less than 4 weeks post discharge) must be ensured for these patients. Patient education on inhaler technique and peak flow diaries may be required and has been shown to reduce hospital admissions.[3]

Key Learning Points

- The decision to intubate a patient with life- threatening asthma and management of the immediate period following needs input from senior critical care clinicians.
- Ventilation strategies need to allow for prolonged expiration and patience is needed to normalise $PaCO_2$ levels and allow bronchospasm to settle.
- Post critical care management needs to be conducted by respiratory specialists and their long-term input must be ensured.

References

1. Royal College of Physicians. *Why asthma still kills: The National Review of Asthma Deaths (NRAD) Confidential Enquiry report.* RCP: London, 2014.

2. Louie S, Morrissey BM, Kenyon NJ, et al. The Critically Ill Asthmatic – from ICU to Discharge. *Clinic Rev Allerg Immunol* 2012;43:30–44.

3. British Thoracic Society. A Clinical Guideline for the management of Asthma. BTS: 2014.

4. Guerra S, Martinez FD. Epidemiology of the Origins of Airflow Limitation in Asthma. *Proc Am Thorac Soc* 2009;6:707–11.

5. Soriano JB, Davies KJ, Coleman B. The proportional Venn diagram of obstructive lung disease: two approximations from the United States and the UK. *Chest* 2004;124:474–81.

6. Tuxen DV. Detrimental effects of positive end-expiratory pressure during controlled mechanical ventilation of patients with severe airflow obstruction. *Am Rev Resp Dis* 1989;140:5–9.

7. Jones AP, Camargo CA, Rowe BH. Inhaled beta2-agonists for asthma in mechanically ventilated patients. *Cochrane Database of Systemic Reviews* 2001;4: CD001493.

8. Ari A, Fink JB, Dhand R. Inhalation Therapy in Patients Receiving Mechanical

Ventilation: An Update. *J Aerosol Med* 2012;6:319–32.

9. Lau TTY, Zed PJ. Does Ketamine have a role in managing severe exacerbation of asthma in adults? *Pharmcotherapy* 2001;9:1100–6.

10. Lim WJ, Mohammed Akram R, Carson KV, et al. Non-invasive positive pressure ventilation for treatment of respiratory failure due to severe exacerbations of asthma. *Cochrane Database Systemic Reviews* 2012;12:CD004360.

Pneumonia

Gerry Lynch

Introduction

Community acquired pneumonia (CAP) accounts for an increasing percentage of admissions to United Kingdom and European intensive care units. Despite advances in care, it still carries a high mortality.[1]

A case of pneumonia in a young man is presented here and relevant learning points highlighted.

Case Description

An overweight 22-year-old man was admitted to a medical admissions ward with a short history of flu-like symptoms; fever, night sweats and diarrhoea. He lived alone, worked as a postgraduate research student and was an occasional smoker and moderate alcohol drinker with no pets. He had recently returned from a two week holiday in Turkey.

On observation, he was febrile at 38°C, tachypnoeic, with a respiratory rate of 30/min: his oxygen saturations on air were 88 percent, improving to 96 percent with 4l/min of inspired oxygen. Examination demonstrated decreased air entry and harsh crackles over the right base. He had a tachycardia of 103 bpm and a blood pressure of 92/45 mmHg, with prolonged capillary refill time of 4 seconds. Abdominal examination was unremarkable.

He was disorientated but cooperative and had no focal neurological deficits or neck stiffness. Urinalysis was normal and urinary catheterisation was performed.

Table 15.1 Initial investigations

Full blood count	Urea and electrolytes	Coagulation profile	Arterial blood gas	Liver function tests
Hb 155 g/L	Na$^+$ 133 mmol/l	APTT 36 s	PaO2 11.5 kPa	Bilirubin 56 mmol/l
WCC 22x10^3 mm^3	K$^+$ 4.6 mmol/l	PT 13.3 s	PaCO2 5.2 kPa	ALT 80 u/l
Platelets 255x10^3 mm^3	Ur 9.5 mmol/l	Fib 5.45	pH 7.38	AST 113 u/l
	Cr 88 mmol/l		Base excess -2.6	Alk Phos 200 u/l
			Lactate 2.0 mmol/l	GGT 60 u/l

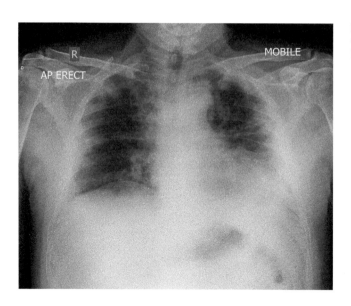

Figure 15.1 Chest radiograph on admission showing predominantly left basal changes.

A diagnosis of community acquired pneumonia was made, with pulmonary embolus (PE) a possibility in view of his recent flight. Blood cultures were sent and treatment commenced with intravenous co-amoxiclav and clarithromycin, with the first antibiotic doses given within 3 hours. Fluid resuscitation with 1000 ml of normal saline given over 4 hours was instituted.

A CT pulmonary angiogram (CTPA) was performed in view of his recent air journey to exclude pulmonary embolus. This showed no evidence of PE, but bibasal consolidation and atelectasis.

Sputum cultures, serum for atypical serology, urine for pneumococcal and legionella antigen were sent and he was transferred to a medical ward. His initial CURB-65 score was 3, indicating severe disease.

Over the next 12 hours, his confusion worsened and a referral for sedation for CT scanning prior to lumbar puncture was made to critical care. Acyclovir was commenced pending CSF analysis.

On review, he was more delirious and looked exhausted with a respiratory rate of 42/min. His inspired oxygen fraction had been gradually increasing to 70 per cent high flow. His systolic blood pressure was 90 mmHg, and urine output had been poor since admission, averaging 25 ml/hr. Repeat arterial blood gas taken at this time showed a PaO_2 of 8.3 kPa with worsening base excess. A decision to intubate and ventilate him on the intensive care unit prior to CT scanning was made. A fluid challenge of 500 ml Hartmanns solution was administered prior to pre-oxygenation using facial CPAP on the intensive care unit (ICU).

Induction of anaesthesia and tracheal intubation were accomplished without incident, and he was started on biphasic positive airway pressure (BiPAP). He required inspiratory pressures of 30/10 cm H_2O and an FiO_2 of 0.8, giving tidal volumes of 550 ml (equivalent to 7 ml/kg ideal body weight). Oxygen saturations were 95 per cent and PaO_2 10.5 kPa. Arterial and central lines were inserted and vasopressor support with a noradrenaline infusion at 0.2 mcg/kg/min was instituted for persistent hypotension after a further infusion of 20 ml/kg of Hartmann's solution.

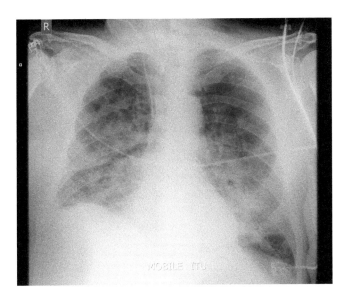

Figure 15.2 Repeat radiograph showing worsening 4 quadrant infiltration.

Transfer to the radiology department was notable for one episode of desaturation requiring manual ventilation prior to the CT head, which was reported as normal. A lumbar puncture showed normal opening pressures and gram stain was negative. CSF for culture and herpes simplex virus/ varicella zoster virus PCR were sent.

Over several hours, with fluid resuscitation and vasopressors guided by cardiac output monitoring via oesophageal doppler, his blood pressure stabilised and lactate improved, but blood gases deteriorated. A repeat chest X-ray film showed worsening four-quadrant infiltration. (Note also NG tube malposition).

After a further recruitment manoeuvre, PEEP was titrated upwards to 14 cm H2O, pressure controlled inverse-ratio ventilation was commenced and prone positioning was considered. The following day, urinary legionella antigen was positive and his antibiotic therapy was changed to ciprofloxacin and clarithromycin.

Over the next 48 hours, his fever settled and gas exchange stabilised. A diuretic infusion was instituted and negative fluid balance maintained.

His subsequent course showed gradual improvement, with a falling C-reactive protein, reduced need for oxygen and tapering ventilator pressures. Daily sedation holds were performed, but ongoing delirium precluded safe extubation. Viral CSF PCR was negative.

Weaning from ventilation was achieved via percutaneous tracheostomy performed on day 7 of admission: his delirium gradually improved and he was subsequently decannulated and discharged from the ICU. He went on to make a full recovery and a follow= up chest X-ray six weeks after discharge showed complete resolution of infiltrates.

Case Discussion

Definition

Pneumonia in the community is defined as an acute illness characterised by:

- Symptoms of a lower respiratory tract infection (cough and at least one other symptom)

Box 15.1   Differential diagnosis of CAP

Pulmonary oedema
Pulmonary embolus
Infective exacerbation of COPD
Tuberculosis
Bronchiectasis including cystic fibrosis
Bronchogenic carcinoma - may coexist
Cryptogenic organizing pneumonia
Eosinophilic pneumonia
Pulmonary vasculitis
Fibrosing alveolitis
Pulmonary haemorrhage

- New focal chest signs on examination
- At least one systemic feature (temp 38°C or flu-like symptoms)
- No alternative explanation, such as pulmonary oedema

In the elderly, however, chest symptoms may be absent and confusion is the only feature that exists.[1] Chest X-ray may show patchy infiltrates, lobar shadowing with air bronchograms or parapneumonic effusions. Other diagnoses to be considered are outlined in Box 15.1, especially in cases where there is failure to improve.

Mortality

Worldwide CAP is the largest single cause of death, killing 3.5 million people every year. In the United Kingdom, the incidence of CAP is 5–11/1000 adults and roughly a third require admission to hospital.[1] Mortality in ICU is up to 30 per cent according to a 2004 analysis of the UK ICNARC database, although recent studies show improved outcomes.

Organisms

Features of pneumonia are traditionally grouped into 'typical' symptoms with fever, pleuritic pain, sputum and local complications and 'atypical' with multisystem problems: skin rashes, metabolic derangement and neurological features. Responsible organisms in non-immunosuppressed adult ICU patients are outlined in descending order of frequency in Box 15.2.[1]

Streptococcus pneumoniae is the commonest bacterial cause of CAP detected in United Kingdom and European studies. Infection occurs predominantly in the winter months:

Box 15.2   Organisms responsible for CAP in ICU patients

Streptococcus pneumoniae
Legionella
Viruses
Staphylococcus aureus
Haemophilus influenzae
Mycoplasma pneumoniae
Others

acute onset, pleuritic chest pain and high fever are characteristic. Ten to twenty-five per cent of pneumococcal pneumonias are bacteraemic and associated with higher mortality.

Legionella pneumophila is a capsulated gram-negative organism spread via colonised water and the second commonest bacterial cause of CAP seen in intensive care units. Serogroup 1 accounts for most infections and is detected by the urinary antigen test. Features of legionellosis overlap with other pathogens, but travel to Mediterranean countries, encephalopathy, deranged liver function tests and myositis, are suggestive of infection. Hyponatraemia is not specific for legionella but reflective of disease severity. Legionellosis is a notifiable condition to the UK Health Protection Authority, and sputum cultures for legionella should be sent in the presence of a positive antigen to assist with typing of an outbreak.

Mycoplasma pneumoniae is a small commensal pleomorphic bacterium, lacking a cell wall. Penicillins are ineffective and agents acting on protein synthesis, such as macrolides, are required. Mycoplasma pneumonia tends to occur in 3 to 4 yearly epidemics.

Haemophilus influenzae is a pleomorphic gram-negative rod which is the commonest bacterial cause of exacerbations in COPD. It also causes epiglottitis and meningitis. Symptoms often mimic a persistent viral upper respiratory tract infection.

Gram-negative bacilli, Klebsiella and anaerobes are commonly found in cases of aspiration and also associated with illness in individuals who abuse alcohol.

MRSA and Pseudomonas are common organisms in ventilator associated pneumonia (VAP), but individuals who have been previously colonised, undergoing dialysis and nursing home patients are also at risk.

Others rarer causative organisms include Moraxhella catarrhalis, Chlamydophila pneumophilia and Coxiella burnetii.

Immunosupression

In cases of immunosuppression, Epstein Barr Virus, Cytomegalovirus, Herpes Simplex Virus, Varicella Zoster Virus, pneumocystis carinii pneumonia caused by Pneumocystis jirovecii, Candida and Aspergillus must be considered and treatment adjusted accordingly.

PVL Staphylococcus

PVL- producing staphylococcus (CA-MRSA) is a form of community-acquired staphylococcus, usually methicillin-resistant, that has emerged as a worldwide threat. Enhanced virulence is coded for largely by Panton-Valentine leukocidin (PVL), a leucocidal and dermo-necrotic toxin. The organism causes skin and soft tissue necrotising infections, but a necrotising pneumonia carrying a high mortality is also seen. It affects children and young adults, usually after viral illness. Septic shock, cavitating multilobar infiltrates, haemoptysis and neutropaenia are seen. Crucially, CURB-65 is likely to underestimate disease severity and refractory hypoxia and pulmonary haemorrhage are particular challenges. Since direct person-to-person transmission has occurred, isolation with barrier precautions including facemasks is indicated if PVL MRSA is isolated. Conventional antibiotic cover is inadequate and a combination of clindamycin, linezolid and rifampicin should be used as they have exotoxin neutralising properties.[2]

Viruses

Viruses are the commonest cause of childhood pneumonia. Respiratory syncytial virus (RSV) is treatable with ribavirin. Rhinovirus and adenovirus are less common causes in adults. Influenza is seen in annual winter epidemics.

Pandemic nfluenza A H1N1 subtype, or swine flu, can cause severe bronchopneumonia with refractory hypoxaemia and renal failure. Secondary bacterial infection with staphylococcus is well described. Over 20,000 confirmed deaths have occurred since 2009 but the fatality rate is very low. Supportive care and rescue oxygenation strategies are mainstays of intensive care management. Doubt has recently been cast on the efficacy of the antiviral oseltamivir.

SARS coronavirus caused a 2003 pandemic in which over 3,000 died. It produced a severe Adult Respiratory Disease Syndrome (ARDS) picture and carried a mortality of about 10 per cent.

MERS (Middle East Respiratory Virus) is a recently identified coronavirus with an animal reservoir in camels and an outbreak centred on Saudi Arabia. It produces a syndrome akin to SARS or H1N1 and thus far carries 50 per cent mortality, but does not easily transmit between individuals.

Microbiological Testing

British Thoracic Society (BTS) guidance recommends sputum for microscopy, gram stain and culture in all hospitalised patients. In intubated patients, a tracheal aspirate may be sent. Bronchoscopy and bronchoalveolar lavage may increase specificity, clear sputum plugs, detect ventilator associated pneumonia or identify bronchogenic carcinoma. For critically ill patients, blood cultures, pneumococcal and legionella urinary antigen should be tested. Viral PCR may be sent where this is suspected and likely to change management (as in this case where the patient's confusion may have had a central cause).

Antibiotics

C-reactive protein measurement is recommended to assist the decision to prescribe antibiotics. Combination therapy with a ®-lactamase stable penicillin and a macrolide is the initial treatment in severe pneumonia and reduces mortality compared to monotherapy.[3] This may reflect anti-inflammatory effects of macrolides or treatment of undiagnosed co-infection.

Due to concern about selection of Clostridium difficile and extended spectrum beta-lactamases (ESBLs), local guidelines may differ. Monitoring of the QT interval on electro-cardiograms is important with the combination of fluoroquinolone and macrolide. At least seven days of treatment is needed, but longer courses may be necessary. Procalcitonin levels have been shown to safely limit duration of antibiotic use, preventing emergence of resistance. Adjunctive steroid therapy is not routinely recommended, unless in proven adrenocortical deficiency, and has no mortality benefit.

Box 15.3   Antibiotic treatment of CAP (adapted from BTS guidance)

Initial therapy of CAP	Co-amoxiclav and clarithromycin
Penicillin allergy (not anaphylaxis)	Cefuroxime or cefotaxime and clarithromycin
Severe penicillin allergy	Vancomycin or teicoplanin and ciprofloxacin
Legionella or mycoplasma	Ciprofloxacin and clarithromycin or rifampicin
PVL MRSA	Clindamycin and linezolid and rifampicin
Aspiration	Augmentin and metronidazole

The Patient Failing to Improve

In the event of failure to improve, the initial diagnosis should be revisited. Risk factors for resistant bacteria, TB or evidence of immunosuppression should be considered. Microbiology assistance to identify pathogens and change antibiotics should be sought. CT of the thorax may be useful to identify complications.

Complications

Local complications include parapneumonic effusion, empyema and lung abscess. Distant complications due to bacteraemia are meningoencephalitis, epidural abscess, endo/pericarditis, osteomyelitis and septic arthritis. A high index of suspicion should be maintained for all of these complications.

Severity and Risk Prediction Systems

An ideal scoring system would identify severe cases in the community and predict need for critical care, mechanical ventilation and mortality on admission. Over 11 scores are described, but commonly used scoring systems are outlined below.

The Pneumonia Severity Index (PSI) is a validated risk scoring instrument that uses 20 variables from history, clinical and laboratory findings. It stratifies patients into five categories, from lowest to highest risk with associated risks of mortality.[4]

CURB-65 is a five point scale scoring for Confusion, Urea greater than 7, Respiratory rate greater than or equal to 30, Blood pressure less than 90 systolic or 60 diastolic and Age over 65.[5] Scores of 3 to 5 indicate severe CAP and referral to critical care is recommended.

The American Thoracic Society/Infectious Diseases Society of America (ATS/IDSA) guidelines mandate critical care admission for self-evident major criteria: patients in septic shock or requiring mechanical ventilation.[6] More than 3 of 9 minor criteria, respiratory rate greater than 30/min, low PaO2/FiO2 ratio, multilobar infiltrates, leucopaenia, thrombocytopaenia, uraemia, confusion, persistent hypotension and hypothermia are also indications.

The Severe Community Acquired Pneumonia (SCAP) score was developed to predict severe adverse outcomes.[7] Severe pneumonia has one or more major criteria of pH less than 7.3 and systolic blood pressure less than 90 mmHg; or greater than or equal to 2 minor criteria: confusion, urea, multilobar infiltrates, PaO2/FiO2 ratio less than 250 mmHg and age greater than 80.

All scores have good sensitivity but lower specificity for poor outcomes. The decisions to admit to ICU and ventilate a patient must be guided by clinical judgment as well as a high score in any scoring system. CURB-65, by virtue of its simplicity and good performance, is endorsed by the BTS.

ICU Management

Whether to offer non-invasive (NIV) or mechanical ventilation encompasses features such as high severity score, comorbidities, severe sepsis, acidosis, worsening oxygenation or fatigue and neurological and multiorgan dysfunction. NIV in pneumonia lacks a strong evidence base, may mask deterioration and make subsequent intubation riskier. BTS guidance suggests it should be offered only in an ICU environment.

Strategies evidenced for ARDS management in invasive ventilation will be needed where there is multilobar involvement rather than shunt due to lobar consolidation.

Box 15.4 Evidence-based strategies for ARDS

Low tidal volumes, limitation of plateau pressure and permissive hypercapnia (ARDSnet 2000)
Limited fluids (FACTT 2006)
Short-term infusion of neuromuscular blockers (ACURASYS 2010)
Prone positioning (PROSEVA 2013 and meta-analysis 2014)
Extracorporeal oxygenation for refractory hypoxaemia (CESAR 2009)

Despite positive trials, a 2013 meta-analysis found no mortality benefit from high as opposed to low peep in ARDS.[9]

General supportive care measures are important. Thromboembolic and stress ulcer prophylaxis, early enteral nutrition, ventilator care bundles, glucose management, daily sedation scores and holds and delirium screening are standard modern ICU management strategies. Weaning from ventilation may be accomplished via extubation +/− NIV or via tracheostomy but daily sedation holds and spontaneous breathing trials are important.[10]

Post discharge from ICU a repeat chest X-ray at six weeks is usual, and vaccination for pneumococcus and Influenza A can be carried out after recovery in elderly or immunosuppressed patients.

Conclusion

Community- acquired pneumonia remains an important cause of mortality in patients admitted to ICU. Effective care requires individualised treatment directed at likely pathogens alongside attention to delivery of evidence based general ICU care packages.

Key Learning Points

- Streptococcus pneumoniae is the most common pathogen in adult patients with CAP.
- Bacteraemic pneumonia is common and use of sepsis bundles and general ICU supportive care packages is best practice.
- PVL-MRSA is a differential diagnosis of importance in young patients with septic shock and multilobar infiltrates.
- Multisystem features are associated with atypical pathogens, but overlap exists.
- Combination therapy with a ®-lactamase stable penicillin and a macrolide is recommended as first line therapy to reduce mortality.
- Viral pneumonias causing ARDS are pandemic threats.
- Severity scoring systems must be combined with clinical judgment in decisions about ICU admission and ventilation.

References

1. Lim WS, Baudouin SV, George RC et al. BTS guidelines for the management of community acquired pneumonia in adults: update 2009. *Thorax* 2009;64(Suppl 3): iii1–55.

2. McGrath B, Rutledge F, Broadfield E. Necrotising pneumonia, Staphylococcus aureus and Panton-Valentine leukocidin. *J Intensive Care Soc* 2008;9(2):170–2.

3. Caballero J, Rello J. Combination antibiotic therapy for community-acquired pneumonia. *Ann Intensive Care* 2011; 1(1):48.

4. Aujesky D, Fine MJ. The pneumonia severity index: a decade after the initial

derivation and validation. *Clin Infect Dis* 2008;47(Suppl 3):S133–9.

5. Lim WS, Van der Eerden MM, Laing R et al. Defining community acquired pneumonia severity on presentation to hospital: an international derivation and validation study. *Thorax* 2003;58(5): 377–82.

6. Salih W, Schembri S, Chalmers JD. Simplification of the IDSA/ATS criteria for severe CAP using meta-analysis and observational data. *Eur Respir J* 2014; 43(3):842–51.

7. España PP, Capelastegui A, Gorordo I et al. Development and validation of a clinical prediction rule for severe community-acquired pneumonia. *Am J Respir Crit Care Med* 2006;174(11): 1249–56.

8. Dellinger RP, Levy MM, Rhodes A et al. Surviving sepsis campaign: International guidelines for management of severe sepsis and septic shock, 2012. *Intensive Care Med* 2013;39(2):165–228.

9. Santa Cruz R, Rojas JI, Nervi R et al. High versus low positive end-expiratory pressure (PEEP) levels for mechanically ventilated adult patients with acute lung injury and acute respiratory distress syndrome. *Cochrane Database Syst Rev* 2013;6: CD009098.

10. Girard TD, Kress JP, Fuchs BD et al. Efficacy and safety of a paired sedation and ventilator weaning protocol for mechanically ventilated patients in intensive care (Awakening and Breathing Controlled trial): a randomised controlled trial. *The Lancet* 2008; 371(9607):126–34.

Interstitial Lung Disease

Zhe Hui Hui and Omar Pirzada

Introduction

Interstitial lung disease (ILD) refers to a heterogeneous group of lung diseases that predominantly affect the interstitium of the lung. They are diagnostically difficult to classify and commonly appear clinically and radiographically indistinguishable yet have highly individual responses to treatment and widely different prognoses. This creates a particular challenge to the intensivist as patients with new disease can present to the intensive care unit (ICU) with rapidly progressive respiratory failure and ideal management requires detailed knowledge of the particular form of ILD.

Individuals with ILD may present to the ICU in one of two characteristic presentations but in general, require different management strategies.

1. *De novo* ILD may present with respiratory failure with the diagnosis hitherto unknown. Early diagnosis is crucial and usually requires invasive investigation followed by immunosuppressive treatment and temporary respiratory support for reversible disease.
2. Known established ILD may suddenly deteriorate presenting with respiratory failure. Multiple specific ILDs, including idiopathic pulmonary fibrosis (IPF), do not respond well to treatment with mechanical ventilation and this disease specific prognostic information allows informed decisions to be made.

The intensivist therefore has the dilemma of making immediate ventilatory and treatment decisions for diseases with very different outcomes sometimes before the final specific diagnosis of ILD is confirmed.

Case Description

A 71-year-old previously fit and well retired electrician presented with a two- month history of worsening cough and severe dyspnoea. There were symptoms of joint pains and a mild difficulty swallowing but no pyrexia, weight loss or other symptoms noted. He had stopped smoking four years previously, having accumulated 20 pack- years of smoking history. On examination, finger clubbing was evident, breathing was laboured, respiratory rate was 25/min, SpO_2 reduced to 78 per cent in air with fine inspiratory bibasal crackles present on chest auscultation. He was in type 2 respiratory failure, with an arterial blood gas showing pH 7.34, $PaCO_2$ 8.5 kPa, PaO_2 7.4 kPa on 40 per cent oxygen. His plain chest radiograph showed multiple peripheral and basal infiltrates consistent with interstitial lung disease.

He was admitted, titrated oxygen was administered and a chest CT was performed demonstrating bibasal subpleural honeycombing with extensive ground glass opacification. Pulmonary emboli were excluded.

He was transferred to the ICU due to increasing oxygen requirements and progressive respiratory failure. A transthoracic echocardiogram showed an elevated systolic pulmonary artery pressure of 35 mmHg with normal left and right ventricular function. Treatment with pulsed intravenous methylprednisolone (1 g/day) and antibiotics was commenced with respiratory support using non-invasive ventilation.

At day three, intubation and mechanical ventilation was required for respiratory support. Bronchoscopy was performed with bronchoalveolar lavage (BAL) isolating no organisms and a transbronchial biopsy was not performed due to the potential risks of pneumothorax in this case. At day 11, clinical improvement was noted after the addition of cyclophosphamide. Extubation was possible shortly after and the patient successfully left the ICU at day 15 on high dose corticosteroids and cyclophosphamide. A diagnosis of connective tissue disease- associated ILD was later confirmed.

Discussion

This case describes *de novo* ILD presenting to the ICU illustrating the diagnostic and management difficulties typically found in ILD patients who progress to respiratory failure. The final diagnosis of ILD is not apparent at presentation and it is exactly this uncertainty that commonly faces the intensivist making important treatment decisions in the patient with ILD and respiratory failure.

Rapidly progressive ILD may present to ICU and is most often caused by either IPF, acute interstitial pneumonitis (AIP) or cryptogenic organising pneumonia (COP).[1]

Idiopathic pulmonary fibrosis is the commonest ILD encountered and is a progressive fibrotic lung condition otherwise known by closely related though confusing nomenclature of cryptogenic fibrosing alveolitis (CFA), usual interstitial pneumonitis (UIP) or even lung fibrosis. Irreversible and inevitable progressive loss of lung function follows and IPF carries a poor prognosis with median survival of 2 to 3 years from diagnosis. Treatment with corticosteroids is usually ineffective and disease-modifying therapeutic options are limited in severe diseases,[2] but recent evidence confirms new treatments such as perfenidone slow forced vital capacity (FVC) decline. In the acute setting though, outcomes using mechanical ventilation are very poor. In contrast, sarcoidosis, carries an excellent prognosis with spontaneous remission rates of up to 60 percent without treatment and a mortality rate due to progressive lung disease of only 1 to 6 percent.[1]

Acute Interstitial Pneumonitis (AIP) is a particularly aggressive ILD, and probably a distinct subtype of IPF and eponymously known as the Hamman-Rich syndrome. Individuals typically describe a viral prodrome followed by severe dyspnoea progressing over days to weeks. Radiology shows ground glass change, with nodules and interlobular septal thickening but the diagnosis is only secured by demonstrating diffuse alveolar damage on biopsy. The survival rate is less than 20 percent.

COP may present as a fulminant ILD in a similar manner to AIP, rendering it potentially indistinguishable until biopsy which confirms an organising pneumonia is present. In contrast, survival rates are very good as COP is treatment sensitive and rapidly responds to corticosteroids.

Other ILDs that are notably treatment- sensitive include sarcoidosis, vasculitis and ILDs secondary to connective tissue disorders. An important aspect of managing ILD is, therefore, making a precise and timely diagnosis of the particular form of ILD. However, making an accurate diagnosis is also difficult and at least 10 per cent of ILD remain 'unclassifiable' even after thorough multi-disciplinary review.[3]

The principles for managing ILD on the ICU should be clearly understood. A CT chest can be extremely helpful in confirming the presence of an interstitial lung disease but the differential diagnosis remains very broad involving primary lung disease, infections and even disseminated cancer. The clinician may be faced with making treatment decisions in the absence of a definitive diagnosis, as in this case, and so management should be directed towards early diagnosis and treatment as this improves survival.[1]

Invasive investigations including bronchoscopy with BAL and surgical biopsy should be considered in the early window of opportunity to secure a precise ILD diagnosis, exclude alternative diagnoses and identify precipitating factors such as infection. However, the risks of invasive investigation have to be weighed carefully in a critically ill patient with respiratory failure against the benefit of an accurate diagnosis leading to very different treatment outcomes and prognoses. Infection must be excluded and is a frequent cause of deterioration in both *de novo* presentations and in patients with known ILD. Thorough evaluation for infection with bronchoscopy with BAL can help isolate pathogens including rare opportunists and aid the clinician in avoiding known diagnostic pitfalls e.g. tuberculosis, HIV and cancer.

Diagnostic Investigations for ILD

An ILD always includes a very broad differential diagnosis. Initially, the history can identify drug induced lung disease, an important reversible cause of ILD, with drugs such as nitrofurantoin and amiodarone commonly implicated. At this initial point, patients do not usually require invasive mechanical ventilation presenting a window of opportunity, where timely diagnostic investigations should be performed, to guide important later management decisions.

High resolution CT chest (HRCT) is an essential component of the diagnostic algorithm for ILD.[1,2]

Although several ILDs can appear clinically, radiographically and even histologically similar, other ILDs show highly characteristic HRCT appearances obviating the need for pathological confirmation if clinical features and laboratory findings are consistent with the HRCT diagnosis.[1] For example, the positive predictive value of a diagnostic HRCT for the commonest ILD encountered, that is IPF, is 90 to 100 percent[2,4]. Diffuse malignant lung disease (lymphangitis carcinomatosis) may mimic the presentation of an apparently acute ILD.

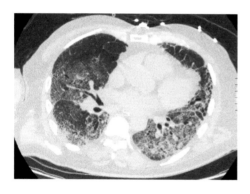

Figure 16.1 Interstitial Lung Disease with typical features of established honeycombing and areas of ground glass consolidation.

A chest CT pulmonary angiogram (CTPA) provides HRCT images and simultaneously excludes pulmonary emboli since there is an increased risk of thromboembolism with certain forms of ILD.[5] The CT images provide not only diagnostic information on the ILD but also provide information on future prognosis and outcome. For example, diffuse ground glass changes are associated with the worst prognosis among IPF patients presenting with acute worsening respiratory failure.[6]

An important consideration concerns the role of biopsy in this population and each case should be considered on individual merits. The investigation of ILD characteristically requires invasive investigation and tissue biopsy may be achievable by bronchoscopic or surgical routes. Although less invasive and safer, a transbronchial biopsy can cause pneumothorax in an individual who may not have sufficient respiratory reserve and biopsy yield rates are much lower than definitive surgical biopsy. Up to 50 percent of IPF patients will not have a 'diagnostic' HRCT appearance,[4] emphasising the utility of surgical biopsy. However, with a median age of presentation of 70 years, many patients with suspected IPF may have substantial co-morbidities, complicating respiratory failure as well as increased risks associated with the presenting ILD. Video-assisted thoracoscopic surgical (VATS) lung biopsy is safer than open thoracotomy, but still carries a morbidity risk of around 20 per cent and a 60-day mortality risk of around 5 per cent.[7] Postoperative risks are highest among hypoxic patients[1,7] but the benefits of surgical biopsy may outweigh the risks in securing the precise diagnosis of ILD and excluding alternative diagnoses such as cancer.

The British Thoracic Society (BTS) ILD guideline recommends that the 'threshold for proceeding to a surgical biopsy is lower when the underlying ILD diagnosis is unknown' in ILD patients with respiratory failure.[1]

Other Investigations for ILD Patients with Acute Respiratory Failure

Patients with known ILD may decompensate due to five common causes easily remembered as the 5 'P's:

1. Progression of the underlying ILD
2. Pulmonary oedema
3. Pulmonary embolism
4. Pneumothorax
5. Pulmonary infection

Investigation of rapid deterioration in ILD is directed towards identification of these five causal factors. A transthoracic echocardiogram is useful to identify overt cardiac decompensation,[1] is readily available and non-invasive. A CTPA excludes significant pulmonary emboli, pneumothorax and can visualise pleural effusions and pulmonary oedema.

Exclusion of infection is an integral part of the workup for all ILD patients and is a common cause of deterioration of established ILD but can seldom be excluded by non-invasive means.[1] Bronchoscopy with BAL should therefore be considered during the early window of opportunity. Patients with established ILD and those with connective tissue disorders are often treated with immunosuppressive agents making them more susceptible to infection including opportunistic infections which bronchoscopy with BAL can identify and guide targeted therapy against.

Two particular infections deserve special consideration as they can themselves present with the radiological appearances of ILD and demand a high index of suspicion for recognition.

Tuberculosis can masquerade as several forms of ILD and occurs in unusual circumstances since the advent of biological therapies, e.g., anti-tumour necrosis factor (TNF) used in treating conditions such as connective tissue disorders. The picture can be further confounded by the finding that the underlying connective tissue disease itself can be a cause of ILD. The effects of immunosupression as potential treatment in the presence of TB would be catastrophic and so exclusion of tuberculosis should be considered in all patients presenting with ILD.

HIV-related disease is protean and it is well recognised that pneumocystis carinii pneumonia (PCP) (now reclassified as *pneumocystis jiroveci*) can appear indistinguishable from NSIP (non-specific interstitial pneumonitis) causing diagnostic confusion but requires specific alternate therapy usually with intravenous co-trimoxazole. HIV testing is simple but easily overlooked in the evaluation of ILD.

The Role of Immunosupression for ILD Patients with Acute Respiratory Failure

Certain types of ILD respond favourably to immunosupression and rapid treatment is essential to reduce mortality with the BTS recommending early treatment for all rapidly progressive primary ILD.[1] Pharmacological therapy for this group of patients generally consists of high dose intravenous corticosteroid given as pulsed methylprednisolone, 750 mg or 1 g on three consecutive days as first line therapy. However, it should be noted that no controlled trials have been performed to judge the efficacy of corticosteroid in the context of rapidly progressive ILD.[1] The response to corticosteroids is not immediate and patients may require temporary ventilatory support for several days with a recommendation to wait 5 to 7 days before assessing response to first line therapy.[1] Second line therapies such as cyclophosphamide may be required later to induce remission.

The Role of Ventilatory Support for ILD Patients with Acute Respiratory Failure

The treatment of respiratory failure in ILD presents a challenging treatment dilemma and the value of early diagnosis cannot be overemphasised in helping to make later ventilatory support decisions. If a precise diagnosis of ILD is established when respiratory failure supervenes, knowledge of the ILD can guide on whether a disorder is treatable, corticosteroid responsive and potentially reversible or conversely corticosteroid non-responsive and therefore mechanical ventilation is unlikely to be beneficial or appropriate.

In contrast, the management of patients with known ILD with sudden decompensation differs and occurs in 5 to 10 per cent of ILD patients per annum. Those with known established ILD, sudden deterioration and acute respiratory failure are often critically ill. The underlying pulmonary process in diffuse ILD causes lung stiffness and clinical studies demonstrate increased susceptibility to ventilator- induced lung injury. During ventilation, higher PEEP settings are required with high tidal volumes (often above 6 to 8 mls/kg of ideal body weight) and therefore overinflation of remaining intact lung units contributes to poor outcome.[8] Consequently, mechanical ventilation is associated with a very high mortality and ranges between 50 to 90 per cent. As a result, the BTS ILD guideline recommends that invasive ventilation is seldom appropriate when the diagnosis is secure.[1] A systematic review of IPF and mechanical ventilation indicated a mortality rate of 87 per cent leading to the American Thoracic Society (ATS) recommendation that the majority of IPF patients should not receive invasive ventilation.[2] This differs substantively to the situation where the ILD is unknown and may be potentially treatment sensitive and reversible, so requiring temporary ventilatory support. There may be exceptions – patients with postoperative respiratory failure after VATS lung biopsy appear to have a better prognosis since their deterioration is likely to be due to reversible operative or anaesthetic complications rather than disease progression.[9]

Risk factors for adverse outcomes from ventilation have been identified and these subgroups are those with extensive fibrotic change (or honeycombing) on CT, co-existing renal impairment or pulmonary hypertension in which mortality is greater when mechanical ventilation is employed.

Non-invasive ventilation (NIV), has the advantage of avoiding the risks of invasive ventilation and is commonly used as an alternative or precursor to invasive ventilation. However, there is no strong evidence that NIV alters the prognosis in this group of patients and overall survival in a NIV treated cohort is similar to an invasive ventilation cohort.[10] The prognosis is particularly poor among patients with fibrosing idiopathic interstitial pneumonia (which consists of IPF and NSIP).[11]

Conclusion

Acute respiratory failure in the context of ILD is a potentially lethal complication that presents a difficult challenge on the ICU especially when the precise ILD is new and unknown. The differential diagnosis is broad and early diagnosis is crucial in determining later ventilatory decisions and treatment escalation. Invasive investigations including bronchoscopy with BAL and surgical biopsy should be considered in the early window of opportunity to secure a precise ILD diagnosis, exclude alternative diagnoses and identify precipitating factors such as infection. Early immunosupression with intravenous methylprednisolone (+/− cyclophosphamide) should not be delayed and is indicated for all rapidly progressive ILD. Although patients may require ventilatory support, there is currently no strong evidence that NIV or invasive ventilation alter the prognosis of this devastating condition so careful consideration of each case on an individual basis is important in deciding whether ventilation should be instituted.

Key Learning Points

- ILD is a heterogeneous group of (predominantly restrictive) lung diseases with individualised treatments and outcomes.
- An accurate diagnosis of the ILD subtype is crucial, but difficult, often requiring invasive investigation with 10 percent remaining 'unclassifiable'.
- ILD patients may present to ICU with acute respiratory failure due to one of the five 'P's.
- Early investigation should be pursued to confirm the precise ILD, exclude serious alternative diagnoses such as cancer and to identify precipitating causes such as infection.
- All rapidly progressive primary ILD should be treated with high dose immunosuppression.

- Certain known ILD including the commonest, IPF, have very poor outcomes with invasive mechanical ventilation making this seldom appropriate as a treatment.

References

1. Bradley B, Branley HM, Egan JJ, et al. Interstitial lung disease guideline: the British Thoracic Society in collaboration with the Thoracic Society of Australia and New Zealand and the Irish Thoracic Society. *Thorax* Sep 2008;63 Suppl 5: v1–58.

2. Raghu G, Collard HR, Egan JJ, et al. An official ATS/ERS/JRS/ALAT statement: idiopathic pulmonary fibrosis: evidence-based guidelines for diagnosis and management. *Am J Respir Crit Care Med* Mar 15 2011;183(6):788–824.

3. Ryerson CJ, Urbania TH, Richeldi L, et al. Prevalence and prognosis of unclassifiable interstitial lung disease. *Eur Respir J* Sep 2013;42(3):750–7.

4. Flaherty KR, Thwaite EL, Kazerooni EA, et al. Radiological versus histological diagnosis in UIP and NSIP: survival implications. *Thorax* Feb 2003;58(2): 143–8.

5. Sprunger DB, Olson AL, Huie TJ, et al. Pulmonary fibrosis is associated with an elevated risk of thromboembolic disease. *Eur Respir J* Jan 2012;39(1): 125–32.

6. Akira M, Kozuka T, Yamamoto S, Sakatani M. Computed tomography findings in acute exacerbation of idiopathic pulmonary fibrosis. *Am J Respir Crit Care Med* Aug 15 2008;178(4):372–8.

7. Kreider ME, Hansen-Flaschen J, Ahmad NN, et al. Complications of video-assisted thoracoscopic lung biopsy in patients with interstitial lung disease. *Ann Thorac Surg* Mar 2007;83(3):1140–4.

8. Baydur A. Mechanical ventilation in interstitial lung disease. *Chest* May 2008;133(5):1062–3.

9. Fernandez-Perez ER, Yilmaz M, Jenad H, et al. Ventilator settings and outcome of respiratory failure in chronic interstitial lung disease. *Chest* May 2008;133(5): 1113–19.

10. Vianello A, Arcaro G, Battistella L, et al. Noninvasive ventilation in the event of acute respiratory failure in patients with idiopathic pulmonary fibrosis. *J Crit Care* Aug 2014;29(4):562–7.

11. Vial-Dupuy A, Sanchez O, Douvry B, et al. Outcome of patients with interstitial lung disease admitted to the intensive care unit. *Sarcoidosis Vasc Diffuse Lung Dis.* Jul 2013;30(2):134–42.

Chronic Pulmonary Hypertension
What Does Critical Care Have to Offer?

Bevan Vickery and Andrew Klein

Introduction

This case study considers a patient with persistent pulmonary hypertension following pulmonary thromboembolism (PTE) and severe haemodynamic compromise. This places the patient at high risk for death and urgent action is required. The case details a patient who has subsequently undergone a pulmonary endarterectomy (PEA) for the treatment of chronic pulmonary hypertension due to PTE.

What follows is a discussion of the initial critical care postoperative management for this patient. Many of the underlying principles are applicable to any critically unwell patient with chronic pulmonary hypertension due to a raised pulmonary vascular resistance.

Case Description

A 67-year-old male has severe pulmonary hypertension secondary to recurrent pulmonary emboli, thought to be associated with his factor V Leiden thrombophilia. This is an inherited condition that causes hypercoagulability. He has been on long term warfarin and had an inferior vena cave (IVC) filter placed two years ago.

He underwent investigation 12 months previously for increasing breathlessness:

- A transthoracic echocardiogram showed a severely dilated and hypertrophied right ventricle with moderate systolic dysfunction, consistent with severe pulmonary hypertension.
- A ventilation perfusion scan showed significant regional perfusion deficits, suggesting the diagnosis of chronic thromboembolic pulmonary hypertension (CTEPH).
- A right heart catheterisation study showed significant pulmonary hypertension with pulmonary arterial pressures of 82/43 mmHg (mean 57 mmHg) and a pulmonary vascular resistance (PVR) of 1200 dyn.s/cm^5. The pulmonary artery occlusion pressure (PAOP) of less than 15 mmHg further demonstrated that this was not due to left-sided heart disease.
- Pulmonary angiography suggested that the majority of disease was surgically resectable.

The overall diagnosis was CTEPH with severe pulmonary hypertension requiring surgical treatment, i.e., pulmonary endarterectomy (PEA).

PEA is a major surgical procedure that can take over eight hours and requires prolonged cardiopulmonary bypass and several episodes of deep hypothermic circulatory arrest. Anaesthetic management is complex, and consists of haemodynamic monitoring, including invasive arterial pressures (radial and femoral), central venous pressure, pulmonary artery pressure and transoesophageal echocardiography (TOE). Near infrared spectroscopy is also used for monitoring of cerebral oxygenation during circulatory arrest.[1] The surgical procedure involves median sternotomy, establishment of cardiopulmonary bypass and incision of the pulmonary arteries. Endarterectomy of the affected pulmonary vasculature is then performed. To facilitate the endarterectomy, brief periods of deep hypothermic circulatory arrest are performed to eliminate bleeding from the bronchial circulation and provide a bloodless field.[1]

During surgery, more severe distal pulmonary disease was found than had been originally diagnosed and not all of the disease could be removed surgically.

Weaning from cardiopulmonary bypass was difficult, and TOE at the time showed severe right ventricular dysfunction, with an underfilled and hyperdynamic left ventricle. Inotropic support included dopamine and noradrenaline. Pulmonary artery catheter studies in theatre revealed significant persistent pulmonary hypertension with a PVR of 600 dyn.s/cm^5.

He has now been delivered to the intensive care unit (ICU). He is in a paced rhythm at 90bpm, with BP of 85/40 mmHg (MAP 55 mmHg), PA pressures of 60/30 mmHg, and a cardiac index of 1.6 l/min. Oxygen saturations are 95 per cent on FiO2 0.8 and PEEP 7 mmHg.

Discussion

Pulmonary hypertension is defined as a mean pulmonary artery pressure greater than 25 mmHg at rest.

A variety of disease processes can result in pulmonary hypertension. The World Health Organization (WHO) has classified the causes of pulmonary hypertension into five groups (Table 17.1).[2]

Table 17.1 WHO classification of causes of pulmonary hypertension

Group	Site/ Mechanism of Disease	Examples
One	Pulmonary Arterial Hypertension	Idiopathic PAH Heritable PAH Drug/ toxin induced Associated with other disease: • Portal Hypertension • Connective Tissue Disease • Congenital Heart disease
Two	Left Heart Disease	Left ventricular systolic or diastolic dysfunction Valvular disease
Three	Lung disease/ Hypoxia	Chronic Obstructive Pulmonary Disease Interstitial lung disease Sleep disordered breathing Chronic exposure to high altitude
Four	Chronic thromboembolic pulmonary hypertension	
Five	Multifactorial/ Unknown	Haematological disease, e.g.: • Splenectomy, • Myeloproliferative disorders Systemic disorders, e.g.: • Sarcoidosis

Patients with chronic pulmonary hypertension may present to the ICU for a number of reasons. Whatever the cause, the presence of pulmonary hypertension carries increased morbidity and mortality. One recent observational study of 99 patients admitted to a medical ICU with pre-existing pulmonary hypertension found a 30 percent ICU mortality and a 40 percent six month mortality.[3] A more detailed analysis of prognosis would depend on the underlying disease process, right ventricular function, functional limitation, rate of progression in chronic symptoms,[4] as well as the nature of the current critical illness.

CTEPH is an important cause of pulmonary hypertension as it is potentially surgically curable. The diagnostic process described in our case is typical. Without surgery, only 10 percent of patients with a mean pulmonary artery pressure greater than 50 mmHg will be alive at five years.[1] Pulmonary endarterectomy has been performed since 1970. In its early years this procedure carried a 16.8 percent mortality; however experienced centres now expect mortality rates as low as 2.2 percent.[5]

Haemodynamic Pathophysiology and Management

In a patient with pulmonary hypertension, the right ventricle is of prime importance in our haemodynamic considerations and management as patients have the potential to decompensate very quickly from right ventricular failure.

Ventricular Interdependence and the Vicious Cycle of Deterioration

Any perturbation that results in right ventricular distension will distort the left ventricular septum. This distortion can impair left ventricular filling as well as contraction, resulting in reduced cardiac output. A vicious cycle may follow with systemic hypotension, hypoperfusion of the right ventricle and further right ventricular impairment with increased distension and distortion of the left ventricle. This interaction between the two ventricles has been termed ventricular interdependence.[6] (Figure 17.1).

Right Ventricular Afterload - The Pulmonary Circulation

The right ventricle is usually a thin walled, compliant structure.[7] It can adapt to pump against a chronically elevated afterload by becoming hypertrophied. Unlike the left ventricle

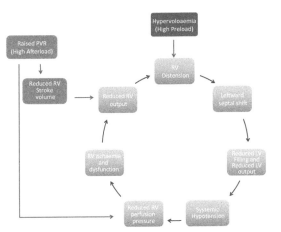

Figure 17.1 Ventricular interdependence and the vicious cycle of deterioration.

however, it responds poorly to an acute rise in afterload. This results in reduced stroke volume and right ventricular distension.[7]

Calculation of Pulmonary Vascular Resistance

The units for pulmonary vascular resistance (PVR) are given in either Woods Units, or dyn.s/cm^5.

PVR is calculated in an equation analogous to Ohm's law:

PVR = Pressure drop across pulmonary vascular bed/ Flow through the pulmonary vascular bed

The pressure drop across the pulmonary circulation is called the transpulmonary gradient (TPG). It is represented by the equation:

TPG = mPAP – PAOP

Here we are using PAOP to estimate left atrial pressure. Patients with a normal TPG (less than 12mmHg), and a raised PAOP (more than 15 mmHg) have pulmonary hypertension due to left-sided heart disease. It is important to note that their management will be different to that described in this chapter.

Overall:

PVR (Woods units) = mPAP (mmHg) – PAOP (mmHg)/ cardiac output (l/min)) PVR (dyn.s/cm5) = Woods units x 80

Determining the above Variables: The Pulmonary Artery Catheter

All patients will have a pulmonary artery catheter placed prior to undergoing a PEA. A pulmonary artery catheter (PAC) allows direct assessment of pulmonary artery pressures, and measurement of the cardiac output through thermodilution. Normally a left atrial pressure can be estimated from the pulmonary artery occlusion pressure (PAOP), allowing calculation of the transpulmonary gradient (TPG) and PVR. Inflation of the PAC balloon in an endarterectomised vessel carries the risk of pulmonary rupture. PAOP is therefore not directly measured, and is assumed to be 10 mmHg in these patients.

The use of the PAC in critically ill patients with pulmonary hypertension who have not undergone PTE, and in centres not familiar with their use, is more controversial. The PAC will provide more accurate and continuous measures of pulmonary artery pressure and PVR than echocardiography, as well as a good estimate of cardiac output. This data will provide valuable feedback on response to management. The PAC, like any monitor, will have a positive effect on management only if interpreted correctly. Potential complications of the PAC are well documented, including infection and pulmonary artery rupture.

Pulmonary Vasodilators

A number of factors can increase PVR, including:
- Intrinsic factors
  . Morphological changes
    - Thickening of the arteriole walls

- . Physiological changes
  - – Circulating catecholamines
  - – Acidosis
  - – Hypoxia
  - – Hypercapnia
- Extrinsic factors
  - . High airway pressures (PEEP)

Before instituting pulmonary vasodilators, it is important to ensure that reversible factors contributing to a raised PVR, such as those described above, are addressed.

Pulmonary vasodilators may reduce PVR if the reduced vessel calibre in the arterial circulation is not corrected. Although a substantial portion of the high PVR in the patient described may be attributed to CTEPH disease within the pulmonary vasculature (which will not respond to vasodilation), there may have been vascular remodelling in the pulmonary vasculature where CTEPH is not present due to chronically raised pulmonary pressures. This may respond to vasodilation.

Enteral Pulmonary Vasodilators

There are a variety of orally administered pulmonary vasodilators, and these can be administered via a nasogastric tube in a critically ill patient. Examples include the phosphodiesterase inhibitor sildenafil, the endothelin antagonist bosentan and the soluble guanylate cyclase stimulator riociguat. There are, however, a number of newer agents becoming available. Many patients with chronic pulmonary hypertension will be taking these medications long term.

These agents will result in systemic vasodilation as well as pulmonary vasodilation. Our patient is unlikely to tolerate this reduction in his right ventricular perfusion pressure. A long half-life will result in administration of this agent not being an easily reversible decision. It is therefore recommended that these agents only be considered once a degree of haemodynamic stability has been achieved, and maintenance of coronary perfusion pressure is no longer an issue.

Intravenous Pulmonary Vasodilators

Intravenous prostacyclin is sometimes used to manage acute pulmonary hypertension. Although it is an effective pulmonary vasodilator, it also results in systemic vasodilation and can compromise right ventricular perfusion. It must be given as an intravenous infusion due to its very short elimination half-life of 3 to 6 minutes. It requires careful dose titration from 1 to 2 ng/kg/min upwards, monitoring pulmonary haemodynamics and side effects (hypotension, jaw pain, headache). Rebound pulmonary hypertension can occur when weaning.[6]

Parenteral agents that have both a vasodilating and inotropic effect are more useful. Commonly used examples include the phosphodiesterase inhibitors (milrinone, enoximone) and dobutamine. These agents will augment right ventricular function by increasing inotropy and at the same time reduce the afterload that it is working against. They will cause a reduction in systemic blood pressure so they will often be administered in conjunction with a vasoconstrictor, such as noradrenaline. Dobutamine has the increased potential for tachyarrhythmias and is often poorly tolerated.[6]

Inhaled Pulmonary Vasodilators

Nitric oxide and prostacyclin (and its analogue iloprost) can both be administered to an intubated patient. The inhalational route is a major advantage because it provides selectivity for the pulmonary circulation. As well as causing pulmonary vasodilatation, they may promote matching of ventilation and perfusion by selectively dilating arterioles of ventilated alveoli. As with most vasoactive therapies in critically ill patients with pulmonary hypertension, there is little evidence supporting their use other than demonstration of improved haemodynamics.

Nitric oxide is a very effective and widely used pulmonary vasodilator. It is, however, an expensive agent. Moreover, a complex delivery system is required to allow for accurate dose administration and to monitor for harmful nitrogen dioxide. It can lead to complications including methaemaglobinaemia and bleeding. Additionally, it can only be administered to patients whose trachea is intubated meaning that it must be weaned prior to tracheal extubation. Weaning nitric oxide can be difficult, due to rebound hypertension that occurs with dose reduction and discontinuation.

Inhaled iloprost is a less expensive alternative to nitric oxide. A 100 mcg ampoule can be diluted into 30 ml of 0.9 per cent sodium chloride, yielding a 3.3 mcg/ml solution. This solution can be refrigerated for 24 hours before expiry. A typical dose range is 3.3 to 9.9 mcg every three hours. If less than 3 ml of the diluted solution is used, then make up to a volume of 3 ml with further 0.9 per cent sodium chloride. It is administered via an ultrasonic nebulizer, and does not require the patient's trachea to be intubated. If not being used as part of a closed circuit, a filter is used in the expiratory limb of the circuit to avoid environmental contamination. Complications include bleeding due to platelet dysfunction and troublesome headaches.

Right Ventricular Preload

In patients with pulmonary hypertension, it is important that intravascular volume is carefully managed.

Hypervolaemia and right ventricular distension results in distortion of the septum and left ventricular geometry. As described above, this can lead to a vicious cycle of haemodynamic deterioration. Aggressive diuresis may be required, targeting a negative fluid balance.

The patient in this case has significant haemodynamic compromise postoperatively. Moreover, his right ventricle is hypertrophied and dilated, meaning it will tolerate hypovolaemia poorly. It is therefore possible that hypovolaemia is contributing to his haemodynamic state. Options for determining if fluid administration is required include a passive leg raise or administration of a cautious fluid bolus, monitoring the haemodynamic response closely. A significant increase in CVP with signs of tricuspid regurgitation may be helpful in diagnosing RV distension. Transthoracic or transoesophageal echocardiography (TOE) is invaluable in monitoring for right ventricular distension and left ventricular filling. Transthoracic echo may be technically difficult in the postoperative patient who requires mechanical ventilation and therefore TOE is preferred.

Tachyarrhythmia will result in reduced right ventricular filling and the potential for rapid decompensation. Sinus rhythm should be maintained if at all possible.

Right Ventricular Contractility

Right ventricular contractility may be impaired in situations such as sepsis or acidosis. Moreover, augmentation of RV contractility may be required to overcome an acute increase in PVR to prevent RV distension and a reduced cardiac output.

In addition to the use of inodilators described above, adrenaline or dopamine by infusion will have a positive inotropic effect. When compared to the inodilators, both have the advantage of not causing systemic hypotension and the disadvantage of not decreasing the ratio of pulmonary vascular resistance to systemic vascular resistance.[7] Other well-known disadvantages of adrenaline include tachyarrhythmias and lactic acidosis, both of which may be poorly tolerated in a patient with pulmonary hypertension.

Right Ventricular Perfusion

Unlike the left ventricle, the right ventricle is perfused throughout systole and diastole.

Right ventricular perfusion pressure in systole will be compromised by a high PVR and consequent raised right ventricular systolic pressure. Systemic hypotension will result in an even lower perfusion pressure.

Right ventricular perfusion in diastole will be compromised by right ventricular distension and increased end diastolic pressure.

Right ventricular hypertrophy, which has developed in response to a chronically raised afterload, increases right ventricular oxygen demand and makes it even more susceptible to ischaemia.[7]

Right ventricular ischaemia will result in reduced contractility and further distension.

It is essential therefore that systemic mean arterial pressure is maintained in order to ensure adequate right ventricular perfusion. Analogous to the detrimental effects of pulmonary vasodilators on the systemic circulation, vasopressors also have the potential to increase pulmonary vascular resistance. In the patient described, with severe haemodynamic compromise due to pulmonary hypertension, both an inodilator and vasopressor can be commenced with the aim that the adverse effects of one are offset by the other. There is very little evidence to guide this practice however.

There is no compelling evidence to guide the choice of vasopressor in this situation. Vasopressin (ADH) may carry a theoretical advantage of causing less pulmonary vasoconstriction than noradrenaline, however evidence here is conflicting.[6]

Mechanical Haemodynamic Support

Right ventricular failure can result in precipitous haemodynamic decompensation. Once this occurs, it can be very difficult to reverse by conventional means. A period of veno-arterial extra corporeal membrane oxygenation (VA-ECMO) will reduce flow through the pulmonary circulation and offload the right ventricle, whilst providing adequate systemic cardiac output and oxygenation. This may provide time for any reversible factors contributing to his haemodynamic compromise to be addressed.[8,9] One published series reported a 57 per cent survival rate for PEA patients with severe haemodynamic compromise requiring VA-ECMO in the immediate postoperative period.[8]

Respiratory Management

Table 17.2 presents physiological considerations and suggestions for an initial management strategy in a patient with pulmonary hypertension.

In routine PEA cases, tracheal extubation usually occurs on the first postoperative day. When a patient with persistent pulmonary hypertension is at the point where tracheal extubation is being considered, this needs to be managed cautiously. Respiratory failure following extubation may result in haemodynamic compromise and rapid deterioration. Our strategy for extubation will therefore include a longer spontaneous breathing trial.

Reperfusion Pulmonary Oedema

Reperfusion pulmonary oedema occurs in up to 15 percent of patients following PEA.[1] Clinical features include hypoxaemia, alveolar infiltrates on chest x-ray in the region of the endarterectomized segments of the lungs, and no other cause for the infiltrate.

Hypoxaemia can be severe, requiring ventilation strategies similar to the management of severe Acute Respiratory Distress Syndrome (ARDS). Lung protective ventilation with

Table 17.2 Ventilation strategy in patients with pulmonary hypertension

Setting	Physiological Considerations	Suggested management
Mandatory vs Spontaneous Mode	A mandatory ventilation mode will minimise the work of breathing and avoid increased cardiovascular demands	Mandatory mode whilst haemodynamically unstable Sedation +/− neuromuscular blockade to facilitate this
Volume or Pressure Control	Hypercapnia will increase PVR	Volume control will allow a guaranteed minute ventilation to be delivered
FiO2	Hypoxia will increase PVR	Target PaO2 > 12 kPa
PEEP	PVR is related to lung volume: PVR lowest at FRC PVR increases below FRC, Larger pulmonary blood vessels are compressed by collapsed lung parenchyma PVR increases above FRC, Raised alveolar pressure and volume compresses smaller vessels associated with the alveoli	PEEP set to 5 – 7 mmHg Careful titration from here to avoid hypoxia, but also avoid unnecessarily raised intrathoracic pressure
Tidal Volume/ Airway pressure	Lower tidal volumes and reduced peak/ plateau airway pressures will help limit the following: Intrathoracic pressure and therefore PVR Alveolar distension and ventilator induced lung injury	Tidal volumes of 6 – 8 ml/kg Peak airway pressures <30 cmH2O (if PCV or PRVC modes) Plateau airway pressures <30 cmH2O (if VCV mode)
Respiratory Rate	Hypercapnia will increase PVR Patients with CTEPH (and low cardiac output) may have a large amount of poorly perfused alveoli (physiological dead space) and require a higher minute ventilation than normal	Titrate to PaCO2 Initial setting of 14 – 18 breaths per minute

Abbreviations used in table: FiO2 – Fractional Inspired Oxygen, PEEP – Positive End Expiratory Pressure, FRC – Function Residual Capacity, PaO2 Partial Pressure of Oxygen in arterial blood, PCV – Pressure Control Ventilation, PRVC – Pressure Regulated Volume Control, VCV – Volume control ventilation.

increased levels of PEEP will be required. Permissive hypercapnia will be poorly tolerated in these patients however, so an adequate minute ventilation is important. Increasing PEEP however will lead to increased PVR (see above), and caution should be applied.

If hypoxaemia is refractory to optimal conventional management following PEA, then Veno-Venous Extra Corporeal Membrane Oxygenation (VV-ECMO) is indicated. This will provide good gas exchange whilst minimising positive airway pressure and ventilator induced lung injury.

Other Organ System Considerations

Pain and anxiety will lead to increased endogenous catecholamines, with an increased pulmonary vascular resistance; adequate analgesia and sedation is therefore important. If his respiratory status remains borderline, a tracheostomy will allow a longer period of mechanical ventilation with reduced need for sedation to facilitate endotracheal tube tolerance.

Continuous renal replacement therapy (CRRT) may be started at a relatively early stage in the advent of acute kidney injury. Oliguria and resultant positive fluid balance will be poorly tolerated. Moreover, acidaemia associated with acute kidney injury has the potential to affect PVR. CRRT will give us good control over both these factors.

Right ventricular failure with increased venous pressures, combined with a period of a low cardiac output state carries the potential for gastrointestinal and hepatic ischaemia. A high index of suspicion for this is needed. Gastrointestinal oedema may result in poor tolerance to enteral nutrition.

Therapeutic anticoagulation in patients with CTEPH is very important. Patients will be commenced on therapeutic low molecular weight heparin subcutaneously once bleeding is not an issue, and lifelong warfarin will be restarted once discharged from the ICU.

Long Term Considerations

If this patient survives the postoperative ICU admission, his persistent pulmonary hypertension requires ongoing management.

He will be established on targeted medical therapy. This will include pulmonary vasodilator therapy such as sildenafil, bosentan, riociguat.

Conclusion

The management of a critically unwell patient with pulmonary hypertension requires a management strategy focussed around ensuring adequate right ventricular function. This has implications for the management of multiple other organ systems.

Key Learning Points

- Pulmonary hypertension is the end result of a number of diverse causes. Each underlying cause will have unique implications on management and prognosis of the patient.
- CTEPH is a potentially curable cause of pulmonary hypertension. Morbidity and mortality from PEA has decreased considerably since it was first performed.
- Haemodynamic considerations can be structured considering right ventricular preload, afterload, contractility and perfusion. Heart rate and rhythm are also important.

- Other organ systems need to be managed in such a way that optimises right ventricular function.
- Perturbations that lead to right ventricular impairment and distension can result in a vicious cycle of haemodynamic deterioration, facilitated by ventricular interdependence.

References

1. Roscoe A, Klein A. Pulmonary endarterectomy. *Curr Opin Anaes* 2008;21:16–20.

2. Simonneau G, Gatzoulis MA, Adatia I, et al. Updated clinical classification of pulmonary hypertension. *JACC* 2013;62:S34–1.

3. Huynh TN, Weigt SS, Sugar CA, et al. Prognostic factors and outcomes of patients with pulmonary hypertension admitted to the intensive care unit. *Crit Care* 2012;27:e7–739.

4. Galie N, Hoeper MM, Humbert M, et al. Guidelines for the diagnosis and treatment of pulmonary hypertension. *Eur Resp J* 2009;34:1219–63.

5. Madani MM, Auger WR, Pretorius V, et al. Pulmonary endarterectomy: Recent changes in a single institution's experience of more than 2,700 patients. *Ann Thorac Surg* 2012;94:97–103.

6. Zamanian RT, Haddad F, Doyle RL, et al. Management strategies for patients with pulmonary hypertension in the intensive care unit. *Crit Care Med* 2007;35:2037–50.

7. Hosseinian L. Pulmonary hypertension and noncardiac surgery: implications for the anesthesiologist. *J Cardiothorac Vasc Anesthes* 2014;28:1076–86.

8. Berman M, Tsui S, Vuylsteke A, et al. Successful extracorporeal membrane oxygenation support after pulmonary thromboendarterectomy. *Ann Thorac Surg* 2008;86:1261–7.

9. Kim NH, Delcroix M, Jenkins DP, et al. Chronic thromboembolic pulmonary hypertension. *JACC* 2013;62:D92–9.

Acute Lung Injury

Gary H Mills

Introduction

Patients who develop respiratory failure, demonstrate a failure of oxygenation or an inability to clear carbon dioxide. This may be in the context of single organ or multi-organ failure and may originate from an acquired or pre-existing respiratory disease or follow surgery[1] or trauma. Some patients may develop mild, moderate or severe adult respiratory distress syndrome (ARDS), which is classified according to the Berlin definition (Table 18.1). There are a number of common risk factors: pneumonia, non-pulmonary sepsis, aspiration of gastric contents, major trauma, pulmonary contusion, pancreatitis, inhalational injury, severe burns, non-cardiogenic shock, drug overdose, multiple transfusions or transfusion-associated acute lung injury (TRALI), pulmonary vasculitis or drowning.[2]

This chapter will illustrate severe respiratory failure and its treatment, using a perioperative case as an example to illustrate the complexities of therapy. Extracorporeal techniques are covered in a subsequent chapter.

Case Description

A 75-year-old male patient presented for repair of a large upper abdominal incisional hernia under general anaesthesia. He was otherwise well. At the end of surgery he was extubated with a working thoracic epidural in situ. Postoperatively, he was placed on CPAP, as a form of prophylaxis to prevent deterioration of perioperative atelectasis.[3]

The patient remained stable and CPAP was discontinued within 24 hours. However, 48 hours later he developed pyrexia, breathlessness, increased white cell count and a climbing lactate. Oxygen saturation began to fall. Clinical examination revealed unilateral crackles and a clinical diagnosis of pneumonia was made. Blood and sputum cultures were

Table 18.1 The Berlin definition of ARDS

Oxygenation	Mild	Moderate	Severe
PaO$_2$/FiO$_2$ (mm Hg)	200 <PaO$_2$/FiO$_2$ ≤300	100 < PaO$_2$/FiO$_2$ ≤200	100 ≤PaO$_2$/FiO$_2$
PEEP/CPAP	PEEP CPAP ≥5 cm H$_2$O	PEEP ≥5 cm H$_2$O	PEEP ≥5 cm H$_2$O

The Berlin definition of ARDS has four main components: timing, chest imaging, aetiology of oedema and oxygenation.
ARDS occurs within one week of a known clinical insult or worsening of symptoms. Chest imaging shows bilateral opacities not fully explained by effusions, lobar collapse or nodules. Pulmonary oedema is not fully explained by cardiac failure or fluid overload and requires objective assessment such as echocardiography.

taken and antibiotics commenced. There was concern as to whether the patient might have developed a pulmonary embolism because of the history of recent surgery, but chest X-ray illustrated an increase in radio density at the right base, consistent with pneumonia. Echocardiography showed normal size heart chambers and the electrocardiogram was normal, other than for a sinus tachycardia. Prophylactic sodium bicarbonate was started to reduce the risk of contrast induced renal damage during CT pulmonary angiography (CTPA).

The CTPA demonstrated signs of bilateral basal pneumonia and no PE was identified. The patient was transferred to the ICU and non-invasive ventilation commenced with pressure settings adjusted to achieve adequate tidal volumes and reduce respiratory rate. Over the course of the next two hours his oxygen requirements increased, respiratory rate climbed and tidal volumes fell. A decision was taken to intubate and ventilate the patient, because he was becoming increasingly breathless and fraction of inspired oxygen (FiO2) had increased to 0.9.

A rapid sequence induction was performed and the patient was intubated using an endotracheal tube equipped with a supraglottic suction port and controlled cuff pressure. Invasive ventilation was commenced, using a pressure controlled mode, with the patient sitting up at 30 degrees. Low tidal volumes were adopted to protect the lungs.[4]

Ventilation parameters consistent with ARDSnet were considered. A tidal volume of 6 ml/kg ideal body weight was commenced. Ideal body weight was based on patient height and gender, because these factors are related to lung size. Initial PEEP was set according to a modified ARDSnet scale. Care was taken to ensure that expiratory flow returned to baseline before the subsequent inspiration, to avoid breath stacking.

The systolic pressure swing on the arterial trace was more than 10 per cent of systolic pressure suggesting fluid responsiveness and fluid boluses and metaraminol were required prior to starting noradrenaline as a vasoconstrictor via a new central line.

Once the patient was more stable, lung recruitment was attempted using a step wise increase in peak pressure and PEEP. Pulmonary compliance was monitored, together with oxygen saturation and arterial blood gases. During the recruitment procedure peak airway pressures were increased to peak 40 cm H2O pressure control with PEEP of 25 in steps of 5 cm H2O and then decreased gradually to establish at which level of PEEP saturations began to fall once again. Once this pressure was determined, the recruitment manoeuvre was repeated and in this case ventilator pressures were set to a pressure controlled peak pressure of 30 and a PEEP of 15.

Arterial PaCO2 was elevated at 8.0 KPa, with a pH of 7.29. This PaCO2 was tolerated (permissive hypercapnia) rather than increasing respiratory rate, because the pH was greater than 7.2.

Because of continued poor basal expansion, attempts were made to encourage diaphragmatic contractility using airway pressure release ventilation (APRV). This mode has the potential advantage of allowing the diaphragm to contract and draw air into the lower zones by generating negative pressure. This also has the useful effect of reducing intrathoracic pressure and so may increase venous return, reduce pulmonary vascular resistance and boost cardiac output. Sedation was decreased slightly to encourage spontaneous breathing with a 6 second plateau, combined with 0.7 second release. APRV effectively allowed a relatively high level of continuous positive airways pressure (CPAP) around which the patient could breathe, combined with a release of this pressure down to zero for a brief period of around 0.5 secs. This release period was short enough to avoid sudden airway collapse, but enough to supplement CO_2 exhalation. Spontaneous breathing around the pressure levels set on the APRV was achieved and both $PaCO_2$ and PaO_2 improved.

However, over the next 24 hours respiratory function deteriorated. A decision was taken to return to pressure controlled ventilation, to paralyse the patient with non-depolarising muscle relaxants and then to place the patient prone. In this case paralysis was produced with an atracurium infusion, with the aim of avoiding patient ventilator asynchrony. The neuromuscular blockade was monitored by peripheral nerve stimulation, to ensure adequacy of paralysis, together with bispectral index monitoring (BIS) monitoring to avoid over or under sedation.

Neuromuscular blocking drugs may improve ventilator patient interaction and if used for 24 to 48 hours may improve survival.[5] The main disadvantages are the importance of deep sedation to avoid awareness whilst paralysed and the potential increase in muscle atrophy due to lack of movement, combined with the impact of sepsis.

Prone ventilation was achieved by a group of nursing and medical staff experienced in turning patients. Care was taken to ensure protection of eyes, pressure points and to minimise stress on limbs and joints. Arterial blood gases were recorded, together with dead space and compliance both immediately before and half an hour after turning. Following the protocol used by Guerin, the patient remained prone for at least 16 hours[6] with mechanical ventilation at low tidal volumes (Vt less than 6 ml/kg).

The lungs were once again recruited and PEEP set at 15 cm H2O. FiO2 requirements began to fall and $PaCO_2$ improved. Compliance was better in the prone position. The process continued for the next 48 hours.

Whilst the patient was in a supine phase, fibre-optic bronchoscopy and lavage was carried out. Sputum samples were sent to microbiology. A throat swab was sent for viral PCR analysis even though a previous sample had been found to be negative. Consideration was given to performing a pleural tap of an effusion to obtain a sample for microscopy and culture, and to look for low pH, high LDH and high protein levels, which would be consistent with empyema. This plan was rejected because a swinging pyrexia and high white cell count and inflammatory markers (CRP) were not present and the effusion was small.

Over this time. liver function tests showed a rising ALT and AST. Concerns were raised as to whether prone ventilation was impairing liver perfusion and so the patient was returned to the supine position. The atracurium infusion was discontinued and the respiratory parameters remained stable. FiO2 had reduced to 0.5. Unfortunately, over the next 48 hours increasing abdominal distension was noted with an IAP elevated at 25 cm H2O. CT scanning of the abdomen and chest was performed and extensive changes were detected in the chest with small pleural effusions, but no abnormality in the abdomen. The surgical opinion was that cause of the distension was thought to be ileus, made worse by gut oedema.

Serum lactate remained normal and creatinine was within normal range. Over the next 48 hours the abdominal distension subsided and liver function returned to normal.

However the decreased compliance of the chest wall, which had been caused by the distended abdomen, had caused a worsening of lung collapse and function. A decision was taken to measure transpulmonary pressure, which is the difference between alveolar pressure and intrapleural pressure.[7] Therefore, an oesophageal catheter was inserted into the lower third of the oesophagus as a proxy measurement of pleural pressure. This would potentially allow a more accurate setting of PEEP to match transpulmonary pressure during expiration to optimise the expansion of the lung to minimise opening and closing of alveoli during the respiratory cycle. If intra-airway pressure during end expiration matched PEEP, then those alveoli that could open would remain open throughout the respiratory cycle. During inspiration, transpulmonary pressure could be set to be less than 20 cm H2O, to reduce overdistension in the non-dependent parts of the lung. Slow pressure volume curves might also allow the visualisation of an improvement in compliance above a certain pressure level, which might also help confirm PEEP settings and show worsening compliance at higher pressure levels. Therefore, the aim was to use the mechanisms to set ventilator pressures, combined with a low tidal volume (Vt 6 to 7 ml/kg IBW), with a relatively low respiratory rate to reduce lung shearing forces, volutrauma and barotrauma. Transpulmonary pressures and the behaviour of the lung is also time dependent as resistive forces are overcome. The impact of this is only just being explored in the damaged and ARDS lung.[8]

Over the next two days FiO2 requirements began to fall and it became possible to once again allow sedation holds, during which spontaneous breathing efforts were detected and the patient was transitioned to a spontaneous breathing mode and the process of weaning from ventilator support commenced.

Discussion

The process of lung injury may begin early. In patients undergoing surgery, lung protective ventilation is important. The IMPROVE study group[9] showed that in patients more than 40 years old with an elevated preoperative risk index of respiratory complications, having surgery of two or more hours in duration, the number of respiratory complications could be reduced significantly by adopting low tidal volumes (6 to 8 ml/kg predicted body weight) plus PEEP 6 to 8 cm H2O and recruitment (30 second, 30 cm H20 airway pressure inspiratory holds). PROVHILO challenged the use of higher levels of PEEP, finding no benefit in 12 cmH_2O versus 0-2 cmH_2O (10). In the postoperative period the avoidance of progressive atelectasis is very important and so patients need to be well analgesed, fully awake and cardiovascularly stable. Urine output should be adequate and fluid overload avoided. CPAP immediately after surgery may help reduce respiratory complications.[3]

Many patients begin with normal or relatively normal lungs and then deteriorate, providing a spectrum of lung damage. On the ICU in ARDS, the ARDSnet research group demonstrated better survival in patients with low tidal volumes (6 ml/kg) compared to the higher level of 12 ml/kg.[11] Subsequently ARDS definitions have been modified to allow three categories of ARDS (Table 18.1) that are designed to fit the definitions, clinical outcomes and the severity of illness. ARDS is a potentially complex disease process with multiple aetiologies and so an easy to use definition is important clinically and vital for discussion of treatment options or research.

In this case, the problems of trying to ventilate a patient with a stiff abdominal wall became apparent. This was caused by a distended abdomen. This adds further complexity to the effectiveness of PEEP and in particular risks increasing intra-thoracic pressure at the expense of reducing cardiac output, whilst making lung expansion difficult. In this situation determining the cause of the stiff chest wall and trying to treat these causes becomes very important. In this case, had the raised intra-abdominal pressure worsened and treatment failed then decompressing the abdomen to protect the chest and abdominal organs could have been required.

The position of PEEP and recruitment is unclear. Radiological studies have shown how atelectasis can be reduced, but have more recently looked at the difficulty of knowing how much lung is recruitable and started to explore the extent to which pressure increases are beneficial or more likely to be harmful.[12,13] PEEP levels were relatively high in the ARDSnet study and many would advocate lower levels.

High frequency oscillatory ventilation (HFOV) was not attempted in this case. Recent large clinical studies have failed to show benefit from HFOV. This is in contrast to some physiological studies and to some clinical experience in respiratory centres prior to extra-corporeal membrane oxygenation (ECMO).[14] However, the OSCILLATE trial showed superior survival using conventional protective ventilation with low tidal volumes.[15]

Prone ventilation was employed. This attempts to reduce the compressing effect of the weight of the lungs, heart and abdominal contents, particularly on the dependent posterior and posterobasal parts of the lung. This makes ventilation perfusion ratios more even throughout the lung and most importantly evens out the effects of over distension, which occurs in the supine patient in the non-dependent parts of the lung. This over distension may cause major volutrauma in these areas. In the past there have been suggestions of improved survival in patients whose PaCO2 improved on turning prone.[16] Recent studies have demonstrated survival benefit using this technique,[6] but close attention to patient care is vital to avoid complications. Prevention of further insults to the lung, such as ventilator associated pneumonia is very important. Hence the use of sitting up to reduce aspiration, together with subglottic suction and mouth care to reduce the pooling of secretions and increased bacterial load entering the lungs.

Reducing fluid overload is important in the inflamed lung, just as it is in avoiding gut wall oedema. There is some evidence that the combination of albumin and furosemide is effective in improving oxygenation, but survival data is not conclusive.

Conclusion

Respiratory disease and respiratory complications are common after surgery and in the critically ill medical patient. It is vital that appropriate ventilatory techniques are used, together with other care adjuncts such as sedation holds and ventilator care bundles in VAP reduction. It is important to minimise the additional damage that lifesaving mechanical ventilation can cause to the lungs and the other organs and to reduce the impact these processes have on the patient's inflammatory response.

Key Learning Points

- Lung protective ventilation is important for at risk patients undergoing surgery of 2 hours or more to reduce the risk of respiratory complications.
- High levels of PEEP (greater than 12 cm H2O) applied routinely in ARDS cases may be harmful and lower levels of PEEP should be considered.
- Prone ventilation may be of survival benefit but carries an associated high degree or morbidity.
- Ventilator care bundles, prevention and treatment of infection, avoidance of fluid overload and reductions in lung water with diuretics +/− albumin prevent further lung damage.

References

1. Canet J, Gallart L, Gomar C, et al. Prediction of postoperative pulmonary complications in a population-based surgical cohort. *Anesthesiology* 2010 Dec;113(6):1338–50. PubMed PMID: 21045639.

2. Ferguson ND, Fan E, Camporota L, et al. The Berlin definition of ARDS: an expanded rationale, justification, and

supplementary material. *Intensive Care Medicine* 2012 Oct;38(10):1573–82. PubMed PMID: 22926653.

3. Squadrone V, Coha M, Cerutti E, et al. Continuous positive airway pressure for treatment of postoperative hypoxemia: a randomized controlled trial. *JAMA: the journal of the American Medical Association* 2 Feb 2005;293(5):589–95. PubMed PMID: 15687314.

4. Gattinoni L, Caironi P. Refining ventilatory treatment for acute lung injury and acute respiratory distress syndrome. *JAMA: The Journal of the American Medical Association* 13 Feb 2008;299(6):691–3. PubMed PMID: 18270359.

5. Papazian L, Forel JM, Gacouin A, et al. Neuromuscular blockers in early acute respiratory distress syndrome. *The New England Journal of Medicine* 16 Sep 2010;363(12):1107–16. PubMed PMID: 20843245.

6. Guerin C, Reignier J, Richard JC, et al. Prone positioning in severe acute respiratory distress syndrome. *The New England Journal of Medicine* 6 Jun 2013;368 (23):2159–68. PubMed PMID: 23688302.

7. Caironi P, Langer T, Gattinoni L. Acute lung injury/acute respiratory distress syndrome pathophysiology: what we have learned from computed tomography scanning. *Current Opinion in Critical Care* 1 Feb 2008 Feb;14(1):64–9. PubMed PMID: 18195628.

8. Stenqvist O, Gattinoni L, Hedenstierna G. What's new in respiratory physiology? The expanding chest wall revisited! *Intensive Care Medicine* Jun 2015;41(6):1110–13. PubMed PMID: 25672279.

9. Futier E, Constantin JM, Paugam-Burtz C, et al. A trial of intraoperative low-tidal-volume ventilation in abdominal surgery. *The New England Journal of Medicine* 1 Aug 2013;369(5):428–37. PubMed PMID: 23902482.

10. Hemmes SN, Gama de Abreu M, Pelosi P, Schultz MJ. High versus low positive end-expiratory pressure during general anaesthesia for open abdominal surgery (PROVHILO trial): a multicentre randomised controlled trial. *Lancet* 2014 Aug 9;384(9942):495–503. PubMed PMID: 24894577.

11. Ventilation with lower tidal volumes as compared with traditional tidal volumes for acute lung injury and the acute respiratory distress syndrome. The acute respiratory distress syndrome network. *The New England Journal of Medicine* 4 May 2000;342(18):1301–8. PubMed PMID: 10793162.

12. de Matos GF, Stanzani F, Passos RH, et al. How large is the lung recruitability in early acute respiratory distress syndrome: a prospective case series of patients monitored by computed tomography. *Critical Care* 2012;16(1):R4. PubMed PMID: 22226331. Pubmed Central PMCID: 3396229.

13. Gattinoni L, Caironi P, Cressoni M, et al. Lung recruitment in patients with the acute respiratory distress syndrome. *The New England Journal of Medicine* 27 Apr 2006;354(17):1775–86. PubMed PMID: 16641394.

14. Camporota L, Sherry T, Smith J, Lei K, McLuckie A, Beale R. Physiological predictors of survival during high-frequency oscillatory ventilation in adults with acute respiratory distress syndrome. *Critical Care* 2013;17(2):R40. PubMed PMID: 23497577. Pubmed Central PMCID: 3733430.

15. Ferguson ND, Cook DJ, Guyatt GH, et al. High-frequency oscillation in early acute respiratory distress syndrome. *The New England Journal of Medicine*. 28 Feb 2013;368(9):795–805. PubMed PMID: 23339639.

16. Gattinoni L, Vagginelli F, Carlesso E, et al. Decrease in PaCO2 with prone position is predictive of improved outcome in acute respiratory distress syndrome. *Critical Care Medicine*. 2003 Dec;31(12):2727–33. PubMed PMID: 14668608.

Chapter 19

The Role of Noninvasive Ventilation Following Extubation of Intensive Care Patients

Alastair J Glossop

Introduction

Endotracheal intubation and mechanical ventilation (MV) are supportive interventions that may be life saving in critically ill patients but also introduce a significant risk of morbidity and mortality to a patient group already at high risk of poor outcomes. Mechanical ventilation introduces the risk of several pathological pulmonary conditions including volutrauma and barotrauma, and all patients who are intubated are at risk of developing ventilator associated pneumonia (VAP) and other complications associated with sedation and MV. In recent years VAP has been demonstrated to be associated with poor clinical and economic outcomes, with a large data registry series from the USA demonstrating rates of VAP in ventilated intensive care unit (ICU) patients of 9.3 percent with increased morbidity and ICU length of stay observed.[1] Timely extubation is one way of minimising this morbidity, but premature or inappropriate extubation may in itself be detrimental, and the need for reintubation is associated with a hospital mortality of up to 40 percent[2] in some patient groups.

The term noninvasive ventilation (NIV) is often used as an umbrella term to describe both continuous positive airway pressure (CPAP) and noninvasive positive pressure ventilation (NPPV). By definition NIV is delivery of ventilatory support via the patient's upper airway using a mask or similar device,[3] and its use has increased considerably over the last 20 years as a viable alternative to MV. Use of NIV in patients as a therapy for acute respiratory failure (ARF) is well established, and NIV has been demonstrated to reduce intubation rates and mortality in patients with exacerbations of chronic obstructive pulmonary disease (COPD), cardiogenic pulmonary oedema and the immunocompromised[4]

More recently NIV has been used in populations of ICU patients who are difficult to wean from MV[5] or have recently been extubated following a period of MV[6] as a form of ongoing ventilatory support following extubation and the cessation of MV. These populations of recently extubated patients are at an increased risk of morbidity and mortality should they develop respiratory failure and require reintubation, and may therefore benefit from the use of NIV to prevent this progression and the deleterious consequences of a further period of intubation and MV.

Several studies examining the use of NIV in these situations have been either inconclusive or have produced conflicting results, and debate continues within the critical care community regarding the optimal use of NIV following extubation. Additionally there is no consensus opinion as to which patient groups may benefit from NIV following extubation or the duration of time for which NIV should be applied to recently extubated critical care patients.

Case Description

A 68-year-old man was admitted to hospital with a three-day history of increasing shortness of breath, lethargy, and cough productive of green sputum. He had a past medical history of COPD, for which he used bronchodilator and steroid inhalers, and hypertension. Additional medications included bendrofluazide, amlodipine, atorvastatin and aspirin and he had no known drug allergies. He was a smoker of 15 cigarettes per day and had been given a course of amoxicillin and prednisolone by his GP two days prior to admission to hospital as treatment for his presumed infective exacerbation of COPD.

It was evident from the history taken at admission that he lived alone in a bungalow but managed to walk distances of several hundred metres on the flat and was independent with all of his activities of daily living. Although he had received short courses of oral steroids in the past for exacerbations of COPD, he had never been admitted to hospital before, and did not require home nebulisers or oxygen to control his disease.

On examination he was found to be tachypnoeic with a respiratory rate of 36 breaths per minute and wheezy, with pronounced crackles over the right lung base on auscultation. He was tachycardic (110 bpm) with a blood pressure of 145/85 and his conscious level was reduced at 13/15. A chest x-ray taken shortly after admission to hospital demonstrated extensive right lower and mid zone lobar consolidation, and an arterial blood gas taken on 60 per cent humidified oxygen showed type 2 respiratory failure with pH 7.12, pCO_2 11.8 kPa, pO_2 7.9 kPa, HCO_3^- 32 mmol/L, lactate 3.7 mmol/L. He was started on bilevel NIV with pressures of 15 over 5, graduated inspired oxygen aiming for saturations of 88 to 92 per cent, IV piperacillin/tazobactam and hydrocortisone and 'back to back' salbutamol and ipratropium nebulisers. His respiratory rate, saturations and conscious level failed to improve after an hour on NIV, at which stage he was requiring 80 per cent oxygen and his GCS had dropped further, so the decision was made to proceed to intubation, invasive ventilation and transfer to the ICU.

After 5 days of MV and treatment with steroids, bronchodilators and piperacillin/tazobactam the patient was felt to be ready for a trial of extubation. He was appropriate on sedation hold and comfortable during a 30-minute trial of zero ASB so was extubated onto 28 per cent low flow oxygen. However following an initial period of stability, his respiratory rate started to increase and 3 hours after being extubated, it was 35 breaths per minute. He was also noted to have a poor cough and was not clearing respiratory secretions effectively. An arterial blood gas taken 12 hours post extubation revealed a respiratory acidosis with pH 7.18, pCO_2 10.4 kPa, pO_2 10.1 kPa, HCO_3^- 36 mmol/l, lactate 5.1 mmol/l on 65 per cent oxygen delivered via a high flow circuit. At this point he was started on bilevel NIV but despite a brief, initial stabilization of his pCO_2 at 9 kPa he became increasingly drowsy and unresponsive and his pCO_2 began to climb again so the decision was taken four hours after starting NIV to reintubate the patient and recommence MV.

Following reintubation, a bronchoscopy and lavage were performed and his antibiotics changed to meropenem. He was quickly changed to a spontaneous breathing mode on the ventilator and his pressure support requirements reduced over the following 48 hours. On day three following his reintubation he was felt to be well enough again to be extubated following a successful sedation hold and spontaneous breathing trial.

On this occasion the patient was extubated directly onto bilevel NIV with pressures of 16 over 6. The NIV was provided continuously for the first 24 hours via a facial mask following his extubation with no deterioration in his gas exchange, respiratory pattern or conscious level. On day two post extubation the patient had four separate two-hour periods off NIV, during which time he received low flow oxygen via nasal cannulae, and these periods were gradually increased in length as his condition improved over the following 48 hours. On day five post extubation, he was deemed well enough to be discharged to the general respiratory ward having been free of the need for NIV for 24 hours, from where he continued to make a good recovery and was subsequently discharged home.

Discussion

Extubation of ICU patients who have received MV carries the risk of extubation failure and the need for a further period of MV. Although the reported rate of extubation failure in the literature varies, it may be as high as 19 per cent in ICU patients.[7] It is also widely acknowledged that failing an extubation is associated with worse outcomes and increased risk of morbidity and mortality, although this may be the result of patients with more severe illness and greater comorbidities having a higher risk of extubation failure rather than a direct effect of reintubation per se.

The use of NIV in recently extubated patients is an attractive treatment option for critical care physicians, as it has the potential to provide ongoing respiratory support to recently extubated patients whose respiratory muscle strength and co-ordination may still be recovering following a period of critical illness and MV, without the attendant risks of endotracheal intubation and MV and associated morbidity and mortality.

There have been several randomised controlled trials (RCTs) examining the use of NIV as a rescue treatment for post extubation respiratory distress. Early work suggested that application of NIV to patients with premorbid cardiorespiratory disease who developed respiratory failure post extubation did not reduce reintubation rates, duration of ventilation (IMV), hospital mortality or length of stay compared to standard therapy.[8] A subsequent multicentre RCT reported that patients who had been extubated following a successful spontaneous breathing trial (SBT) but then developed post extubation respiratory failure had an increased ICU mortality if then treated with NIV compared to standard medical therapy.[9]

There has been some criticism of this trial and it is important to note that the patients who failed on NIV and went on to require intubation had received long periods of ineffective NIV before reintubation – on average 9 hours longer than the controls – which is likely to have contributed to their worse outcomes. Additionally, post hoc analysis of patients with COPD in this study suggested that use of NIV may still be warranted if used judiciously in post-extubation respiratory distress. However in general the onset of post extubation respiratory failure is an ominous development and delaying reintubation by any means risks potential harm and detriment to the patient.

Following these findings several studies have examined the earlier use of NIV post extubation as a preventative or prophylactic measure in high risk patients before the development of respiratory distress. In an early landmark study by Nava and colleagues, NIV was assessed as a preventative strategy following extubation. Patients who had been ventilated for greater than 48 hours and deemed suitable for extubation – but had risk factors for reintubation such as age greater than 65, poor cough, cardiac and respiratory co-morbidity and hypercapnia (whilst ventilated or pre-existing) – were randomised to receive either prophylactic NIV or standard medical therapy once extubated following a successful spontaneous breathing trial. The study group had NIV applied within 1 hour of extubation for periods of 8 hours or more per day for the first 48 hours following extubation. This early use of NIV was demonstrated to reduce reintubation rates by 16 percent and mortality by 10 percent when compared to controls who received standard medical therapy alone.[6]

These findings were supported by research published by Ferrer and colleagues, in which NIV used prophylactically was demonstrated to reduce the incidence of respiratory failure post extubation when used for up to 24 hours post extubation.[10] It was noted by the authors that patients with chronic respiratory disease derived greater benefits from prophylactic NIV than other subsets of patients included in the analysis. A later study by the same authors demonstrated that prophylactic NIV used for 24 hours following extubation significantly reduced respiratory failure and 90 day mortality (11 percent versus 31 percent in controls) when compared to standard medical therapy alone.[11] Of note in this study, all patients enrolled had chronic respiratory disease and had been hypercarbic during their period of MV and received early NIV for an average of 18 hours during the first 24 hours post extubation, suggesting a possible benefit for early and longer periods of application of NIV in patients with chronic chest disease.

These findings have been largely echoed by a recent meta analysis of studies that pooled data from 10 trials and 1382 patients who received NIV following extubation to prevent the onset of post extubation respiratory failure and reintubation.[12] The authors concluded that use of NIV as a prophylactic treatment post extubation conferred significant benefits in terms of mortality and reintubation rates that were not seen if NIV was used as a treatment for post extubation respiratory distress. Therefore it seems that NIV has an important role to play in the prevention of post extubation respiratory failure and requirement for reintubation, but that vigilance is required for the onset of respiratory failure and caution should be taken to not allow NIV to delay reintubation once post extubation respiratory failure is established.

Conclusion

The use of NIV in recently extubated ICU patients remains a contentious area as the success and validity of treatment is highly dependant on timing of intervention and patient selection. It is evident from the literature that early, prophylactic use of NIV is preferential to treatment of established respiratory failure post extubation; indeed, using NIV as a rescue therapy may be detrimental to patient outcomes and should be avoided in this patient group.

It is also apparent that patients with risk factors for reintubation or, in particular chronic respiratory disease, are the most likely to benefit from prophylactic NIV post extubation, and thus efforts should be made to identify these patients prior to extubation so that prophylactic therapy can be instituted in a timely fashion to prevent the development of further morbidity.

There is no consensus regarding the optimal time period for which NIV should be provided following extubation of ICU patients, although a stronger signal for beneficial effects with NIV was seen in a study that used NIV prophylactically for 48 hours post extubation, suggesting that this longer time period may be optimal.

Key Learning Points

- Using NIV prophylactically requires investment of time, resources and occupancy of critical care bed space in the short term and the benefits may not be immediately apparent.

- In some patient groups, e.g., those with chronic respiratory disease use of NIV post extubation, improves endpoints such as patient mortality and need for reintubation.
- There is an important distinction between use of NIV for prophylaxis and for treatment of post-extubation respiratory failure.
- Applying NIV early post extubation proactively is preferable to its use in a reactive fashion when respiratory failure develops.
- It is vitally important to recognise the patient who is developing respiratory failure post extubation and not delay reintubation if necessary, as this is associated with a significant risk of increased mortality.
- It is important for ICU physicians to appreciate the limitations of NIV as an intervention and a possible alternative to MV in certain clinical situations rather than a universally applicable treatment.

References

1. Rello J, Ollendorf DA, Oster G, et al. Epidemiology and outcomes of ventilator-associated pneumonia in a large US database. *Chest* 2002;122(6):2115–21.

2. Epstein SK, Ciubotaru RL. Independent effects of etiology of failure and time to reintubation on outcome for patients failing extubation. *American Journal of Respiratory & Critical Care Medicine* 1998;158(2):489–93.

3. British Thoracic Society Standards of Care C. Non-invasive ventilation in acute respiratory failure. *Thorax* 2002;57(3): 192–211.

4. Hill NS, Brennan J, Garpestad E, Nava S. Noninvasive ventilation in acute respiratory failure. [Review] [60 refs]. *Critical Care Medicine* 2007;35(10):2402–7.

5. Ferrer M, Esquinas A, Arancibia F, et al. Noninvasive ventilation during persistent weaning failure: a randomized controlled trial.[see comment]. *American Journal of Respiratory & Critical Care Medicine* 2003;168(1):70–6.

6. Nava S, Gregoretti C, Fanfulla F, et al. Noninvasive ventilation to prevent respiratory failure after extubation in high-risk patients.* *Critical Care Medicine* 2005;33(11):2465–70.

7. Thille AW, Harrois A, Schortgen F, Brun-Buisson C, Brochard L. Outcomes of extubation failure in medical intensive care unit patients. *Critical Care Medicine* 2011;39(12):2612–8.

8. Keenan SP. Noninvasive Positive-Pressure Ventilation for Postextubation Respiratory Distress: A Randomized Controlled Trial. *JAMA: The Journal of the American Medical Association* 2002; 287(24):3238–44.

9. Esteban A, Frutos-Vivar F, Ferguson ND, et al. Noninvasive positive-pressure ventilation for respiratory failure after extubation.[see comment]. *New England Journal of Medicine* 2004;350(24): 2452–60.

10. Ferrer M, Valencia M, Nicolas JM, Bernadich O, Badia JR, Torres A. Early noninvasive ventilation averts extubation failure in patients at risk: a randomized trial. *American Journal of Respiratory & Critical Care Medicine* 2006;173(2): 164–70.

11. Ferrer M, Sellares J, Valencia M, et al. Non-invasive ventilation after extubation in hypercapnic patients with chronic respiratory disorders: randomised controlled trial. *Lancet* 2009;374(9695): 1082–8.

12. Lin C, Yu H, Fan H, Li Z. The efficacy of noninvasive ventilation in managing postextubation respiratory failure: a meta-analysis. *Heart & Lung: The Journal of Critical Care* 2014;43(2):99–104.

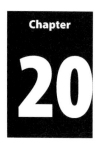

Chapter 20

Valvular Heart Disease and Endocarditis: Critical Care Management

Jonathan H. Rosser and Nick Morgan-Hughes

Introduction

Infection of the endocardium can be a devastating condition that, without prompt treatment, confers a very high mortality. The incidence is approximately 1.7 to 6.2 cases per 100,000 patient years.[1] It is characterised by the development of vegetations that consist of micro-organisms, platelets, fibrin meshes and inflammatory cells which adhere to the endocardial surface. Infective endocarditis (IE) may affect heart valves, atrial or ventricular septal defects, the mural endocardium or prosthetic material contained within the heart. The disease may manifest through valvular destruction and valvular insufficiency, infective emboli, sepsis and various immunological phenomena.

Over the last 40 years, the epidemiological profile of IE has shifted from disease mainly in a younger population with either rheumatic or congenital heart disease to an older cohort without known valve disease.[2] The presentation of IE is varied and diagnosis requires a high index of suspicion especially given the complexities of many critically ill patients.

Case Description

A 70-year-old man was admitted to the emergency department with a history of back pain which had increased dramatically over the preceding 24 hours. He was conscious but confused, hypotensive with a blood pressure of 68/42 mmHg, tachycardic at 125 beats per minute and had a distended abdomen. He was afebrile and had oxygen saturations of 96 per cent whilst breathing air. Arterial blood gas analysis revealed good gas exchange but a metabolic acidosis with a lactate of 6.5 mmol/l and a haemoglobin of 121 g/l. The emergency department physicians diagnosed a ruptured abdominal aortic aneurysm (AAA) based on the history, examination and the results of a targeted abdominal ultrasound examination.

The patient was transferred urgently to theatre for repair of the ruptured AAA following a review by the vascular surgeons. At laparotomy the abdominal aorta was found to be normal with a diameter of 2.2 cm. The rest of the intra-abdominal contents were also noted to appear normal. The patient was transferred sedated and ventilated to the general intensive care unit following the negative laparotomy. Over the next eight hours, he became progressively more haemodynamically unstable with increasing requirements of noradrenaline up to 0.70 mcg/kg/min whilst concomitantly on a vasopressin infusion at 2 iu/hr and 200mg of hydrocortisone daily in divided doses. His lactate remained at between 4–8 mmol/l despite adequate volume loading with crystalloid solutions and a calibrated arterial waveform analysis cardiac output monitor suggested a good cardiac index (CI) with a low systemic vascular resistance index (SVRI). He had received cefuroxime and metronidazole intra-operatively but this was changed to piperacillin with tazobactam following the drawing of peripheral blood cultures. Sputum and urine were also sent for microbiological analysis. His post-operative bloods revealed a urea of 27 mmol/l and a creatinine of 374 mmol/l. He was oligo-anuric so a vascath was placed and he was commenced on continuous veno-venous haemofiltration (CVVH) at a dose of 30 ml/kg/hr.

He had been febrile on the intensive care unit with tympanic temperatures recorded as high as 38.9 °C. His CRP was 512 mg/l and his white cell count (WCC) was 31 x 10^9/l with a predominate neutrophilia. During this period, the intensive care physicians had updated the family and gleaned further information about his background. He was independent with daily activities and could walk about a mile on the flat. He lived independently in a house with his wife and could climb the stairs easily. He had had an out of hospital arrest at home five years before this episode due to a myocardial infarction that was investigated with an angiogram, but no coronary intervention was performed at the time. Before hospital discharge an implantable cardiac defibrillator (ICD) had been inserted and he had been started on secondary prophylaxis for his heart attack. He also suffered with dyspepsia for which he took a proton pump inhibitor. His wife said that he had suffered with back pain for the last six to twelve months and that it had gradually worsened.

Both the clinical state and inflammatory markers pointed to a diagnosis of severe sepsis with multiple organ failures but the source was unclear. It was felt his chest or urinary tract was an unlikely source. Given the history of longstanding back pain a presumptive diagnosis of discitis with epidural or spinal abscess formation was made. He was too unstable for magnetic resonance imaging (MRI) so he underwent spinal CT on his second day on ITU with the administration of iodinated contrast. This revealed no evidence of discitis, spinal or epidural collections but did show bibasal consolidation of the lungs. The CT also demonstrated multiple sclerotic vertebral lesions (Figure 20.1) most likely in

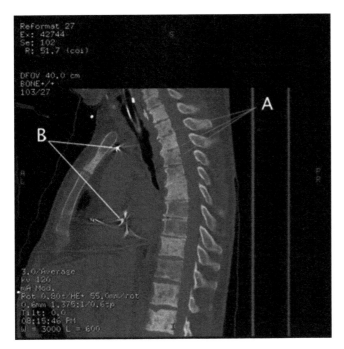

Figure 20.1 Computed tomography of the chest, sagittal section. The red-lines marked with the letter 'A' highlight some of the multiple sclerotic lesions demonstrated by the scan felt to be in keeping with metastatic prostate disease. The yellow lines from letter 'B' point to the ICD device, seen entering the heart. The endotracheal tube can also be seen in situ. A black and white version of this figure will appear in some formats. For the colour version, please refer to the plate section.

keeping with prostatic malignancy. A subsequent prostate specific antigen (PSA) was markedly raised at 480 ng/ml. The urologists were consulted and agreed this likely represented a prostatic malignancy. They stated he would probably have a good long-term prognosis and would investigate further following resolution of his critical illness with a view to starting anti-androgen therapy.

On his second ITU day, both sets of blood cultures that had been sent grew a streptococcal species. The piperacillin with tazobactam was continued, with the addition of vancomycin, to treat possible community acquired pneumonia though the history and presentation were not convincing for this diagnosis.

On his third day on ITU the microbiologists phoned through results that the streptococcus was, a group G streptococcus fully sensitive to penicillin. Antibiotics were changed to a high dose benzylpenicillin infusion at a dose of 14.4 grams daily. A transoeophageal echocardiogram (TOE) was also performed.

The results of the TOE showed a cystic mobile mass 12 mm by 44 mm, contained in the right atrium associated with the ICD. All valves were free of vegetation and the biventricular systolic function was normal. A referral to cardiology and the infectious diseases specialists (ID) was made and it was agreed by both teams that the device should be removed.

The ID team wanted six to twelve weeks of antibiotics to be administered post device removal. Unfortunately, the cardiology team felt that the ICD could not be removed percutaneously because the vegetation was too large and posed substantial risk of embolising to the lungs on extraction. The patient was therefore referred to the cardiothoracic surgeons for consideration of surgical removal of the device. The patient was anticoagulated with heparin as he was still receiving CVVH, though he was now on minimal cardiovascular and respiratory support. Another TOE assessment was made at the request of the surgeons to assess the burden of thrombus in the superior vena cava (SVC). If the SVC had been involved the vessel can become inflamed and friable which can make extraction difficult. The patient also underwent computed tomography pulmonary angiography (CTPA) looking for pulmonary septic emboli or abscesses. The CTPA did not show emboli and the SVC had a low burden of thrombus and was patent. In view of these findings, he underwent open surgical removal of the infected ICD under the care of the

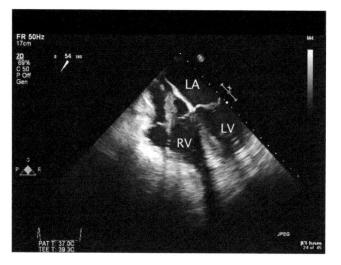

Figure 20.2 A transoesophageal echocardiogram showing the mid-oesophageal four-chamber view. The ICD can be seen entering the right atrium, passing through the tricuspid valve and continuing into the right ventricle. A large vegetation can clearly be seen attached to the ICD contained within the right atrium. The tricuspid valve was clear of vegetation as were the other remaining valves, There were no atrial or ventricular septal defects and biventricular function was normal. RV – right ventricle, LA – left atrium, LV – left ventricle. A black and white version of this figure will appear in some formats. For the colour version, please refer to the plate section.

cardiothoracic surgeons. The surgery was relatively uneventful and the device was successfully removed. Peri-operative vancomycin and gentamicin were administered to cover the extraction. Post-operatively, he had a prolonged ITU stay but was eventually discharged to the ward for investigation of his possible prostatic disease.

Discussion

This patient's initial presentation was one of hypotension and shock. Broadly, this may be due to hypovolaemia or vasodilatation, or be of neurogenic or cardiogenic origin. The back pain in this instance was a 'red herring' but this was compounded by a false positive result from the targeted abdominal ultrasound scan, leading to the incorrect diagnosis of a ruptured AAA. Once the patient was admitted to ITU. it became clear from the fever, high inflammatory markers and circulatory picture that he had severe sepsis. Antibiotic administration prior to obtaining blood cultures may make diagnosis of IE more difficult but in critically ill patients with severe sepsis, the benefits of early broad-spectrum antibiotic coverage far outweigh the risks of withholding therapy as outlined by the surviving sepsis guidelines.[3] At risk groups for IE consist of intravenous drug users, patients with prosthetic valves or intra-cardiac devices and those with degenerative valve sclerosis.

Group G β-haemolytic streptococci (GGS) are found in the normal flora of the skin, oropharynx, gastro-intestinal and genitourinary tracts. The organism may cause pharyngitis, puerperal and neonatal sepsis, septic arthritis and endocarditis. Group G streptococcal endocarditis tends to occur in older individuals. Native and prosthetic valves may be affected, with left sided lesions tending to be more common, unlike in this case.[4]

The practice for prophylaxis against endocarditis for certain patient groups has recently changed. National Institute for Clinical Excellence (NICE) guidance in the United Kingdom recommends against the use of antibiotic prophylaxis for dental, upper and lower gastro-intestinal, urinary tract and respiratory tract procedures.[5]

As infective endocarditis may present in a variety of ways and it continues to be a diagnostic challenge. The Modified Duke Criteria[6] (Table 20.1) may be used to aid the diagnosis of IE, but clinical experience and judgment are crucial given the diversity of presentation.

Table 20.1 Modified Duke Criteria adapted from Li et al.[6] Diagnosis of IE is definite in the presence of either: 2 major criteria, 1 major and 3 minor criteria or 5 minor criteria. IE is possible with 1 major and 1 minor criterion or 3 minor criteria

Major Criteria	Minor Criteria
Positive blood culture (typical causative organism)	Fever
Echocardiogram consistent with endocarditis	At-risk patient
New valvular regurgitation	Vascular phenomena (emboli, mycotic aneurysm, intra-cranial haemorrhage, conjuctival haemorrhage, Janeway's lesions)
	Immunologic phenomena (Osler's nodes, Roth's spots, rheumatoid factor positive, glomerulonephritis)
	Positive microbiology not meeting major criteria

The European Association of Echocardiography has published comprehensive guidance for the role oechocardiography in the diagnosis of IE.[7] Transthoracic echocardiography (TTE) is the initial imaging investigation of choice but in patients with poor views (high body mass or in ventilated patients) it is reasonable to proceed directly to TOE, as occurred in this case. In situations with a low clinical suspicion of IE a negative TTE is usually adequate to exclude the diagnosis. However, if the clinical suspicion is high and the initial TTE is negative, TOE should be performed. If the initial TOE is negative but clinical suspicion remains high, then the TOE should be repeated after one to two weeks. A positive echocardiogram may display an oscillating or non-oscillating intra-cardiac mass consistent with a vegetation. Other features consistent with IE include intra-cardiac abscesses, pseudoaneurysms, fistulae or mycotic valve aneurysms. Echocardiographic diagnosis of IE may be difficult with prosthetic valves but dehiscence and new paravalvular regurgitation may signify an infected prosthesis.

Staphylococcus aureus, coagulase negative staphylococcus, streptococci and enterococci were found to be the most common causative organisms in the 2009 International Collaboration on Endocarditis study which enrolled 2781 patients with definite IE across 25 countries.[8] Fungi and yeasts are potential pathogens and occur more frequently in patients with pre-disposing risk factors including previous surgery, indwelling devices and lines, broad spectrum antibiotic use, prosthetic heart valves, structural heart disease and in immunocompromised individuals.[9]

Several causative organisms of IE may be associated with frequently or persistently negative blood cultures. This may occur with fastidious gram-negative bacilli of the HACEK group (Haemophilus parainfluenzae, H. aphrophilus, H. paraphrophilus, H. influenaze, Actinobacillus actinomycetemcomitans, Cardiobacterium hominis, Eikenella corrodens, Kingella kingae and K. dentrificans) or intracellular bacteria such as Coxiella burnetti, Bartonella, Chlamydia and Tropheryma whipplei.[7]

The cornerstone of treatment for IE is appropriate antimicrobial therapy supplemented with surgical source control. Long-term (6 weeks or longer) antimicrobial therapy is required though completion of courses can occur in the community.

When considering the role of surgery with IE, it is useful to classify the site of infection as left-sided lesions, right-sided lesions and infections associated with implantable devices.

Implantable devices will need to be removed, either percutaneously or surgically. Vegetations may extend from the right heart through the SVC to the subclavian vein. Generally, the more thrombus there is in the large veins, the more friable they will be and, therefore, will pose a greater risk of damage on removal of the device. In this case, although the SVC was free of thrombus, the vegetation was larger, risking embolisation with potential percutaneous extraction.

Left-sided lesions represent a high risk of systemic embolisation. Anticoagulation should be avoided, given the risks of cerebral emboli and subsequent secondary haemorrhage. Surgery may be considered if the risk of embolisation is high as demonstrated by multiple embolic episodes or large vegetations (greater than 10 to 15 mm). Other indications for surgery include infective source control (for abscesses, fistulae or resistant organisms) and cardiac failure. Cardiac failure may manifest as refractory pulmonary oedema or cardiogenic shock due to severe valvular regurgitation or the vegetation may cause partial or complete valvular obstruction.

Right-sided IE has a lower mortality than left-sided IE and will more often be managed conservatively. Pulmonary septic emboli are a risk but the risk – benefit of anticoagulation is less clear than for left-sided lesions. In this case, the patient was therapeutically anti-coagulated with unfractionated heparin at the surgeon's request. Surgical treatment may be considered for right-sided lesions in patients with resistant causative organisms, recurrent pulmonary emboli with large vegetations or refractory right heart failure secondary to severe tricuspid regurgitation.

Conclusion

Infective endocarditis is a disease entity that is difficult to diagnose, requires long-term and often complex treatment, and is associated with significant morbidity and mortality. The patient in this case study was initially misdiagnosed. This highlights the need for intensivists to maintain a high index of suspicion for the disease in a variety of different patient groups and presenting features. Close liaison with cardiology, cardiothoracic surgery and infectious disease specialists is essential for successful treatment of this diverse disease.

Key Learning Points

- The Modified Duke Criteria provide a framework for diagnosis of infective endocarditis.
- Infective endocarditis should always be considered with the growth of associated microorganisms from the blood.
- A significant proportion of causative organisms may be difficult to detect by blood culture.
- Transthoracic echocardiography is the initial imaging investigation of choice though transoesophageal echocardiography may be more suitable in certain patient groups.
- Appropriate antimicrobial therapy is the mainstay of treatment but surgical therapy should be considered in specific patient groups.

References

1. Mylonakis E, Calderwood SB. Infective Endocarditis in Adults. *N Engl J Med* 2001;345:1318–330.

2. Hoen B. Epidemiology and antibiotic treatment of infective endocarditis: an update. *Heart* 2006;92(11):1694–700.

3. Dellinger RP, Levy MM, Rhodes A et al. Surviving Sepsis Campaign: Guidelines for the Management of Severe Sepsis and Septic Shock: 2012. *Crit Care Med* 2012; 41(2):580–637.

4. Rolston K. Group G Streptococcal infections. *Arch Intern Med* 1986; 146(5):857–58.

5. NICE guidelines [CG64] March 2008 available at www.nice.org.uk/guidance/cg64

6. Li JS, Sexton DJ, Mick N et al. Proposed modifications to the Duke Criteria for the diagnosis of infective endocarditis. *Clinical Infectious Diseases* 2000;30:633–38.

7. Habib G, Hoen B, Tornos P et al. The Task Force on the Prevention, Diagnosis and Treatment of Infective Endocarditis of the European Society of Cardiology. Guidelines on the Prevention, Diagnosis and Treatment of Infective Endocarditis. *Eur Heart J* 2009;30:2369–413.

8. Murdoch DR, Corey R, Hoen B et al. Clinical presentation, etiology and outcome of infective endocarditis in the 21st century: the international collaboration on endocarditis:prospective cohort study. *Arch Intern Med* 2009; 169(5):463–73.

9. Baddley JW, Benjamin DK, Cabell C. Candida infective endocarditis. *Eur J Clin Microbiol Infect Dis* 2008;27 (7): 519–29.

Cardiac Failure Management and Mechanical Assist Devices

Miguel Garcia and Julian Barker

Introduction

Cardiac failure is a clinical syndrome characterised by the inability of the heart to supply the metabolic demands of the body.

Approximately 900,000 patients in the United Kingdom currently have a diagnosis of cardiac failure. The estimated mortality of this condition within the first year of diagnosis is around 40 per cent and around 10 per cent per year in subsequent years.[1] The main cause in the United Kingdom is ischaemic heart disease. Patients can present with a spectrum of symptoms ranging from a reduction in exercise tolerance, fatigue and malaise to acute pulmonary oedema and cardiogenic shock which is the most severe form of cardiac failure.

Mortality in cardiogenic shock remains extremely high at around 40 percent compared with other acute diseases such as sepsis. The mortality of cardiogenic shock associated with multi-organ failure, including acute kidney injury and ischaemic hepatitis with liver failure is unknown but based on scoring systems such as the sequential organ failure assessment (SOFA), it is probably close to 100 per cent.[2] The most common cause of cardiogenic shock in the United Kingdom is acute myocardial infarction.

Diagnosis of cardiogenic shock includes haemodynamic and clinical criteria. The haemodynamic criteria are: systolic blood pressure less than 90 mm Hg for more than 30 minutes or requirement for catecholamines to maintain systolic pressure greater than 90 mmHg, cardiac index less than 2.2 l/m^2, pulmonary capillary wedge pressure greater than 18 mmHg. Clinical signs include pulmonary congestion and organ hypoperfusion manifested by one of following criteria (i) altered mental status (ii) cold, clammy skin and extremities (iii) oliguria with urine output less than 30 mls per hour or (iv) serum lactate greater than 2 mmol /l.[3]

The management of patients with cardiogenic shock includes pharmacological therapy with inotropic and vasopressor drugs, percutaneous and/or surgical revascularisation procedures. It may also involve valve replacement and mechanical support with the temporary use of intra-aortic balloon pumps or ventricular assisted devices including venous-arterial extracorporeal membrane oxygenation (V-A ECMO).

Case Study

A 47-year-old caucasian male presented to the emergency department with a history of 4 days of general fatigue and increasing shortness of breath that had deteriorated in the past 24 hours. There was no history of chest pain or productive cough. Past medical history included essential hypertension diagnosed at 42 years of age and controlled with amlodipine 10 mg/day. There was no history of travel abroad, use of recreational drugs or excessive alcohol intake.

On admission to hospital, his vital signs were BP 80/40 mmHg, HR 110 bpm, RR 24 bpm, O_2 saturation of 86 per cent on air and temperature of 36.2 °C. He was peripherally and centrally cyanosed, had cold extremities and a capillary refill time greater than 5 seconds. Chest examination revealed bilateral fine crackles extending from the bases to the mid zones. The heart sounds were abnormal, given by a pan systolic murmur radiating to the axilla and audible third heart sound. Abdominal and neurological examinations were normal and there was no peripheral oedema.

Initial blood gases performed on air showed a pH of 7.33, PaO_2 8kPa, $PaCO_2$ 4.5 kPa, bicarbonate 17 mmol/l, lactate 3.1 mmol/l, Na 128 mmol/l, K 5.1 mmol/l and Cl 104 mmol/l. ECG showed sinus tachycardia and chest radiography showed cardiomegaly and bilateral lung infiltrates consistent with pulmonary oedema and/or pneumonia. Blood results reported a serum creatinine of 160 micromol/l, urea 18 micromol/l, albumin 22 g/dl, alkaline phosphate 300 IU, alanine transaminase 80 IU, bilirubin 42 IU and INR 1.2.

The patient was admitted to the high dependency unit (HDU) with a diagnosis of cardiogenic shock and pulmonary oedema. Invasive monitoring was sited, including central venous access and arterial line insertion.

The initial management included an intravenous infusion of furosemide started at 10 mg/hr, noradrenaline at 0.2 micrograms/kg/min and adrenaline 0.05 micrograms/kg/min. Respiratory support was given with CPAP at a level of 7.5 cm H_2O with an FiO_2 of 0.8.

Bedside echocardiogram showed severe systolic impairment with an ejection fraction of 20 per cent, normal valves, no pericardial effusion and conserved right ventricular function with a TAPSE (Tricuspid Annular Plane Systolic Excursion) of 18 mm (within the published normal range).

Further investigations reported a troponin T level within the normal range, a WCC 12 x 10^9/l, Hb 136 g/l and platelets 110 x 10^9/l.

The patient continued to deteriorate developing hypoxic / Type I respiratory failure requiring intubation and positive pressure ventilation.

A transoesophageal echocardiogram (TOE) performed soon after intubation showed deterioration in the systolic function compared with the initial echocardiogram. Continuous hemodiafiltration was started and an intra-aortic balloon pump (IABP) was inserted.

Due to the need for increasing inotropic support with noradrenaline 0.8 mcg/kg/min, adrenaline 0.2 mcg/kg/min and milrinone 0.5 mcg/kg/min after a loading dose of 50 mcg/kg, the patient was referred to a quaternary referral centre with the facility to provide further invasive cardiovascular support.

On arrival to the referral centre the patient's initial blood gases showed a pH of 7.1, $PaCO_2$ 4.0 kPa, PaO_2 10 kPa, bicarbonate of 14 mmol/l and a lactate of 6.0 mmol/l. Initial biochemistry was reported as creatinine 240 micromol/l, urea 25 mmol/l, alanine transaminase 200 IU and INR 3.5, indicative of worsening multiorgan failure.

Following the assessment by the acute heart failure team, the patient was classified as INTERMACS Class I (Table 21.1). The decision was made to transfer to the operating theatre where central venous-arterial extra corporeal membrane oxygenation (V-A ECMO) was implanted through a median sternotomy. Two cannulae were placed, the outflow cannula was placed in the right atrium and the inflow cannula was implanted in the ascending aorta, providing a cardiac output (or flow) of 4.5 litres a minute, which led to rapid, progressive weaning of inotropic and vasopressor support. The IABP was kept in place and the patient required coagulation support with fresh frozen plasma, cryoprecipitate and platelets.

Table 21.1 INTERMACS® Patient Profile at time of implant: Select one. These profiles will provide a *general* clinical description of the patients receiving primary LVAD

Profile	Profile Description	Features
1	Critical cardiogenic shock describes a patient who is 'crashing and burning'	Patient has life-threatening hypotension and rapidly escalating inotropic pressor support, with critical organ hypoperfusion often confirmed by worsening acidosis and lactate levels.
2	Progressive decline	Patient who has been demonstrated 'dependent' on inotropic support but nonetheless shows signs of continuing deterioration in nutrition, renal function, fluid retention, or other major status indicator. Patient profile 2 can also describe a patient with refractory volume overload, perhaps with evidence of impaired perfusion, in whom inotropic infusions cannot be maintained due to tachyarrhythmias, clinical ischemia, or other intolerance.
3	Stable but inotrope dependent	Patient who is clinically stable on mild-moderate doses of intravenous inotropes (or has a temporary circulatory support device) after repeated documentation of failure to wean without symptomatic hypotension, worsening symptoms or progressive organ dysfunction (usually renal).
4	Resting symptoms	Patient who is at home on oral therapy but frequently has symptoms of congestion at rest or with activities of daily living (ADL). He or she may have orthopnea, shortness of breath during ADL such as dressing or bathing, gastrointestinal symptoms (abdominal discomfort, nausea, poor appetite), disabling ascites or severe lower extremity oedema.
5	Exertion intolerant	Patient who is comfortable at rest but unable to engage in any activity, living predominantly within the house or housebound. This patient has no congestive symptoms, but may have chronically elevated volume status, frequently with renal dysfunction, and may be characterized as exercise intolerant.
6	Exertion limited	Patient who is comfortable at rest without evidence of fluid overload, but who is able to do some mild activity. Activities of daily living are comfortable and minor activities outside the home such as visiting friends or going to a restaurant can be performed, but fatigue results within a few minutes of any meaningful physical exertion.
7	Advanced NYHA class 3	Patient who is clinically stable with a reasonable level of comfortable activity, despite history of previous decompensation that is not recent. This patient is usually able to walk more than a block.

In the cardiothoracic intensive care unit, continuous support was provided via a V-A ECMO circuit, hemodiafiltration and intra-aortic balloon pump. There was progressive improvement of both renal and liver function and on day 6 the renal support was stopped.

A biopsy taken during the implantation of V-A ECMO demonstrated lymphocytic infiltration of cardiomyocytes suggestive of a viral cardiomyopathy. All serological tests were negative.

TOE performed on day five after ECMO implantation showed no improvement of the ejection fraction of the left ventricle but there was marked improvement of the right ventricular function compared with the previous TOE examination.

After seven days of V-A ECMO support a multidisciplinary meeting took place where the following options were considered:

1   To wean V-A ECMO support and continue with inotropic support and IABP. This option was considered unlikely to be successful because of persistent poor left ventricular function.
2   To remove the V-A ECMO support and change it to a temporary left ventricular assist device (L-VAD), giving the left ventricle an opportunity to recover. The main limitation of this option was the limited lifespan of 30 days of the circuit and pump.
3   To remove the VA ECMO support and change it to a long term L-VAD as a bridge to recovery or transplant.

The third option was considered the most appropriate option for this patient because of his potential for full recovery with an unpredictable time course. It also gave time to have the relevant investigations and assessments performed for a potential transplant. On day eight the patient was taken to theatre and a long term L-VAD was implanted with no complications. A tracheostomy was performed on day nine due to extreme generalised muscle weakness and the failure of several spontaneous breathing trials. Following further weaning of respiratory support, the patient was discharged to the ward on day 21 to continue rehabilitation. He went home on day 35 to continue management as an outpatient. Whilst still supported by the L-VAD device, he had the relevant investigations completed in order to fully assess him as a candidate for cardiac transplantation. After six months of support under the care of the heart failure and L-VAD service, the patient showed improvement in his left ventricular function and the L-VAD was explanted with no complications.

Management

Only a minority of patients with viral cardiomyopathy will present with progressive deterioration after optimal care has been given. The need for an increasing dose of vasopressors and inotropes with no response to IABP dictates appropriate referral to a quaternary facility. The objective assessment of progressive multi-organ failure using recognised scoring systems such as the sequential organ failure assessment (SOFA) score will help to decide whether early referral and transfer are required and where further support can be provided.

This type of patient with refractory cardiogenic shock and a potentially reversible cause is the ideal candidate for mechanical circulatory support. Whether or not a patient is a candidate for circulatory support is determined mainly by whether there is any contraindication to cardiac transplant in case there is no recovery of the native heart.[4]

There are many different mechanical support devices: in the United Kingdom the most frequently used device is IABP followed by V-A ECMO and temporary VADs.

V-A ECMO support is a recognised rescue therapy for cardiogenic shock that is unresponsive to conventional therapy. It is used as a bridge to decision-making, recovery or transplantation. The most common causes for its use include myocardial infarction, viral and non-viral acute cardiomyopathy and post cardiotomy. In recent years it has also been used in cases of refractory septic shock with myocardial depression, pulmonary embolism, cardiac toxicity secondary to drug overdose, hypothermic cardiac arrest and has been used for extra-corporeal support during cardiopulmonary resuscitation (CPR), so called E-CPR.[4]

Absolute contraindications for V-A ECMO include patients who are not candidates for transplant or long term ventricular assist devices, advanced age, and chronic organ dysfunction with considerable additional burdens such as emphysema, cirrhosis and renal failure.

Data from the Extracorporeal Life Support Organisation (ELSO) registry that included V-A and V-V ECMO, reported 58,842 cases internationally in 2013. Of these, 4,042 cases represented V-A ECMO in adults.[5] There is no data available from the United Kingdom. Currently V-A ECMO in the United Kingdom is limited to adult transplant centres.

Data from retrospective cohort studies suggest that outcomes in extracorporeal support therapies including V-V ECMO and V-A ECMO are related to the number of patients treated per year. It is generally accepted that the minimum number of patients treated per year in any particular centre should be around 20 in order to achieve good outcomes.

The National Institute for Health and Care Excellence (NICE) issued procedure guidance on V-A ECMO for acute heart failure in adults in March of 2014 and it concluded that there is evidence that V-A ECMO is effective in supporting patients with acute heart failure. There is uncertainty around which patients benefit the most and at which point in the natural history of acute heart failure this therapeutic intervention should be used. NICE recommends that only clinical teams with specific training and expertise should carry out V-A ECMO for treating acute heart failure in adults.

There are no randomised controlled trials comparing V-A ECMO to conventional therapy or comparing V-A ECMO to miniaturised ventricular support devices. In 2014, a meta-analysis by Cheng included 170 patients with severe myocarditis complicated by cardiogenic shock or cardiac arrest, who received V-A ECMO. The studies included in this meta-analysis were published between 2000 and November 2012 and only studies with more than 10 patients were included. The pooled survival rate to discharge was 67 percent (95 percent CI 57 percent to 75 percent) (I2 = 17.0 percent). This result compares favourably with historical mortality rates in patients in cardiogenic shock secondary to severe myocarditis.[6]

The evidence for V-A ECMO in patients with acute STEMI complicated with cardiogenic shock is less conclusive. There is one study by Sheu et al in 2010 comparing retrospective data in one institution from two time periods, the first period from 1993 to 2002 and the second from 2002 to 2009. Following the introduction of V-A ECMO there was a significant difference in 30 day mortality of 61 percent vs 28 percent p = 0.008 with an absolute risk reduction of 33 percent.[7]

Outcomes in patients who received V-A ECMO post cardiotomy are less favourable. A study by Rastan et al. in 2010 looked at the outcomes in patients with refractory post-cardiotomy cardiogenic shock. In this retrospective analysis of 517 patients requiring V-A ECMO to wean from cardio-pulmonary bypass, the rate of survival to discharge was 25 percent: one-year survival was 17 percent and 5-year survival was 14 percent.[8]

There are other devices on the market which can support the circulation when cardiogenic shock is refractory to pharmacological therapy. These include the intra-aortic balloon pump (IABP) and percutaneous left ventricle assist device (L-VAD) such as the Tandem Heart percutaneous L-VAD system (Cardiac Assist, Inc., Pittsburgh, PA, USA), the Impella LP2.5 and the Impella CP (Abiomed Europe GimbH, Aaachen, Germany). Recent trials comparing IABP with other percutaneous L-VADs such as the ones mentioned above have shown no mortality improvement at 30 days.[3,9]

Worldwide, the IABP is the most commonly used mechanical assist device in refractory cardiogenic shock. The main limitation of the IABP is that it relies on the residual function of the left ventricle. The effectiveness of the IABP has been tested in the IABP-SHOCK II trial that unfortunately did not show a significant reduction in 30-day mortality in patients with cardiogenic shock and STEMI. A systematic review published by Cochrane reported a hazard ratio of 1.04 (95 percent CI 0.62–1.73) for all-cause mortality in patients with myocardial infarction. Recent international guidelines have downgraded the recommendation for the use of IABP in cardiogenic shock secondary to myocardial infarction to grade IIa or IIb.

Patients in cardiogenic shock INTERMACS class I are not candidates for long term L-VAD support because of their poor outcome. The International Society for Heart and Lung Transplantation guidelines recommend the use of temporary support such as V-A ECMO or short-term VAD for patients in multi organ failure, with sepsis or on mechanical ventilation, to allow neurological assessment and optimisation and subsequent improvement of multi organ failure before considering long term VAD support.[10] This makes the choice of long term L-VAD in this case unusual.

There are two main ways of providing VA ECMO support: peripheral and central. Peripheral V-A ECMO requires venous cannulation of the femoral vein and cannulation of the femoral artery. Central V-A ECMO requires venous cannulation of the right atrium and arterial cannulation of the aorta through a median sternotomy as in this case.

The main advantage of central over peripheral V-A ECMO is the effective decompression of the heart, avoiding further dilatation when native function is extremely poor and therefore reducing the risk of hydrostatic pulmonary oedema, particularly in patients with torrential mitral regurgitation. A significant disadvantage of central V-A ECMO is the need for a sternotomy with the concomitant risk of major haemorrhage and tamponade. In addition the scar tissue will increase the risk substantially for subsequent procedures like VAD implantation or heart transplantation.

One of the advantages of peripheral V-A ECMO is the easy deployment by the bedside in different environments including intensive care, the emergency department, and the catheterisation laboratory or during CPR. Further potential problems with peripheral V-A ECMO are leg ischaemia and the increased incidence of hydrostatic pulmonary oedema.[4]

The ECMO circuit is composed of an inflow cannula, an outflow cannula, a centrifugal pump, an oxygenator and a heat exchanger (Figure 21.1). The configuration is flexible in order to adapt to the particular needs of different patients.

At our institution, we prefer central V-A ECMO as emergency support for severe heart failure. The patient is continually reassessed to look for a period of stability, improvement in tissue perfusion and to see whether the heart function is improving and in particular whether the right ventricle is compromised. After a period of stability (generally less than a week), support is generally switched to temporary right and left mechanical assist devices (bi-VAD support). This has the advantage of allowing normal blood flow through the lungs and hence improving pulmonary function. In some circumstances, support will be switched to a long term L-VAD if there is substantial improvement of the right ventricle. Rarely the magnitude of improvement in heart function is such that it allows the removal of V-A

(a)   (b)

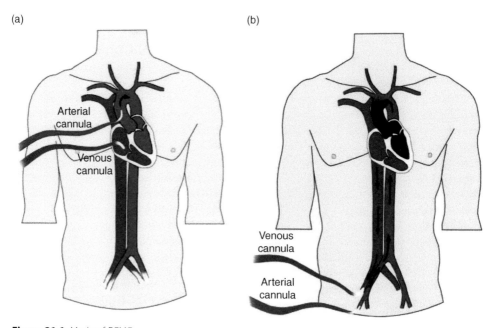

Figure 21.1 Mode of ECMO.
Ho-Ki Min and Young Tak Lee (2011). *Role of Percutaneous Cardiopulmonary Support (PCPS) in Patients with Unstable Hemodynamics during the Peri-Coronary-Intervention Period*, Prof. Baskot Branislav (Ed.), *Coronary Angiography: The Need for Improvement in Medical and Interventional Therapy*, ISBN: 978-953-307-641-6, InTech, DOI: 10.5772/20969. Available from: www.intechopen.com/books/coronary-angiography-the-need-for-improvement-in-medical-and-interventional-therapy/role-of-percutaneous-cardiopulmonary-support-pcps-in-patients-with-unstable-hemodynamics-during-the1. With permission.

ECMO without the requirement for further mechanical support. In patients who do not recover right and left ventricular function the only option will be cardiac transplantation.

Conclusion

Cardiogenic shock can be the clinical manifestation of a variety of pathologies but is a serious diagnosis with a high mortality at present. Initial management should be tailored to the individual patient. Patients in cardiogenic shock and multi-organ failure with no contraindications for cardiac transplant should be referred to centres where further extra-corporeal support can be provided.

IABP might be used as initial mechanical support in cardiogenic shock when there is still some ventricular function. Based on current practice, patients with cardiogenic shock that is not responsive to IABP and high doses of vasopressors and inotropes could be salvaged with V-A ECMO support.

Current evidence does not support using percutaneous mechanical devices instead of IABP and further research is warranted before the widespread adoption of these devices.

V-A ECMO is a complex and expensive intervention that is effective in treating cardiogenic shock. It is unknown whether V-A ECMO reduces mortality compared with standard treatment because there are no randomised controlled trials in the literature that answer this question. All the evidence for its use comes from observational data and registries from around the world with a wide variability in medical practice and resources.

Further research is needed to recognise which patients will benefit the most.

Key Learning Points

- Mortality in cardiogenic shock is around 40 percent.
- Cardiogenic shock can be the manifestation of multiple primary pathologies affecting the myocardium.
- The INTERMACS classification is a useful tool to assess patients in cardiogenic shock because it provides a scale to stratify risk in patients who may be candidates for mechanical support.
- IABP is the first option for mechanical support in cardiogenic shock.
- There is no evidence to support percutaneous assist devices instead of IABP.
- V-A ECMO is an effective therapy to reverse multi-organ failure in patients with cardiogenic shock as a bridge to short term VAD support followed by long term VAD implantation, recovery or transplant.
- V-A ECMO should only be offered in centres that provide more than 20 cases a year.

References

1. NICOR. National Heart Failure Audit 2013 at www.ucl.ac.uk/nicor/audits

2. Combes A, Leprince P, Luyt CE, et al. Outcomes and long-term quality-of-life of patients supported by extracorporeal membrane oxygenation for refractory cardiogenic shock. *Crit Care Med* 2008 May;36(5):1404–11.

3. Werdan K, Gielen S, Ebelt H, Hochman JS. Mechanical circulatory support in cardiogenic shock. *Eur Heart J* 2014 Jan;35 (3):156–67.

4. Shekar K, Mullany DV, Thomson B, Ziegenfuss M, Platts DG, Fraser JF. Extracorporeal life support devices and strategies for management of acute cardiorespiratory failure in adult patients: a comprehensive review. *Crit Care* 2014;18 (3):219.

5. Paden ML, Conrad SA, Rycus PT, Thiagarajan RR. Extracorporeal life support organization registry report 2012. *ASAIO J* 2013 May–Jun;59(3):202–10.

6. Cheng R, Hachamovitch R, Kittleson M, et al. Clinical outcomes in fulminant myocarditis requiring extracorporeal membrane oxygenation: a weighted meta-analysis of 170 patients. *J Card Fail* 2014 Jun;20(6):400–6.

7. Sheu JJ, Tsai TH, Lee FY, et al. Early extracorporeal membrane oxygenator-assisted primary percutaneous coronary intervention improved 30-day clinical outcomes in patients with ST-segment elevation myocardial infarction complicated with profound cardiogenic shock. *Crit Care Med* 2010 Sep;38 (9):1810–17.

8. Rastan AJ, Dege A, Mohr M, et al. Early and late outcomes of 517 consecutive adult patients treated with extracorporeal membrane oxygenation for refractory postcardiotomy cardiogenic shock. *J Thorac Cardiovasc Surg* 2010 Feb;139 (2):302–11, 11 e1.

9. Massetti M, Bruno P. Mechanical circulatory support for acute heart failure in 2013: an update on available devices, indications and results. *Minerva Anestesiol* 2014 Mar;80(3):373–81.

10. Stevenson LW, Pagani FD, Young JB, et al. INTERMACS profiles of advanced heart failure: the current picture. *J Heart Lung Transplant* 2009 Jun;28(6):535–41.

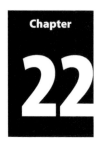

Chapter 22

Management of Common Overdoses
A Severe Case of Amitriptyline Overdose

Ascanio Tridente

Introduction

Tricyclic antidepressant (TCA) overdose is an important cause of mortality and morbidity among those taking intentional overdoses.

This case presents a patient with predominantly cardiac and neurological toxic features and the management and evidence base for currently recommended practice when treating TCA overdose is discussed.

Case Description

A 56-year-old woman with a past medical history of ischaemic heart disease, hypertension, depression, type II diabetes mellitus and morbid obesity presented to the Accident and Emergency department (A&E) having ingested an estimated total dose of approximately 56 x 50 mg tablets (2800 mg in total, more than 20 mg/kg) of amitriptyline, approximately two hours prior to arrival. The lady was known to the emergency services due to several prior overdoses of amitriptyline. Following this ingestion, the emergency services had been called and, on arrival at the scene, no other substances had been found.

On examination she was markedly tachycardic (heart rate 176 bpm) with a blood pressure of 112/65 and tachypnoeic (respiratory rate approximately 24 breaths/min). Her blood pressure had been unrecordable prior to resuscitation with 2 litres of colloids and crystalloids initiated in A&E. Her current Glasgow Coma Scale was 9/15 (E = 2, M=5, V=2) and pupils were noted to be dilated at 6 mm. Tympanic membrane temperature was 38.3 °C. Heart sounds were normal but she had a prolonged capillary refill time, with relatively cold peripheries, easily palpable femoral arterial pulses, but peripheral pulses that were difficult to feel. Respiratory examination was unremarkable apart from decreased air entry bilaterally at the lung bases; the abdomen was mildly distended, slightly and diffusely tender but otherwise soft and not peritonitic.

Abnormal initial investigations were a raised white cell count (WCC) to 21.2×10^9/l with marked neutrophilia, and blood glucose of 18.4 mmol/l. The remaining full blood count profile, electrolytes and liver enzymes were within normal ranges. Arterial blood gases (ABGs) showed type I respiratory failure and a mild metabolic acidosis: pH 7.32 base excess (BE) −7 mmol/l, lactate 3.9 mmol/l, $PaCO_2$ 4.3 kPa and PaO_2 11.4 kPa on FiO_2 0.8 via a non-rebreathing face mask. Paracetamol and salicylate were not detected and blood alcohol levels were not measured.

Chest radiograph was unremarkable, but the electrocardiogram (ECG) showed a ventricular tachycardia (HR of 170 to 180 bpm), with broad QRS complexes with a right bundle branch block mimicry pattern (QRS width of 209 ms, RSR' pattern) (see Figure 22.1).

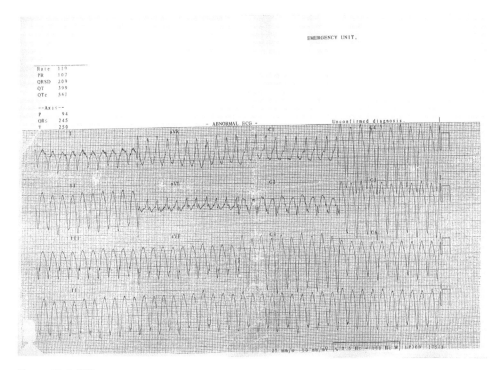

EMERGENCY UNIT,

Rate   119
PR   107
QRSD   209
QT   399
QTc   561

--Ax i s--
P   94
QRS   245
T   250

- ABNORMAL ECG -

Unconfirmed diagnosis

Figure 22.1 ECG.

Initial Management

Further intravenous fluids were administered as a temporising measure (to a total of 3 l during resuscitation) and an intravenous dose of 100 mmol of sodium bicarbonate was administered in A&E to achieve alkalinisation and increase the extracellular sodium concentration, for the purposes of reversing the cardiotoxic effects of the TCAs.

While being monitored in the resuscitation area, the patient became progressively less responsive, more drowsy and less cooperative, attempting to remove peripheral cannulae and pulling on the oxygen face mask. Attempts to deliver further treatment were being hampered and so she underwent controlled rapid sequence induction with endotracheal intubation and controlled ventilation. Sedation was achieved using propofol and alfentanil infusions.

Shortly after induction, the patient received direct current cardioversion (DCCV) which was successful in restoring sinus rhythm from the ventricular tachycardia. A subsequent ECG revealed sinus rhythm with a broad QRS of 189 ms and prolonged QTc of 563 ms. At this stage the blood pressure had improved to 146/86 mmHg with the help of peripherally infused vasoconstrictors (metaraminol boluses). A urinary catheter was inserted.

ICU Management

Once she was transferred to the intensive care unit (ICU), a central (internal jugular) venous catheter and a radial arterial line were inserted to allow infusion of noradrenaline as pressor, with initial doses of approximately 0.15 to 0.25 micrograms/kg/min required to maintain a mean arterial pressure of around 75 mmHg. A sodium bicarbonate infusion (150 mmol in 1l of 0.9 percent sodium chloride) was also started at a rate of 250 ml/hour. The ventilation was adjusted with the aim of maintaining a slight respiratory alkalosis. Daily ECGs were obtained to monitor progress of the electrical changes and regular blood gases to ensure maintenance of pH within a range of 7.50 to 7.55.

Over the course of her ICU stay (a total of three days) the patient remained intubated, invasively mechanically ventilated and on the noradrenaline infusion for 2 days, having been assessed neurologically each day during regular sedation holds. ECG changes, metabolic and respiratory states, together with electrolytes and other routine measurements in the ICU were kept under strict monitoring.

She was eventually successfully extubated and weaned off the vasopressors on day three, when neurologically appropriate. The patient survived the overdose without any significant sequelae and was discharged to a level 1 ward with a planned review by the psychiatry team.

Discussion

Amitriptyline is one of the most commonly prescribed tricyclic antidepressants and one of the commonest medications taken in overdose for self–harm.[1] This case exemplifies many of the features of toxicity from TCA overdose, which are listed in Table 22.1. The predominant features of this case of poisoning were those related to cardiovascular compromise and neurological involvement.

The important effects of amitriptyline toxicity are a direct consequence of its pharmacological actions, which include serotonin and noradrenaline reuptake inhibition at a presynaptic level, anti-histamine action, blockade of cardiac fast sodium channels (His-Purkinje

Table 22.1 Features of TCA toxicity

Organ/system affected	Clinical manifestations
Central Nervous System	Sedation Confusion Agitation Delirium Seizures Coma
Cardiac/Vascular	Sinus tachycardia Hypotension Ventricular tachycardia/fibrillation Ventricular conduction delay Prolongation QT/QTc intervals
Gastro-intestinal	Ileus
Urinary	Urinary retention
General and Metabolic	Metabolic acidosis Hyperthermia Flushing Dilated pupils Blurred vision Dry and warm skin

system and myocardium), peripheral alpha-adrenoreceptor blockade, muscarinic receptor blockade and central nervous system gamma-aminobutyric acid A receptor inhibition. Amitriptyline, like any TCA, has a high volume of distribution as it is lipophilic and is highly protein bound; the primary site of metabolism is the liver, via CYP2D6 and glucuronidation. The half life of elimination in therapeutic doses, is 31 to 46 hours.[1]

The pharmacokinetics of TCAs in overdose is unpredictably altered, with potentially significant delay in elimination. Patients ingesting significant tricyclic overdoses may have detectable levels of the medications for days. When excessive doses are ingested, absorption may be delayed due to decreased intestinal motility as a consequence of the anticholinergic effects of the drugs and the first pass hepatic metabolism may be overwhelmed by the large quantities of the medication ingested (as the hepatic enzymes become saturated). Another factor which could potentially significantly alter the drugs' pharmacokinetics is the effect of enterohepatic recirculation, with consequent delay in the elimination of a proportion of the medication. Furthermore, the proportion of TCA not bound to plasma proteins (and hence toxic) can increase as a consequence of acidaemia, which will be contributed to by the overdose induced respiratory depression with consequent respiratory acidosis and any metabolic acidosis caused by seizures or tissue hypoperfusion secondary to cardiovascular compromise. Concomitant ingestion of ethanol further reduces metabolism of TCA by limiting its oxidation, and therefore blood alcohol levels should be measured in cases of self-harm from drug ingestion.[2,3]

Ingestion of amitriptyline can be potentially life-threatening, especially where more than 20 mg/kg body weight is ingested, such as in this case.[1]

The initial assessment of the patient with TCA toxicity follows a standard 'ABCDE' approach and testing for concomitant ingestion of other substances, including paracetamol and salicylate levels, routine blood tests, serial ABGs and ECGs with QRS duration monitoring. An attempt should be made to determine the time and amount ingested of the medication, the circumstances and whether concomitant consumption of alcohol or other substances has occurred.

Monitoring of unstable patients with significant overdoses should be in a high dependency/critical care area, where continuous ECG and vital parameter monitoring are available and where, if necessary, adequate airway management and organ support can be provided.

Higher serum drug levels have been associated with higher mortality risk, increased risk of cardiac arrest, unconsciousness, need for respiratory support, seizures, QRS complex prolongation, interventricular conduction delay and ventricular tachyarrhythmias.[4]

There is conflicting evidence as to the utility of QRS duration for predicting outcome. In a prospective study performed on 49 patients with a TCA overdose, no seizures or ventricular arrhythmias occurred where the QRS duration was shorter than 100 ms, but there was a 34 percent risk of seizures and a 14 percent risk of ventricular arrhythmias in the group with QRS duration above 100 ms. Serum drug levels, were poor predictors of the risk of seizures or ventricular tachyarrhythmias, while widening of the QRS above 160 milliseconds was associated with a 50% risk of malignant ventricular dysrhythmias.[5] The reliability of the QRS complex duration as a marker of severity of TCA overdose has subsequently been questioned by another study, which failed to replicate these findings.[6]

Although prolongation of the PR and QT intervals has also been advocated as potential markers of cardiac toxicity, the QRS complex duration is generally regarded as a better marker of toxicity and is more commonly used in clinical practice. The measurement of TCA serum concentrations are not regarded as of prognostic utility and usually the results of such tests are not available to the bedside clinician in a timely fashion.

Management of TCA toxicity includes ensuring airway protection, adequacy of ventilation with supplemental oxygen as required and cardiovascular stability. Fluid resuscitation should be started with crystalloids, such as 0.9 per cent sodium chloride, which can be administered in 250 to 500 millilitres boluses as clinically indicated. Sodium bicarbonate can be used to treat cardiac toxicity. The initial doses of bicarbonate can be administered as a series of slow intravenous boluses in the form of 8.4 per cent bicarbonate from 50 ml pre-filled syringes. An infusion can be set up with 100 to 150 mEq/l of sodium bicarbonate in 1 l of 0.9 per cent sodium chloride solution, and run at 250 ml/hour as here. Experimental evidence would suggest that the beneficial effects of sodium bicarbonate are a consequence of both the process of alkalinisation and the increase in the extracellular concentration of sodium.[7] Further alkalinisation may be achieved, if appropriate, by manipulating the ventilator settings to achieve a slight respiratory alkalosis where patients are invasively mechanically ventilated.

Activated charcoal can be administered if ingestion has happened within 1 hour of presentation, or later if delayed gastric emptying or absorption is suspected.

Seizures can be controlled with the use of benzodiazepines, such as intravenous lorazepam (1 mg) or diazepam (5 mg), which can be repeated at 5 to 10 minute intervals as clinically indicated.

In cases of acute malignant dysrhythmias, the relevant management protocol should be followed, including DCCV where cardiovascular instability is present, along with administration of sodium bicarbonate. Where cardiac toxicity and haemodynamic compromise remain refractory to bicarbonate treatment, the use of vasopressors such as noradrenaline may be required.

The use of any drugs with the potential to prolong the QT interval should be avoided; these include phenytoin, amiodarone and most other anti-arrhythmics, apart from magnesium and lignocaine, which can be used as a second line treatment for ventricular arrhythmias resistant to treatment with bicarbonate.[8]

Lipid rescue has also been used as second line therapy, where sodium bicarbonate has failed. Cases have been reported of successful use in adults and children, allowing treatment of comatose and cardiovascularly unstable patients where treatment with first line standard therapies has failed to achieve haemodynamic stabilisation. The use of such therapy may make the patients' laboratory tests results difficult to interpret and is potentially associated with the development of pancreatitis.[9,10]

Conclusion

Ingestion of amitriptyline for the purposes of self-harm is not uncommon and can be potentially life-threatening, especially where more than 20 mg/kg body weight is ingested. Cardiac and neurological features of toxicity are the predominant aspects of such overdoses, with altered mental state, seizures and cardiac dysrhythmias being the main concerns. Monitoring of severe cases should be in a high dependency area. Management is predominantly supportive and follows the ABC approach, with controlled ventilation, vasopressors and sodium bicarbonate as first line therapies. Seizures can be controlled with benzodiazepines and drugs prolonging the QT interval should be avoided.

Key Learning Points

- Potentially life threatening amitriptyline overdose is more likely when a dose of more than 20 mg/kg body weight is ingested.
- Cardiac toxicity, central nervous system involvement and potential airway compromise are the life-threatening features of amitriptyline toxicity.
- The QRS complex duration, together with other ECG changes, is deemed to be the most clinically relevant and most readily available marker of toxicity severity.
- Emergency management should be based on the standard 'ABCDE' approach.
- The mainstay of treatment is predominantly supportive; management of the cardiotoxic effects including alkalinisation with sodium bicarbonate infusion, mild hyperventilation and control of seizures with benzodiazepines.
- QT prolonging medications should be avoided.
- Psychiatric assessment should be performed in cases of self-harm.

References

1. Kerr GW, McGuffie AC, Wilkie S. Tricyclic antidepressant overdose: a review. *Emerg Med J* 2001;18(4):236–41.

2. Jarvis MR. Clinical pharmacokinetics of tricyclic antidepressant overdose. *Psychopharmacol Bull* 1991;27(4):541–50.

3. Spiker DG, Biggs JT. Tricyclic antidepressants. Prolonged plasma levels after overdose. *Jama* 1976;236(15):1711–12.

4. Petit JM, Spiker DG, Ruwitch JF, Ziegler VE, Weiss AN, Biggs JT. Tricyclic antidepressant plasma levels and adverse effects after overdose. *Clin Pharmacol Ther* 1977;21(1):47–51.

5. Boehnert MT, Lovejoy FH, Jr. Value of the QRS duration versus the serum drug level in predicting seizures and ventricular arrhythmias after an acute overdose of tricyclic antidepressants. *N Engl J Med* 1985;313(8):474–9.

6. Foulke GE, Albertson TE. QRS interval in tricyclic antidepressant overdosage: inaccuracy as a toxicity indicator in emergency settings. *Ann Emerg Med* 1987;16(2):160–3.

7. Sasyniuk BI, Jhamandas V. Mechanism of reversal of toxic effects of amitriptyline on cardiac Purkinje fibers by sodium bicarbonate. *J Pharmacol Exp Ther* 1984;231(2):387–94.

8. Pentel PR, Benowitz NL. Tricyclic antidepressant poisoning. *Management of arrhythmias. Med Toxicol* 1986;1(2):101–21.

9. Kiberd MB, Minor SF. Lipid therapy for the treatment of a refractory amitriptyline overdose. *Cjem* 2012;14(3):193–7.

10. Levine M, Brooks DE, Franken A, Graham R. Delayed-onset seizure and cardiac arrest after amitriptyline overdose, treated with intravenous lipid emulsion therapy. *Pediatrics* 2012;130(2):e432–8.

Chapter 23

Necrotising Soft Tissue Infections in the Intensive Care Unit Setting

Jane Cunningham and Dave Partridge

Introduction

Necrotising soft tissue infections are characterised by extensive rapid soft tissue destruction, systemic toxicity and are associated with high mortality if untreated. Recent Public Health England (PHE) data estimates that in the United Kingdom there around 500 cases of necrotising fasciitis annually.[1] Although the images portrayed in many textbooks are dramatic, early clinical signs and superficial appearances are often atypical making the initial diagnosis easy to overlook thereby delaying effective intervention. A high index of suspicion should be maintained in soft tissue infections where pain or parameters of systemic sepsis are out of proportion to the clinical appearances.

The term necrotising soft tissue infection encompasses necrotising infections of the skin (necrotising cellulitis), subcutaneous tissues and fascia (necrotising fasciitis), or muscle (necrotising myositis). The terminology surrounding this group of infections is complex as clinical classification pre-dates comprehensive understanding of the pathological and microbiological agents involved.[2]

Microbial aetiology of necrotising fasciitis can be divided into two distinct syndromes. Type 1 necrotising fasciitis includes a mixed microbiological picture including at least one anaerobe (e.g. Bacteroides or Peptostreptococcus) in addition to facultative anaerobes such as Streptococci or coliforms.[2] Patients developing this condition may have an array of predisposing factors including diabetes, obesity, immunosuppression or recent surgery/trauma.

Type II necrotising fasciitis is caused by Group A Streptococcus (GAS) in isolation or in conjunction with other species. The presence of pre-disposing factors is less salient in this cohort.[3] Strains of toxin producing Staphylococcus aureus (both methicillin sensitive and resistant) termed Pontine-Valentine leukocidin (PVL) strains can also present with a necrotising picture.

Fournier's gangrene is the term used to describe necrotising fasciitis of the genitals. Craniofacial necrotising fasciitis refers to a rare form of disease usually associated with group A Streptococci and cervical necrotising fasciitis which is associated with polymicrobial infection from a dental source.[3]

Necrotising myositis or spontaneous gangrenous myositis is necrotising infection of skeletal muscle by GAS or other beta haemolytic streptococci. This differs from clostridial myonecrosis, also termed gas gangrene, as there is no evidence of gas in the soft tissues. Additional differentials include pyomyositis in which the predominant organism is Staphylococcus aureus with the pathophysiology being mainly of abscess formation as opposed to muscle necrosis.

Case Description

A 35-year-old woman with a history of mild eczema and no other significant past medical history presented to the Accident and Emergency department with right-sided shoulder pain. Her observations were unremarkable and clinical examination revealed a decreased range of movement with no apparent superficial skin abnormalities. She lived with her partner and young son who had recently contracted chicken pox. There was no recent travel history or contact history of note. After undergoing a shoulder X-ray, she was diagnosed with a frozen shoulder and discharged on oral analgesia.

She re-presented 24 hours later complaining of shortness of breath in conjunction with severe pain and swelling of the right chest wall. She was profoundly septic with a pyrexia of 38.9°C, systolic blood pressure of 75 mmHg and a sinus tachycardia of 134/minute. Crepitus was noted over her anterior chest wall and her skin was described as mottled. Initial investigations revealed a C reactive protein (CRP) of 675 mg/l (normal range (NR) 0 to 5), lactate of 63 mmol/l (NR less than 2.3) in conjunction with an elevated creatinine of 193 micromol/l (NR 44 to 80) and a urea of 10.9 mmol/l (NR 2.5 to 7.8). She was markedly acidotic with a pH of 7.29 (NR 7.35 to 7.45) and bicarbonate of 20 mmol/L (NR 18 to 23). Haematological parameters were grossly deranged, consistent with overwhelming sepsis. Results included a WCC of 1x 10^9/l (NR 3.5 to 9.5) with neutrophils of 0.8 (NR 1.7 to 6.5) and associated lympopenia, haemoglobin of 95 g/l (NR 110 to 147) and platelets of 49 x10^9/l (NR 150 to 400). Her clotting was markedly abnormal with a PT of 14.9 seconds (NR 9.4 to 11.2) and Fibrinogen 5.3 g/l (NR 2.0 to 4.0).

A presumptive diagnosis of necrotising fasciitis was made and appropriate fluid resuscitation and empirical antimicrobial therapy commenced whilst definitive, emergency surgical management was awaited. Antimicrobials included meropenem and clindamycin that were administered in conjunction with intravenous immunoglobulins. Appropriate infection control measures were also implemented.

While the patient was route to the operating theatre, a computerised tomography (CT) of the chest revealed tissue oedema and gas within the tissue consistent with a diagnosis of necrotising fasciitis.

Emergency surgical debridement was undertaken. Extensive subcutaneous tissue was removed with initial sparing of pectoralis major and minor as the underlying muscle tissue appeared uninvolved. Samples were processed urgently within the microbiology laboratory

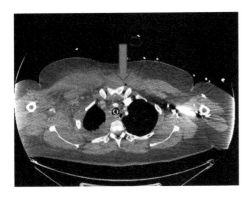

Figure 23.1 CT scan demonstrating free air in the soft tissue. A black and white version of this figure will appear in some formats. For the colour version, please refer to the plate section.

and gram staining of the intra-operative samples revealed gram positive cocci. Following surgical intervention, she was transferred to a side room on the intensive care unit (ICU), requiring noradrenaline and dobutamine infusions having commenced renal support in the form of continuous veno-venous haemofiltration (CVVH).

Once the diagnosis was clinically suspected, the case was referred to the Public Health Specialists with a view to appropriate provision of prophylactic anti-microbials to family members and identification of any potential source. Confirmatory culture results were conveyed as soon as available.

After 24 hours of therapy the patient, remained profoundly septic and required an escalation of inotropic support with the addition of adrenaline to noradrenaline and dobutamine to optimise cardiovascular function. In view of the haemodynamic instability, she was returned to theatre for further surgical exploration. This revealed additional chest wall involvement with non-viable pectoralis major and minor muscles. Further debridement was performed under platelet cover, although peripheral perfusion remained poor with digital ischaemia of both hands and feet. Investigations at this stage were consistent with overwhelming sepsis and an on-going pancytopenia, although biochemistry showed marginal improvement with a falling lactate and CRP of 286 compared to admission. Antimicrobials were continued.

By day four her haemodynamic parameters had improved and inotropic support was weaned. Further debridement of non-viable tissue was undertaken and a vac pump was applied.

However by day five, despite clinical improvement she was noted to have persistent pyrexia. Further imaging of the chest revealed a right-sided pleural effusion and a pigtail chest drain was inserted to drain 1300 mls of brown exudative fluid. The fluid contained leucocytes but no organisms were seen on gram film or subsequently cultured. She improved post chest drainage with resolution of her pyrexia, although CRP remained elevated above 100 mg/l. At day six she continued to wean inotropic support and stopped CVVH. Antimicrobials were rationalised to benzyl penicillin and clindamycin in the context of an isolated sensitive group A streptococcus being identified from multiple perioperative samples and sputum.

Fourteen days after presentation, she developed a deterioration of respiratory parameters and relapse of pyrexia. Repeat CT chest revealed a persistent loculated pleural effusion requiring a video-assisted thoracoscopic surgery (VATS) procedure. Further samples taken at the time of intervention were culture negative. Fourteen days of anti-microbials were completed after the definitive VATS intervention was performed.

She continued to make a good recovery with gradual resolution of her inflammatory markers and normalisation of physiological parameters. At day twenty post initial presentation, a skin graft was performed of the chest wall. The patient was extubated and care stepped down to level 2 high dependency support for on-going care.

Discussion

Clinical Considerations

This lady's initial presentation was relatively nonspecific with few apparent clinical signs. Factors at early presentation suggestive of a necrotising soft tissue infection included pain out of proportion to apparent tissue involvement, pyrexia without obvious underlying aetiology and often, a raised creatinine kinase (CK) and CRP. Skin anaesthesia may also be present due to thrombosis of superficial blood vessels and destruction of superficial nerves. This can precede apparent skin necrosis. There is also an association with recent chicken pox and group A streptococcal infection.[4] In this case, it may be that the patient acquired the infection from her son.

The subsequent re-presentation with profound sepsis and subcutaneous crepitus within 24 hours illustrates the rapid progression of untreated disease. It is essential that once the diagnosis is reached, appropriate therapy is rapidly instituted. Imaging can contribute to the diagnosis and CT is advocated in this context where expedient, but should not delay surgery. Free gas within the fascial planes as seen in Figure 23.2 is highly specific of necrotising infection; however, it has a low sensitivity.

Emergency surgical intervention and debridement is the definitive therapy and has been shown to enhance survival.[2,3] This should be accompanied by aggressive fluid resuscitation and supportive therapy. The aim of debridement is removal of all necrotic tissue as occurred in this case. Current recommendations[5] are that patients should return to theatre 24 to 36 hours after initial debridement and daily thereafter until there is no further evidence of necrotic tissue at operation. It is essential to ensure that intra-operative tissue samples are sent for microbiological culture to enable rationalisation of anti-microbial therapy. Blood cultures are a further useful adjunct to identifying the pathogen with a high positivity rate.

Previous publications have suggested an association between the use of non-steroidal anti-inflammatory drugs and an increased risk of necrotising fasciitis, although this has been discounted in current literature.[2] The role of hyperbaric oxygen in the management of necrotising fasciitis remains uncertain with limited evidence available.[2] The lack of availability of hyperbaric oxygen facilities and unstable nature of the patients involved often means that the practicalities of appropriate management make it unfeasible in the majority of cases.

Antimicrobial Therapy

Initial anti-microbial therapy is empirical and serves as an adjunct to surgery. As the infection can be polymicrobial, therapy should remain broad until microbiological culture results are available. Empirical antibiotic selection should include agents active against gram

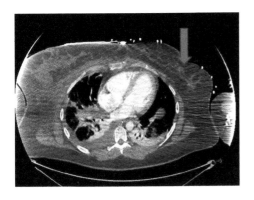

Figure 23.2 CT scan demonstrating soft tissue inflammation. A black and white version of this figure will appear in some formats. For the colour version, please refer to the plate section.

negative, anaerobic and Gram positive isolates. Agents covering gram-positive isolates should have efficacy against streptococci and staphlococci. Local resistance rates of strepto-cocci against erythromycin / clindamicin should contribute to decisions regarding the empirical selection of anti-streptococcal therapy.

In hospitalised patients and those residing in areas with endemic-community associated methicillin resistant Staphylococcus aureus (MRSA), empirical therapy should include an active anti-MRSA agent. These include vancomycin and linezolid. In the event that linezolid is used, it is imperative that drug interactions known to predispose to serotonin syndrome are considered, e.g., antidepressants.

Individuals with severe penicillin allergy can be treated with clindamycin and metroni-dazole in conjunction with an aminoglycoside or fluroquinolone.[5] Despite a theoretical cross reactivity of sensitivity between penicillins and meropenem, there is increasing evidence supporting the safety of meropenem in individuals with a documented penicillin hypersensitivity reaction.[12] The use of meropenem in this context would need to be considered on an individual patient basis.

In addition to broad spectrum antimicrobial cover, therapy should encompass an agent acting at the ribosomal subunit able to reduce bacterial toxin production. Both clindamycin and linezolid are used for this purpose. Current combinations in common use in the United Kingdom include meropenem or piperacillin-tazobactam in conjunction with clindamycin or linezolid. Once definitive microbiology and sensitivities are available, this broad spec-trum approach can be rationalised.

The optimal duration of antimicrobial therapy is as yet unknown. Consensus maintains that this should be tailored to the individual's specific clinical picture. Evidence for the role of continuous infusion of a beta lactam in this context is limited. The theoretical advantage of a continuous infusion would be increased time above the mean inhibitory concentration (MIC) of the isolates.

Immunoglobulin Therapy

Intravenous immunoglobulin therapy (IVIG) has been used as an adjunct in the manage-ment of necrotising skin infections, as in this case. Proposed mechanisms of intravenous immunoglobulin activity in the treatment of necrotising fasciitis include neutralisation of clostridial toxins and streptococcal superantigens by antibodies, modulation of the Fc–receptor blockade, complement activation and opsonisation of GAS.[5]

The relative rarity of the condition limits the strength of the available evidence with regard to treatment however it falls increasingly in favour of the use of both clindamycin and IVIG. Current provision of IVIG in the United Kingdom is in accordance with existing Department of Health guidance due to the cost implications and limitations of supply.[11] Existing guidance supports the use of IVIG in necrotising staphylococcal disease in addition to staphylococcal and streptococcal septic shock syndrome.

A comparative observational study which evaluated the effect of IVIG and clinda-mycin in patients with invasive streptococcal disease reviewed outcomes in 67 patients. 23 patients received IVIG and 44 did not. The results revealed a significant reduction in 28 day mortality in patients who had received IVIG and clindamycin.[6] A further prospective observational study which included 84 cases of invasive group A streptococ-cal disease concluded that those who received IVIG had a reduced fatality rate of 7 per cent and that the adjusted point estimate of the odds ratio (OR) for mortality was lower in clindamycin-treated patients (0.31; 95 percent CI, .09 to 1.12) and clindamycin plus IVIG-treated patients (0.12; 95 percent CI, .01 to 1.29) compared with clindamycin-untreated patients.[7]

Further trials include a European double-blind placebo controlled study which revealed no statistically significant improvement in twenty eight day survival and a statistically non-significant reduction in the median time to limit progression of necrotising fasciitis in the group receiving IVIG vs placebo. It should be noted that this study was terminated prematurely due to slow patient recruitment and only included 21 patients. The mortality rate was 3.6 fold higher in the placebo group versus those receiving IVIG.[8]

Previous evidence has highlighted the batch to batch variation of IVIG in terms of quantifiable neutralising antibodies and this in turn may have a confounding effect on trial outcome data[2] and explain some of the heterogeneity of previous data sets.

Public Health Considerations

In the UK setting, all cases of necrotising fasciitis attributable to Group A Streptococcus should be notified to Public Health England. A recent publication from Australia reported that the incidence rate of invasive group A Streptococcal disease in contacts was 2011 (95 percent CI, 413 to 5929) times higher than the incidence in the general population in Victoria.[7] On the basis of this evidence there is support for the role of prophylaxis for household contacts. Current Public Health England guidance limits prophylaxis to mother and baby (if either develops invasive disease in the neonatal period), symptomatic household contacts and the entire household if there are two or more cases of invasive group A streptococcal disease within a thirty-day time period.

Appropriate infection control should be implemented as soon as the diagnosis is suspected. This entails isolation in a side-room in conjunction with universal control precautions and barrier nursing. Theoretically patients should become non-infectious after 48 hours of anti-microbial therapy; however, decisions to deescalate precautions should be made in conjunction with the infection control and microbiology teams.

Conclusion

The initial clinical presentation of necrotising soft tissue infections can be atypical, with few overt clinical signs beyond a toxic septic picture. Definitive management entails emergency surgical debridement with broad spectrum antimicrobial therapy and immunoglobulins serving as adjuncts.

Key Learning Points

- Necrotising soft tissue infection encompasses necrotising fasciitis, myositis, cellulitis, myonecrosis and pyomyositis.
- Patients with necrotising infections may have limited clinical signs at initial presentation. A high index of suspicion should be maintained in cases where pain or parameters of systemic sepsis are out of proportion to the clinical appearances of a suspected soft tissue infection.
- Predisposing factors to Type 2 necrotising fasciitis include diabetes, drug use, obesity, immunosuppressants, recent surgery and traumatic wounds.[2] Predisposing factors are less salient in Type 1 disease.

- Definitive therapy for necrotising soft tissue infection is surgical debridement and should be undertaken as a surgical emergency. Anti-microbial therapy and IVIG serve as adjuncts to debridement.[10]
- Broad spectrum antimicrobial therapy should be started in conjunction with clindamycin or linezolid which are able to inactivate toxin production.[7] Further anti-microbial therapy can be tailored once culture results and sensitivities are available.
- The role of adjunctive intravenous immunoglobulin has not been evaluated in a large scale randomised control study setting due to the rarity of the condition. The weight of current evidence supports its use.[7] It is postulated that the IVIG contains antibodies to clostridial toxins and streptococcal superantigens.
- Invasive group A strep is a notifiable disease in the United Kingdom. The role of post exposure prophylaxis should be discussed with the public health team.

References

1. Public Health England. General information: necrotising fasciitis. www.hpa.org.uk/Topics/Infectious Diseases/InfectionsAZ/Necrotising Fasciitis/GeneralInformation NecrotisingFasciitis/.

2. Mandell GL, Bennett JE, Dolin R. *Principals and Practice of Infectious Diseases* Seventh Edition. Churchill Livingstone 2009.

3. Torok M, Cooke. *Oxford Handbook of Infectious diseases and Microbiology.* Oxford University Press 2009.

4. Laupland KB. Invasive group A streptococcal disease in children and association with varicella-zoster virus infection. Ontario Group A Streptococcal Study Group. *Paediatrics* 2000 May;105(5):E60.

5. Stevens L. Practice guidelines for the diagnosis and management of skin and soft tissue infections: 2014 update by the infectious diseases society of America. *Clinical Infectious Diseases* 2014 July 15;59 (2):10–52.

6. Linner A. Clinical efficacy of polyspecific intravenous immunoglobulin therapy in patients with streptococcal toxic shock syndrome- a comparative observational study. *Clinical Infectious Diseases* 2014 June;59(6):851–7.

7. Carapetis JR. Effectiveness of clindamycin and intravenous immunoglobulin, and risk of disease in contacts, in invasive group A streptococcal infections. *Clinical Infectious Diseases* 2014 Aug 1;59 (3):358–65.

8. Darenberg J. Intravenous immunoglobulin G in streptococcal toxic shock syndrome: a European randomized, randomised, double-blind, placebo controlled trial. *Clinical Infectious Diseases* 2003;37:333–40.

9. Raithatha AH, Bryden DC. Use of intravenous immunoglobulin therapy in the treatment of septic shock, in particular severe invasive group A streptococcal disease. *Indian Journal of Critical Care Medicine* 2012 Jan;16(1):37–40.

10. Stevens DL. Dilemmas in the treatment of invasive Streptococcus pyogenes infections. *Clinical Infectious Diseases* 2003;37:341–3.

11. *Department of Health Clinical Guidelines for Immunoglobulin Use.* Second Edition. www.ivig.nhs.uk/documents/dh_129666.pdf

12. Wall GC et al. Assessment of hypersensitivity reactions in patients receiving carbapenem antibiotics who report a history of penicillin allergy. *Journal of Chemotherapy* 2014 Jun;26 (3):150–3.

Chapter 24

Fungal Infections

Rachel Wadsworth and Dave Partridge

Introduction

Admission to the intensive care unit has been identified as a risk factor associated with invasive fungal infection.[1] Renal dialysis patients are also at higher risk of invasive fungal disease by the nature of their underlying condition, use of indwelling catheters to facilitate renal replacement therapies and by the use of immunosuppressant therapies to support solid organ transplants. Diagnosis of fungal infection can be challenging because conventional culture is often slow, insensitive or simply unavailable. Molecular tests are evolving and improving our ability to detect fungal disease, especially mould and *Pneumocystis jirovecii* infections.

Case Description

This case is of a 75-year-old woman with a history of previous renal transplant, and immunosuppressed with tacrolimus and low dose prednisolone. The transplant had failed and she had required renal replacement therapy in the form of haemodialysis via a forearm fistula for the past five months. Her background was of hypertensive renal disease, hypo-thyroidism, hypercholestrolaemia, a stroke three years previously and she was anticoagu-lated with warfarin for atrial fibrillation.

She presented to hospital with a painful left arm, and was found to have a thrombosed arterio-venous fistula. During her hospital admission she had a new tunneled vascular access catheter (vascath) for haemodialysis inserted by the renal physicians. She developed a cough productive of sputum, fever and difficulty breathing, and was treated with intraven-ous piperacillin-tazobactam for a left lower lobe hospital-acquired pneumonia, a diagnosis supported by evidence of consolidation on a chest X-ray image.

She deteriorated with increasing oxygen requirements, partly due to fluid overload resulting from her inability to undergo haemodialysis due to cardiovascular instability and hypotension. The critical care team reviewed her for the first time at this stage, due to a significant type I respiratory failure. She presented with respiratory distress, a respira-tory rate of 33/min, SpO_2 of 99% on FiO_2 0.8, HR 123 bpm irregularly irregular, BP 101/67 mmHg and temperature of 37.9°C. Chest radiography was performed showing widespread air space shadowing throughout both lung fields, which had progressed significantly since the initial imaging six days earlier (Figure 24.1). Inflammatory markers on presentation to the ICU were a white cell count of 7×10^9/l, neutrophil count of 6.14×10^9/l and C Reactive Protein (CRP) of 376 mg/l.

She was admitted to the intensive care unit for treatment with CPAP via a hood to maintain adequate oxygenation and insertion of an arterial catheter to aid blood gas moni-toring. A femoral central line was inserted to provide access for vasopressor support for

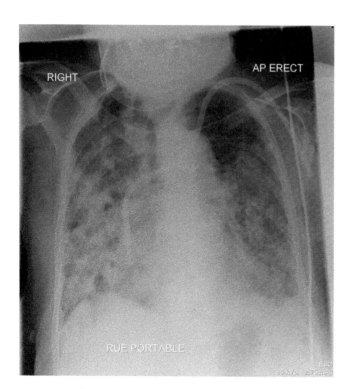

Figure 24.1 Chest X-ray from Day 1 of ICU admission. Image shows bilateral widespread air space shadowing.

treatment of the hypotension. With this she was able to commence renal replacement therapy with continuous veno-venous haemofiltration and fluid removal via the tunneled vascath.

Chest X-ray appearances, although suggestive of pulmonary oedema and initially treated as such, were worsening within 48 hours following the admission to critical care despite removal of fluid. Clinical deterioration and further increase in oxygen requirements led to discussion with the microbiology team regarding alternative diagnoses. At this stage the white cell count had risen to 10.4 x 10^9/l and neutrophil count to 8.83 x 10^9/l. CRP had initially fallen to 98 but then had risen again to 152 mg/l.

The differential diagnosis of infection causing type 1 respiratory failure in an immuno-compromised patient such as this is large, and includes hospital-or community- acquired bacterial pathogens, including 'atypical' agents such as *Legionella pneumophila*, viruses including common respiratory viruses such as influenza but also agents such as adenovirus and cytomegalovirus, and fungi, especially *pneumocystis jirovecii* pneumonia (PCP), given the chest X-ray appearance.

Investigations for the above were arranged. Unfortunately, she was not fit enough to undergo a bronchoscopy and lavage or induced sputum without the significant risk of requiring intubation and ventilation at this stage, so was maintained on treatment with CPAP with a view to bronchoscopy if her clinical state improved enough to safely do so. A further chest X-ray was taken at this stage (Figure 24.2) demonstrating a worsening of consolidation bilaterally. In view of the inability to get a deep respiratory sample, she was commenced on treatment with co-trimoxazole (trimethoprim – sulfamethoxazole), steroids and caspofungin for possible PCP. A serum beta-D-glucan test was requested. This showed a strongly positive result with concentration of Beta glucan of more than 500 pg/ml (normal reference range less than 80 pg/ml), consistent with PCP.

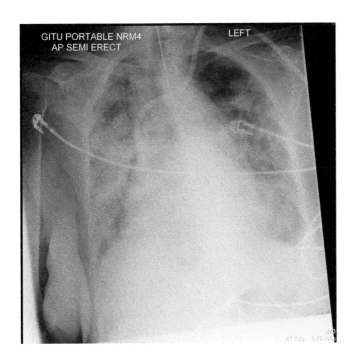

GITU PORTABLE NRM4
AP SEMI ERECT
LEFT

Figure 24.2 Chest X-ray from Day 7 of ICU admission. Worsening of bilateral consolidation.

After a further six days on the intensive care unit, she was well enough for discharge to the renal ward for ongoing treatment, with critical care outreach follow up. She completed a total of 21 days therapy with co-trimoxazole for PCP. CT scan of the chest showed full resolution of changes four months later.

Discussion

Risk factors for fungal infections in intensive care patients include immunocompromise, chronic lung disease, patients with invasive devices including central venous catheters and other generalised risk factors such as broad spectrum antibiotic therapy, intravenous drug misuse and gut lumen contamination of body compartments, e.g., faecal peritonitis or oesophageal perforation. *Candida* species are the most common invasive fungal infections in the ICU and are primarily associated with invasive devices or abdominal pathology. *Aspergillus* infections are an emerging cause of invasive pulmonary disease in the critically ill, having previously been primarily recognised in patients with haematological malignancy. *Pneumocystis jirovecii* causes a pneumonitis and is associated with cellular immune deficits, particularly due to HIV infection, chemotherapy or steroids.

Pneumocystis was first classified as a protozoan around 100 years ago and reclassified in 1988, due to the analysis of the small ribosmal ribonucleic acid (rRNA) establishing a phlyogenetic linkage to the fungal kingdom.[2] Originally thought to be a single species, it has subsequently been recognised that many distinct species of *Pneumocystis* exist with remarkable host specificity. As a result, nomenclature changed and *Pneumocystis carinii* was assigned to the species infecting rats with the human specific organism labelled *Pneumocystis jirovecii* after Otto Jirovec, who first described it as a cause of human disease. Serological evidence in young children suggests that exposure is ubiquitous and nosocomial transmission has been demonstrated. As with many fungal infections, *Pneumocystis* can be considered an opportunistic microorganism causing severe and often fatal pneumonia in immunocompromised patients.

A mortality rate of between 20 percent and 60 percent has been reported.[2] In the 1980s and 1990s, the disease was most frequently recognised in the HIV positive patient but improvements in HIV treatment and rising numbers of patients receiving immunosuppressive therapies for malignancies, allogenic organ transplantations and autoimmune diseases have resulted in a greater proportion of cases now being detected in non-HIV immunosuppressed individuals.[4] A possible association with sudden infant death syndrome has been reported.

The organism's unique cell biology makes it stand out from the other fungi. *Pneumocystis* lacks ergosterol in its cell membrane and thus drugs such as amphotericin and azoles, which bind ergosterol or inhibit its synthesis respectively, are ineffective against it. It exists in distinct trophic and cystic forms, leading to its initial misclassification as a protozoan. Organism attachment to alveolar epithelial cells is essential for *pneumocystis* infection and propagation, invasion of host cells is uncommon and extrapulmonary pneumocystosis occurs very rarely.[4] The cell wall of the cystic form contains abundant beta-glucans, and this may have a role in pathogenesis through the production of TNF-α and generation of macrophage-inflammatory protein-2 by alveolar macrophages.[3] Neutrophils subsequently recruited into the lungs release reactive oxidant species, proteases and cationic proteins which directly injure capillary endothelial cells and alveolar epithelial cells,[2] and it is this host response that appears to lead to the consequence of impaired alveolar-capillary function in gas exchange.

Pneumocystis classically presents as the subtle onset of progressive dyspnoea, nonproductive cough, low-grade fever and malaise. Complications such as pnuemothorax may add to the symptomatology with features of pleuritic chest pain. Development of worsening pneumonia with respiratory failure is the most common reason for these patients to be admitted to the intensive care unit. Non-HIV infected patients usually have a more rapid onset of symptoms.

Chest X-ray findings usually begin with bilateral and symmetrical interstitial infiltrates particularly in the perihilar regions, which may be very subtle initially but which develop into more homogenous and diffuse infiltrates as the disease progresses.

Pneumocystis cannot be cultured and other techniques are required for diagnosis. Microscopy can be performed with identification of the small trophic forms and the larger cysts using conventional cytochemical or immunofluorescence staining. These methods are useful when the organism burden is relatively high but are insufficient for reliable detection when the load is small and are thus less sensitive in non-HIV cases. Polymerase chain reaction (PCR) based diagnosis has provided increased sensitivity and specificity but distinguishing patients who are colonized from those infected with *pneumocystis* can be challenging. Appropriate samples for the above tests include bronchoalveolar lavage fluid, lung biopsy and hypertonic saline induced sputum.

Unfortunately many patients, such as the lady described here, are unfit for bronchoscopy or sputum induction at presentation. The measurement of serum 1,3-beta-D-glucan, a cell wall component of most pathogenic fungi, can be useful for establishing a diagnosis of *pneumocystis* in such patients.[5] Notable exceptions to the presence of 1,3-beta-D-glucan in the cell wall are in *Cryptococcus* and mucoraceous moulds but it has a high sensitivity for the diagnosis of invasive candidiasis and PCP, with a recent meta-analysis reporting a sensitivity of around 95 per cent for the latter.[6]

The test relies upon the induction of the coagulation cascade of the horseshoe crab by beta-D-glucan and is able to detect picogram levels. The test is prone to contamination and specimens require careful handling to prevent this. The fact that it is not specific for any individual species also makes it challenging to interpret if the clinical picture would be compatible with multiple fungal pathogens. If used in the correct clinical context, the test can be very useful in supporting the diagnosis of PCP in patients who are unfit for invasive respiratory sampling.

Trimethoprim–sulfamethoxazole with adjunctive corticosteroid therapy to suppress lung inflammation in patients with severe infection remains the preferred treatment for PCP. In the absence of corticosteroid therapy, early deterioration in the first 3 to 5 days of therapy is typical, and patients generally improve after 4 to 8 days of therapy. Therefore, changes in treatment due to lack of efficacy should rarely be made prior to 4 to 8 days of initial treatment.[4] Side effects of co-trimoxazole therapy include rash (30 to 50 percent), fever (30 to 40 percent), leucopenia (30 to 40 percent) and less commonly hepatitis and thrombocytopenia. Stevens-Johnson syndrome has also been reported and although a rare complication should be closely monitored as it can be life threatening.

The initial dose of co-trimoxazole is usually 120 mg/kg/day in 3 to 4 divided doses. This can be reduced to 90 mg/kg/day after four days therapy[7] and treatment should be continued for 21 days. Oral therapy can be used in mild or moderate cases if gastro-intestinal absorption is adequate as oral bioavailability is good. Caution should be taken in patients who are elderly and in those with renal impairment and severe liver disease, where a dose reduction may be more suitable. In patients who are pregnant and those who are breastfeeding caution should also be used, as there is a risk of teratogenicity in the first trimester and neonatal haemolysis and methaemoglobinaemia in the third trimester and in neonates.[8]

Despite these cautions, co-trimoxazole remains the first line therapy for *pneumocystis jirovecii*. Adjunctive steroids for those with HIV infection and severe disease can be used, with doses up to 80 mg prednisolone in two divided doses in the first five days of treatment reduced to 40 mg daily on days 6 to 10 and further reduction from day 11 onwards, again to complete 21 days. Although less data exists on steroid use in PCP patients without HIV, many centres follow the same regimen.

If the patient has an adverse reaction or is unsuitable for treatment with co-trimoxazole, alternative second-line therapies include clindamycin plus primaquine, IV pentamidine or, for mild disease only, atovaquone or trimethoprim plus dapsone.[1,4] Glucose 6 phosphate dehydrogenase (G6PD) testing should be performed before patients receive primaquine or dapsone which can provoke an acute haemolytic crisis in susceptible patients. Salvage therapy through addition of caspofungin, which is active against the cystic form of the organism, has shown some promise.[9]

Predictors of mortality for PCP include older age, recent injection drug use, increased total bilirubin, low serum albumin and alveolar–arterial oxygen gradient more than 50 mmHg.[10] Among events occurring during hospitalisation, admission to the intensive care unit, requirement for mechanical ventilation and development of pneumothorax were all associated with higher mortality.[10] Non-HIV patients present more acutely with fulminant respiratory failure and frequently require mechanical ventilation.[4]

Primary or secondary prophylaxis with either low-dose co-trimoxazole or nebulized pentamidine is routine for HIV-infected patients with a CD4 count less than 200 cells/mm^3 with prophylaxis continued until adequate and sustained response from highly active antiretroviral therapy (HAART).[11] Prophylaxis is also given to other patients at high risk of disease such as transplant recipients.

Conclusion

Our patient was treated with a high index of suspicion for *pneumocystis* pneumonia allowing early therapy to be instituted, which then could be confirmed once laboratory results became available. At risk patients can deteriorate quickly and irreversibly and so this approach can be adopted to prevent such events in the critically ill immunocompromised patient.

Key Learning Points

- Clinicians should have a high index of suspicion of *Pneumocystis* pneumonia in immunocompromised patients at risk.
- Prompt therapy is crucial early in the disease process.
- Beta-D-glucan has a role in the diagnosis of PCP in patients who are unfit for bronchoalveolar lavage or induced sputum.
- Close liaison with the microbiology team regarding testing and treatment is very useful.
- Prophylaxis for *Pneumocystis* should be considered for at risk patients.

References

1. Beed M, Sherman R, Holden S. Fungal infections and critically ill adults. *Continuing Education in Anaesthesia, Critical Care and Pain* 2014;14:262–7.

2. Thomas Jr CF, Limper AH. Pneumocystis pneumonia. *The New England Journal of Medicine* 2004;350:2487–98.

3. Vassallo R, Standing JE, Limper AH. Isolated Pneumocystis carinii cell wall glucan provokes lower respiratory tract inflammatory responses. *Journal of Immunology* 2000;164:3755–63.

4. Calderón EJ, Varela JM, Durand-Joly I, Dei-Cas E. Pneumocystis jirovecii Pneumonia In: *Pneumonia: Symptoms, Diagnosis and Treatment*. Editors: M.L. Suarez and S.M. Ortega, pp 1–36.

5. Desmet S, Van Wijngaerden E, Maertens J, et al. Serum (1,3)-β-D-Glucan as a tool for diagnosis of Pneumocystis jirovecii pneumonia in patients with human immunodeficiency virus infection or haematological malignancy. *Journal of Clinical Microbiology* 2009;47:3871–4.

6. Karageorgopoulos DE, Qu J–M, Korbila IP, Zhu Y–G, Vasileiou VA, Falagas ME. Accuracy of β-D-glucan for the diagnosis of Pneumocystis jirovecii pneumonia: a meta-analysis. *Clin Microbiol Infect* 2013;19:39–49.

7. Dockrell DH, Breen R, Liipman M, Milller RF. Pulmonary opportunistic infections, In: British HIV Association and British Infection Association guidelines for the treatment for opportunistic infection in HIV-seropositive individuals 2011. *HIV Medicine* 2011;12(Suppl. 2):25–42.

8. British National Formulary. www.bnf.org

9. Armstrong-James D, Stebbing J, John L, et al. A trial of caspofungin salvage treatment in PCP pneumonia. *Thorax* 2011;66:537–8.

10. Fei MW, Kim EJ, Sant CA, Jarlsberg LG, et al. Predicting mortality from HIV-associated Pneumocystis pneumonia at illness presentation: an observational cohort study. *Thorax* 2009;64:1070–6.

11. Schneider MME, Borleffs JCC, Stolk RP, Jasper CAJJ, Hoepelman AIM. Discontinuation of prophylaxis for Pneumocystis carinii pneumonia in HIV-1-infected patients treated with highly active antiretroviral therapy. *Lancet* 1999;353:201–3.

Chapter 25

The Acutely Jaundiced Patient

25 Autoimmune Hepatitis

Lin Lee Wong and Dermot Gleeson

Introduction

Jaundice is yellow discolouration of the sclera and skin due to deposition of bilirubin. When clinically detectable, serum bilirubin is usually more than 50 µmol/l. Onset of jaundice is usually due to impairment of bile production or flow, called cholestasis, which can be due either to acute liver cellular injury or to biliary obstruction. Most patients with cholestatic jaundice (both those with liver injury and with biliary obstruction) report dark urine and sometimes also pale stools and itching.

Diagnosing the cause of jaundice can be challenging. The first question to address is whether there is biliary obstruction. If this can be excluded (by the absence of intrahepatic biliary dilation on ultrasound, or, in cases of doubt, magnetic cholangiography), the patient has liver cellular injury and the cause needs to be established as it is often reversible if diagnosed and treated early. This case describes the processes of investigation and treatment of jaundice in a non-critically unwell patient to inform the choice of differentials and selection of tests in such a patient presenting to critical care.

Case Description

A 57-year-old man presented acutely to hospital with a three-month history of worsening jaundice, itching, fatigue and reduced appetite. He had been travelling in the southern hemisphere for the past nine months. For several years he had taken amlodipine and ramipril for hypertension. Around the time of onset of jaundice, he had been given another unidentified painkiller for acute backache and had been told to stop drinking alcohol (his previous consumption had been 60 units/week). He smoked 10 cigarettes per day.

On examination, he was jaundiced with smooth non-tender palpable hepatomegaly. There were no signs of chronic liver disease, oedema or ascites. The other systems were normal.

His liver function tests (LFTs) were as follows:

Blood tests	Results	Reference range
Bilirubin	115 µmol/l	3–17 µmol/l
ALT	1054 IU/l	3–35 IU/l
AST	500 IU/l	3–35 IU/l
ALP	150 IU/l	30–200 IU/l
gGT	690 IU/l	0–51 IU/l

(cont.)

Blood tests	Results	Reference range
Globulin	**46 g/l**	23–35 g/l
Albumin	36 g/l	35–50 g/l
Prothrombin time (PT)	11 s	10–12 s
INR	1.0	0.9–1.1

Renal function tests and blood count were normal.

The initial differential diagnosis included alcoholic hepatitis, drug-induced liver injury and viral hepatitis. An acute 'non-invasive liver screen' was performed. The results were as follows:

Blood test	Result	Reference range
Virology		
Hepatitis A IgM	Negative	N/A
Hepatitis B surface Antigen & core IgM antibody	Negative	
Hepatitis C antibody	Negative	
Hepatitis E IgM antibody	Negative	
CMV IgM antibody	Negative	
EBV IgM antibody	Negative	
Immunology		
Immunoglobulins		
IgG	**32 g/L**	5–16 g/L
IgM, IgA	Normal	
Anti-nuclear antibody (ANA)	Negative	
Anti-mitochrondrial antibody (AMA)	Negative	
Anti-smooth muscle antibody(sMA)	**POSITIVE**	
Anti-liver-kidney microsomal antibody (a-LKM)	Negative	

An abdominal ultrasound scan showed possible mild dilatation of the left intrahepatic duct with no other abnormality and patent portal and hepatic veins on Doppler examination. Magnetic resonance cholangiopancreatogram (MRCP) showed a normal biliary tree.

Often at this stage, serum bilirubin and transaminases improve either spontaneously (as in viral infections) or follow withdrawal of alcohol or medications. Because this patient's results did not improve, a liver biopsy was performed. This showed interface hepatitis (Figure 1), plasma cell infiltrate (Figure 2), rosettes (Figure 3) and severe active chronic hepatitis with stage 3 fibrosis. At the weekly clinico-pathological meeting the features were thought to be consistent with autoimmune hepatitis (AIH).

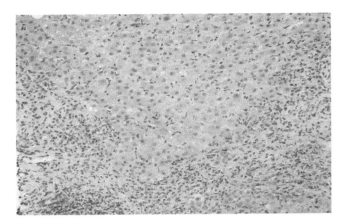

Figure 25.1 Liver biopsy showing interface hepatitis (inflammation of hepatocytes at the junction of the portal tract and hepatic parenchyma). A black and white version of this figure will appear in some formats. For the colour version, please refer to the plate section.

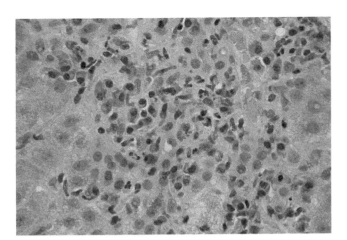

Figure 25.2 Plasma cell infiltrate. A black and white version of this figure will appear in some formats. For the colour version, please refer to the plate section.

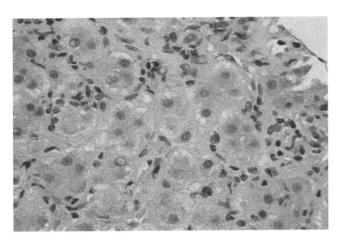

Figure 25.3 Rosettes (clusters of reactive hepatocytes surrounded by inflammatory cells). A black and white version of this figure will appear in some formats. For the colour version, please refer to the plate section.

Following an explanation of the diagnosis and proposed management plan, the patient was started on prednisolone 30 mg once daily as immunosuppressant. His liver enzymes improved within a few days (ALT falling to 280 u/l). Although his baseline bone density (DEXA) scan was normal, he was also started on calcium and vitamin D supplements (AdCal D3 1 tablet twice daily) because he was likely to need steroids for at least two years, and was at risk of developing osteoporosis. Over the next six weeks, his serum transaminases and bilirubin fell gradually to normal and his prednisolone dose was gradually tapered down.

Activity in red blood cells of the azathioprine metabolising red cell enzyme thiopurine methyl transferase (TPMT) was checked and was normal. This excludes severe TPMT deficiency, associated with high sensitivity to azathioprine induced bone marrow suppression. Therefore, after 8 weeks, azathioprine was introduced at 1mg/kg and prednisolone was maintained at 10mg once daily. Random blood glucose levels remained normal. He continued to feel well, so that seven months after presentation, he was able to travel abroad having been given advice on monitoring his liver enzymes and full blood count every three months (with the results being emailed back to the liver unit). A further liver biopsy is planned to take place two years after starting treatment, to confirm histological remission of AIH.

Discussion

This man presented with jaundice, fatigue and anorexia and had markedly elevated serum transaminase enzymes (ALT greater than 1000 u/l). Despite the history of excessive alcohol intake, this liver enzyme pattern is atypical of alcoholic liver disease, in which serum ALT rarely exceeds 200 u/l and in over 90 percent of cases, is less than the serum AST. Other possible diagnoses include various hepatitis and other viruses, which were excluded by serum testing. Drug related liver injury, whilst possible here, usually follows a relatively short (less than 3 months) period of exposure to a drug known to cause injury. The many drugs that can cause such injury include antibiotics, anti-epileptics, antipsychotic drugs and some NSAIDS (such as diclofenac). There were no obvious such candidates here.

Ischaemic liver damage would be unusual in an otherwise healthy 57-year-old and rarely causes jaundice lasting three months. Hepatic venous obstruction (Budd-Chiari syndrome) was excluded by Doppler examination. Finally, a first presentation of Wilson's disease (hepaticolenticular disease due to copper accumulation), although possible, would be very rare in someone over 50.

However, the raised serum globulin and IgG and the presence in serum of smooth muscle antibodies raised the possibility of autoimmune hepatitis. This was confirmed by liver biopsy and enabled prompt initiation of effective treatment.

Evaluation of Jaundice

Bilirubin (see Figure 25.4) is the breakdown product of haem (mostly derived from haemoglobin). This binds to albumin to form unconjugated bilirubin. Unconjugated bilirubin is taken up by the liver in a conjugation process by glucoronyl transferase to form conjugated bilirubin. Conjugated bilirubin is then excreted into bile. In the colon, it is deconjugated and reduced by bacteria to urobilinogen and stercobilinogen (which provides normal colour to faeces). Urobilinogen is either partly reabsorbed (hepatobiliary recirculation) or excreted in the urine and faeces.[1–2]

Jaundice can be either pre-hepatic, hepatic or post-hepatic. The term *cholestatic jaundice* incorporates both hepatic and post hepatic jaundice (see Table 25.1).[1]

Table 25.1 Classification of jaundice

Prehepatic (c)	Hepatic	Post hepatic
Neonatal	Viral hepatitis (A-E, CMV, EBV) (a)	Bile duct stones (a,b)
Haemolysis	Alcoholic hepatitis (a,b)	Intrinsic biliary stricture (b)
Gilbert's	Drug induced liver injury (DILI) (a,b)	Cholangiocarcinoma (b)
syndrome	Autoimmune hepatitis (a)	Pancreatic carcinoma (b)
Crigler-Najjar	Ischaemic liver injury (a)	Extrinsic biliary compression (aneurysm,
syndrome	Wilson's disease (a,b)	hilar nodes) (b)
	Total parenteral nutrition (b)	Acute or chronic pancreatitis (b)
	Primary biliary cirrhosis (b)	Biliary atresia (b)
	Intrahepatic primary sclerosing	Extrahepatic primary sclerosing
	cholangitis (b)	cholangitis (b)
	Cholestasis of pregnancy (a,b)	HIV cholangiopathy (b)
	Granulomatous liver disease (b)	
	Malignant infiltration (b)	
	Bacterial sepsis (a,b,c)	
	Graft-versus-host disease (b)	
	Severe heart failure (a,b)	
	Budd-Chiari syndrome (a,b)	
	Alpha-1-antritypsin deficiency (b)	
	Dubin-Johnson Syndrome (b,c)	

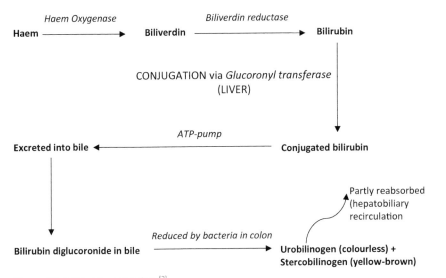

Figure 25.4 Bilirubin metabolism.[2]

History

The duration of jaundice and associated symptoms should be ascertained. The absence of dark urine, pale stools or itching suggests pre-hepatic jaundice. However, the presence of one or more of these cannot distinguish hepatic from post-hepatic jaundice. Unless the diagnosis is already known, the following points should be addressed:

- Associated symptoms of biliary pain, rigors, weight loss, abdominal or leg swelling
- Past history of malignancy, gallstones or biliary surgery and other autoimmune disease
- Drugs (conventional or alternative) started over the few months before onset of jaundice. Recent paracetamol ingestion.
- Potential hepatitis contact (including irregular sexual contact which is the most common source of acute HBV infection in adults)
- Alcohol consumption

Physical examination may reveal signs suggesting chronic liver disease (spider naevi, leuconychia, palmar erythema, splenomegaly, ascites, muscle wasting, loss of axilliary/pubic hair, gynaecomastia, testicular atrophy). None of these is sensitive and their absence does not exclude chronic liver disease, Other signs to look for include Kayser-Fleischer rings at the corneoscleral junction (indicative of Wilson's disease), liver flap and confusion/drowsiness (hepatic encephalopathy).[1]

Investigations

Abnormal liver function tests are often categorised thus:

Hepatocellular pattern: serum transferases (ALT, AST) are elevated proportionately more than serum alkaline phosphatase (ALP). This may be accompanied by elevated bilirubin

Cholestatic pattern: ALP is elevated proportionately more than serum transaminases; Isolated hyperbilirubinaemia: elevated bilirubin with normal serum aminotransferases and alkaline phosphatase

The pattern(s) most commonly associated with the various aetiologies are included in Table 25.1. Note that there is an imperfect correlation with the hepatic/post-hepatic categorisation. For example, the pattern may be 'hepatocellular' in jaundice due to bile duct stones (although transaminases usually fall rapidly) and is 'cholestatic' in many intrinsic liver diseases.

An urgent ultrasound scan of the liver with Doppler of the hepatic vessels should always be obtained. If the scan shows dilated bile ducts, suggesting biliary obstruction, an MRCP should be obtained to elucidate the site and cause. Occasionally, biliary obstruction does not cause intrahepatic dilatation (for example, if it is intermittent, as sometimes occurs with bile stones, or if there is cirrhosis, which may reduce liver compliance). In cases of doubt, an MRCP should be performed to exclude the possibility of biliary obstruction.

Following exclusion of obstruction, investigations to determine the cause of jaundice include:

Hepatitis A IgM, hepatitis B surface antigen, hepatitis C antibody, CMV IgM, EBV IgM

Hepatitis E serology if ALT exceeds 1000 or if other tests are negative

Serum immunoglobulins and liver autoantibodies: anti-nuclear antibody (ANA), anti-smooth muscle antibody (A SMA), anti-mitochondrial antibody (AMA) and anti-liver kidney microsomal antibody (LKM) to evaluate the possibility of autoimmune liver conditions

Caeruloplasmin and 24-hour urine copper (to evaluate the possibility of acute Wilson's disease in younger patients)

In cases of severe liver injury, hepatitis B virus (HBV) IgM core antibody should be measured as in some cases of severe hepatitis B, HBV surface antigen may be absent from serum.

When there is a suspicion of acute hepatitis C, viral PCR level should be obtained as serological seroconversion can take up to 8 weeks. If the history is indicative of recent ingestion, paracetamol levels should always be measured. A clotting profile helps to establish the degree of liver function impairment.

When these investigations do not yield a diagnosis, a liver biopsy is needed. Apart from aiding diagnosis, this allows assessment of the grade (degree of inflammation) and stage (degree of fibrosis) of liver injury. When there is more than mild thrombocytopenia or coagulopathy, biopsy should be performed by the trans-jugular route.

Autoimmune Hepatitis

Autoimmune hepatitis (AIH) is a chronic liver disease affecting 6000 to 10,000 people in the United Kingdom. Seventy to seventy-five per cent of cases are women and all ages and races may be affected. Usually there is no apparent precipitant but occasionally, AIH is triggered by certain drugs or by viral hepatitis. About 40 per cent of patients also have another autoimmune disorder (e.g Hashimoto thyroiditis, vitiligo, coeliac disease, inflammatory bowel disease), and others have a family history of autoimmune disease. Presenting symptoms include fatigue and general ill-health.[3–4] About 40 percent of patients present with acute hepatitis and 1 percent with acute liver failure. AIH accounts for 5 percent of patients presenting with jaundice.[5] Older patients can present with decompensated cirrhosis (including ascites and encephalopathy). One third of patients have already developed cirrhosis by the time of presentation. About 20 percent of patients are asymptomatic and are found incidentally to have abnormal liver tests.[3–4]

Serum antibodies (antinuclear, smooth muscle or liver-kidney-microsomal) are found in about 75 percent of patients and a raised serum immunoglobulin G in 85 to 90 percent. Diagnosis of AIH can be challenging because of its diverse clinical presentations and the absence of a single decisive diagnostic test. A scoring system, devised by the AIH International Group and was simplified in 2008 (see Table 25.2) and is based on four criteria: presence of serum autoantibodies, elevated immunoglobulin G or gamma globulins, liver histology and absence of viral hepatitis.[6]

However, about 10 percent of patients with treatment-responsive AIH do not meet the simplified criteria and ultimately diagnosis is based on clinical judgement.

AIH is sometimes subdivided on the basis of serum antibodies: type-1 AIH (with associated positive ANA and SMA), type-2 AIH (positive liver-kidney microsomal [LKM] antibody and type-3 AIH (soluble liver antibody). The differences among these types are subtle and may not be clinically important.

Treatment of AIH

Treatment is usually instituted after liver biopsy, starting with prednisolone (30 mg/day), and then introducing azathioprine (1 mg/kg) a few weeks later. Budesonide can be used if patients develop severe steroid-related side effects such as psychosis or poorly controlled diabetes, or have osteoporosis. Azathioprine can cause marrow depression in some patients therefore the full-blood count needs to be monitored regularly upon starting therapy as in this case. Thiopurine methyltransferase (TPMT) enzyme levels should be checked before starting azathioprine as patients with low levels are at risk of serious bone marrow toxicity. Mycophenolate may be used in these patients or in those with azathioprine side effects. Patients should be maintained on a low-level of prednisolone (5 to 10 mg/day) with

Table 25.2 Simple diagnostic criteria (2008) adapted from Hennes et al.[6]

Criteria		Points
Autoantibodies	ANA or SMA or LKM ≥1:40	1
	ANA or SMA or LKM ≥1:80	2
	SLA + any titre	2
IgG (or gamma globulins)	Upper normal limit	1
	>1.1x normal limit	2
Liver histology*	Compatible with AIH	1
	Typical for AIH	2
Absence of viral hepatitis	Yes	2
	No	0

Points: 7 points: definite AIH; 6 points: probable AIH; ANA, antinuclear antibody; LKM, liver kidney microsomal antibody; SLA, soluble liver antigen; SMA, smooth muscle antibody
* Liver histology:
Typical:
  (1) Interface hepatitis, lymphocytic/lymphocyte or plasma cell-rich infiltrates in portal tracts, extending into the lobule; Figures I and 2
  (2) emperipolesis (active penetration of one cell by another cell)
  (3) hepatic rosette formation (Figure 3).

Compatible: Chronic hepatitis with lymphocytic infiltration without features considered typical. Atypical: Showing signs of another diagnosis like non-alcohol fatty liver disease (NAFLD).[6]

azathioprine 1 mg/kg/day for a minimum of two years. About 80 percent of patients will achieve normal serum ALT and about 60 percent achieve histological remission (no or minimal hepatitis of follow up biopsy).[7] Because of the risk of osteoporosis, patients should also be started on calcium and vitamin D supplements and have a bone density DEXA scan done every 1 to 2 years while on prednisolone treatment.[3] Patients with osteopaenia and osteoporosis should receive bisphosphonates to reduce the incidence of fractures.

In about 10 percent of patients, there is no or very little fall in serum transaminases after 1 to 2 weeks of prednisolone therapy. Therapeutic options include increasing the dose of prednisolone, or using other drugs such as tacrolimus or infliximab. However, these patients are at risk of liver failure and referral (or at least discussion with) a liver transplant centre should be considered.

In patients in whom serum transaminases normalise, repeat liver biopsy should be considered after treatment for 2 to 3 years to check for histological remission (no or minimal hepatitis) and to inform decisions on continuing or altering immunosuppression therapy.

AIH often has a chronic relapsing course which can progress to cirrhosis and liver failure requiring liver transplantation. Such progression is more likely in patients who do not attain remission or who have multiple relapses. Although the outcome of treated disease was previously thought to be good, recent studies involving longer follow up suggest a substantial excess mortality, due to liver disease.[8] Hepatocellular carcinoma may develop in patients with cirrhosis and therefore, surveillance is recommended.[9]

Key Learning Points

- Evaluation of the acutely jaundiced patient should include a detailed history (with particular focus on medications taken over the previous 3 months) and examination.

- The first aim of investigating jaundice is to exclude the possibility of biliary obstruction followed by tests for all causes of acute liver injury.
- A liver biopsy can be useful in differentiating causes of acute hepatitis if the patient is well enough to undergo it.
- Autoimmune hepatitis can present with acute hepatitis. Diagnosis is based on relevant immunological blood tests, histology and exclusion of other causes
- Management of autoimmune hepatitis involves immunosuppression usually with prednisolone and azathioprine. Response to treatment is evaluated by monitoring serum ALT and IgG and by repeat liver biopsy

Acknowledgement: We are grateful to Drs Asha Dube and Patricia Vergani, histopathologists at Sheffield Teaching Hospitals for providing and interpreting the histology slides.

References

1. Friedman LS. Approach to the patient with abnormal liver biochemical function tests. UpToDate 2014. Accessed: 21 Sep 2014. URL: www.uptodate.com/contents/ approach-to-the-patient-with-abnormal-liver-biochemical-and-function-tests

2. Dooley JS, et al. Sherlock's Diseases of the Liver and Biliary System. *Jaundice and Cholestasis*. 12th ed. Oxford. Wiley-Blackwell Publishing 2011, 234–40.

3. Gleeson D and Heneghan MA. British Society of Gastroenterology (BSG) Guidelines for management of autoimmune hepatitis. *Gut* 2011; 60:1–19.

4. Werner M, et al. Epidemiology and the initial presentation of autoimmune hepatitis in Sweden: a nationwide study. *Scand J Gastroenterol* 2008;43: 1232–40.

5. Panayi V, et al. The natural history of autoimmune hepatitis presenting with jaundice. *Eur J Gastroenterol Hepatol* 2014;26:640–5.

6. Hennes EM, et al. Simplied criteria for the diagnosis of autoimmune hepatitis. *Hepatology* 2008;48:169–76.

7. Soloway RR, et al. Clinical, biochemical and histological remission of severe chronic active liver disease: a controlled study of treatments and early prognosis. *Gastroenterology* 1972;63:820–33.

8. Hoeroldt B, et al. Long term outcomes of patients with autoimmune hepatitis managed at a non-transplant centre. *Gastroenterology* 2011;140(7):1980.

9. Yeoman AD, et al. Evaluation of risk factors in the development of hepatocellular carcinoma in autoimmune hepatitis: Implications for follow-up and screening. *Hepatology* 2008;48:863–70.

Chapter 26

Massive Haemorrhage

Sarah Linford and Thearina de Beer

Introduction

Major trauma accounts for the deaths of five million people per year worldwide.[1] Up to 40 per cent of these deaths are as a result of uncontrolled haemorrhage. The evidence base for the pathophysiology, monitoring and management of massive blood loss associated with trauma will be evaluated in this case review.

Case Description

A fifty-six-year-old, previously fit and well, man presented to the emergency department of a major trauma centre as a pre-alerted trauma call. He had fallen off a ladder from a height of three metres; his vital signs on scene were stable.

On arrival in the emergency department, he underwent a primary survey by the attending trauma team which revealed a patent airway, cardiovascular stability, a Glasgow coma scale of fifteen and no immediately life threatening injuries. He was complaining of pain in the pelvic region. The decision was made to arrange a CT scan of his head, spine and pelvis and the trauma team were dismissed. The CT revealed no head or spinal injury, but demonstrated an isolated pelvic fracture and associated haematoma with no signs of acute bleeding. He returned to the emergency department for a secondary survey, during which his cervical spine was cleared. He remained cardiovascularly stable and was transferred to the major trauma ward to await surgical fixation of the pelvic fracture.

Six hours following admission to the ward, he suffered a seizure and cardiac arrest. He was attended by the arrest team who rapidly established that he was in haemorrhagic shock and resuscitation with fluids re-established a spontaneous circulation. The hospital's major haemorrhage protocol was activated and he received a total of ten units of packed cells, six units of fresh frozen plasma, four units of cryoprecipitate and one pool of platelets over the course of the following two hours. During this time, he was intubated and ventilated and transferred to interventional radiology where he underwent embolisation for his exsanguinating pelvic haemorrhage.

He was admitted to intensive care following this procedure where his resultant acidosis, hypothermia and coagulopathy continued to be corrected. Three days after admission, he deteriorated and a chest X-ray revealed features consistent with acute respiratory distress syndrome, most likely secondary to a combination of trauma and massive transfusion. He was extremely difficult to ventilate requiring an FiO_2 of 1.0, PEEP of 15 cmH$_2$O, high inspiratory pressures and inverse ratio ventilation. He gradually improved to the point that he could undergo a percutaneous tracheostomy and subsequent surgical fixation of his pelvis.

On cessation of sedation he was slow to wake and it was clear that he had critical illness polymyopathy. He went on to wean slowly from ventilatory support.

Discussion

Massive blood loss or massive transfusion is defined as a requirement for transfusion of more than ten units of packed red blood cells in 24 hours, or five units over three hours. Massive blood loss is not common in civilian trauma but when it does occur it carries significant morbidity and mortality.

Trauma Induced Coagulopathy

In the last decade, understanding of the pathophysiology of trauma related major haemorrhage has changed with the traditional theory of blood loss, acidosis, haemodilution and hypothermia leading to coagulopathy being replaced. It is now recognised that an acute traumatic coagulopathy (ATC) exists that is specific to trauma patients. Brohi et al.[2] conducted a prospective observational study to evaluate the incidence of coagulopathy following trauma and analyse any effect on mortality. They found that 25 per cent of 1,088 patients were coagulopathic (laboratory values greater than 1.5 normal) on arrival to hospital. Those who were coagulopathic on arrival had a mortality rate of 46 percent compared to 10.9 percent in those with normal coagulation profiles. Pre-hospital fluids were minimal, with the coagulopathic patients receiving less on average than those with normal clotting. The increase in mortality was greater than that associated with severity of injury. Frith et al.[3] went on to further clarify the definition of acute traumatic coagulopathy with a retrospective, multicentre cohort study of 3,646 patients. They found that even with a prothrombin time ratio (PTr) of 1.3, mortality was double that of patients with a PTr of 1.2 or less. In addition, blood transfusion was three times more likely with a PTr of over 1.2. Further to this they found that significant injury load in isolation (without hypoperfusion) and hypoperfusion in isolation (without significant injury) were not associated with an increase in PTr. Only the two in combination (injury severity score greater than 15 and a base deficit greater than 6 mmol/L) were associated with coagulopathy. This paper redefined the threshold for acute traumatic coagulopathy as a ratio of 1.2 or above.

The exact mechanisms by which ATC occurs are not fully understood. Theories include isolated factor V inhibition, systemic anticoagulation perhaps due to activated protein C, impaired platelet function and hyperfibrinolysis, all driven by tissue damage and tissue factor release combined with hypoperfusion. The subsequent addition of acidaemia, hypothermia and haemodilution lead to established trauma induced coagulopathy. The associated mortality however, is clear, probably mediated in part by blood loss and increased transfusion requirements, creating an area of practice in which improving care will save lives.

Bedside Testing of Coagulopathy: TEG®/ROTEM®

Thromboelastography (TEG®) and thromboelastometry (ROTEM) are methods of performing viscoelastic haemostatic assays. They test whole blood to give a bedside evaluation of coagulation including speed and quality of clot formation, clot strength and rate of fibrinolysis.[1] Interest in its use in trauma has arisen as it has been shown to reduce transfusion requirements in liver and cardiac surgery. In addition, the traditional laboratory based tests, prothrombin and activated partial thromboplastin time (PT and APTT), have never been validated in major haemorrhage but were developed as monitoring tests for anticoagulant therapy. PT and APTT only test initiation of clot formation in the plasma and are not tests of whole blood, so do not reflect platelet or fibrinogen function. Therefore, it is possible for PT and APTT to be normal when whole blood coagulation is anything but.[1] Another disadvantage is the time it takes for these laboratory values to be analysed often meaning that the results, when they are available, reflect what was happening 45 minutes ago: a significant amount of time during trauma resuscitation.

The most recent European guidelines on management of bleeding in trauma recommend the use of TEG®/ROTEM® alongside established laboratory tests.[1] They point out the limitations of the technique including its inability to detect the effect of antiplatelet agents and the lack of randomised controlled trials of the technique in trauma associated bleeding. An additional limitation is in interpretation of the complex graphs generated.

The body of evidence to date predominantly evaluates the comparability of TEG®/ROTEM® with laboratory tests. One of the recent studies, conducted by Tauber et al.[4] evaluated the impact of abnormal ROTEM® assays in a prospective cohort study of 334 patients. The study analysed standard laboratory tests and ROTEM® on patients with severe blunt trauma as defined by ISS looking at transfusion requirements, early and 30-day mortality. ROTEM® values were found to correlate well with standard tests and certain abnormalities on ROTEM®, such as mean clot firmness (MCF), were associated with higher mortality. They also identified that hyperfibrinolysis, especially fulminant, was associated with higher mortality (56.6 percent compared to 20 percent overall). They felt that their findings support previous evidence for the benefit of ROTEM®/TEG® in acute resuscitation of trauma by providing additional prognostic information. As pointed out by the EU guidelines,[1] the biggest limiting factor with the research is study design.

The study that needs to be conducted is a randomised controlled trial directly comparing resuscitation by major trauma protocol (to be discussed later) and resuscitation guided by TEG®/ROTEM® with primary outcomes being number of units of blood or products transfused, type of products administered and mortality. If it can be proven that TEG®/ROTEM® reduces the number of blood products given, thereby reducing the adverse effects and cost associated with transfusion, these techniques may become commonplace. Tapia et al.[5] have gone some way in attempting to answer this question by conducting a retrospective cohort study comparing resuscitation of major trauma patients using TEG® guided transfusion with the major trauma protocol. The methodology of the study is somewhat unclear but they do show that patients with penetrating injury and requirement for more than ten units of blood have higher mortality if resuscitated using the major trauma protocol. In addition, there was a higher incidence of late deaths in the blunt trauma group. What is interesting is that they do not show any difference in the total volume of blood and products used between the groups. The study also demonstrates the impact that the major trauma protocols have had on reducing clear fluid resuscitation, with all groups receiving significantly less crystalloid.

Fibrinogen and Antifibrinolytics

Hyperfibrinolysis is a recognised feature of acute traumatic coagulopathy, and as noted earlier is associated with increased mortality.[4] Tranexamic acid, an antifbrinolytic, is recommended by the EU guidelines[1] and is cemented in major haemorrhage protocols following the CRASH2 trial.[6] CRASH2 is a large (n is greater than 20,000), multicentre, randomised placebo controlled trial which evaluated tranexamic acid in adult trauma patients who had, or were at risk of, significant bleeding; looking at in-hospital mortality. They found that all-cause and bleeding related mortality was significantly reduced with tranexamic acid. The initial analysis looked at the use of tranexamic acid in an eight hour window after trauma but subsequent exploratory analysis revealed that the effects were greatest within the first three hours after injury and that treatment beyond this window could actually be harmful.

The role of fibrinogen itself in traumatic coagulopathy has attracted attention. The EU guideline recommends replacing fibrinogen with either cryoprecipitate or fibrinogen concentrate if there is significant bleeding associated with thromboelastometric evidence of fibrinogen deficiency.[1] Good quality evidence for fibrinogen replacement is lacking. A prospective cohort study of 517 patients was conducted by Rourke et al[7] evaluating the role of fibrinogen in bleeding trauma patients. They found, on multiple logistic regression models, that a low fibrinogen level on admission was an independent predictor of mortality at 24 hours and 28 days. Interestingly, they found that the administration of cryoprecipitate did not significantly alter mortality but that fibrinogen administration overall (calculated from typical amounts in platelets, plasma and cryoprecipitate) and thereby an increasing fibrinogen level, was associated with better outcomes. Further studies are needed to evaluate the role of aggressive fibrinogen replacement further.

Major Trauma Protocols: Damage Control Resuscitation

Guidance of resuscitation in the immediate few minutes following a patient's arrival in hospital is predominantly clinical. A rapid and reliable test that correlates with tissue hypoperfusion and severity of haemorrhagic shock is serum lactate. Multiple studies have shown that high lactate on admission and delayed clearance correlate with post-traumatic organ failure and increased mortality.[1] An important caveat to this is that alcohol ingestion will raise lactate levels and so in alcohol associated trauma base deficit may be more reliable.[1]

The change in pathophysiological understanding has led to change in approach to resuscitation. Damage control resuscitation aims to treat acute traumatic coagulopathy by replacing clotting factors early[1] Much evidence for predetermined protocols for blood and product transfusion has come from military studies. Cotton et al.[8] published a prospective cohort study with historical controls to evaluate the introduction of a major haemorrhage protocol in their trauma centre. Severely injured patients (n equal to 211) were compared to historical controls, finding that use of a major haemorrhage protocol reduced 30 day mortality, produced lower overall transfusion requirements and a higher percentage of unexpected survivors, despite the presence of higher ISS scores overall. This, alongside military and other civilian studies, has led to the advent of major haemorrhage protocols in trauma centres worldwide to ensure that blood, plasma, cryoprecipitate and platelets are available for patients with life threatening traumatic haemorrhage. The protocols generally consist of a stepwise supply of packs, the preparation of which commences as soon as the protocol is activated.

What remains unclear is the ratio in which blood and products should be given to the patient and there is significant variation in practice.[1] Holcomb et al.[9] conducted a prospective observational cohort study to assess the association between timing of blood and blood product administration and in-hospital mortality. The number of patients included was 905 and there was significant variability in transfusion ratios. A positive correlation was found between survival at 6 hours following admission and higher early infusion ratios of plasma and platelets (1:1 blood to plasma/platelets). This benefit did not continue beyond 6 hours for platelets or 24 hours for plasma, most likely because peak time for haemorrhagic death was 3 hours, and other causes started to become more prominent. The results of a randomised multicentre trial commissioned on the basis of this study are awaited.

A common consequence of major haemorrhage and massive transfusion is depletion of ionised calcium. European guidelines[1] recommend maintenance of ionised calcium of greater than 0.9 mmol/l on the basis that studies have shown low ionised calcium to be predictive of massive transfusion and mortality. There is no evidence to date, however, that preventing low ionised calcium reduces mortality. Other complications of massive transfusion can be seen in Box 26.1.

Box 26.1 Complications of massive transfusion

- Respiratory system
  - Volume overload and pulmonary oedema
  - TRALI (transfusion related acute lung injury)
- Circulatory system
  - Air embolism
  - Microemboli (increase risk with age of blood)
- Metabolic
  - Hyperkalaemia
  - Hypocalcaemia (secondary to citrate toxicity)
  - Hypothermia
  - Febrile reactions (non-haemolytic)
- Haematological
  - Haemolytic reactions
  - Coagulopathy
- Immunological
  - Immune sensitisation (Rhesus D antigen)
  - Protein related allergic reactions
  - Increased risk of tumour recurrence
- Infective
  - Bacterial contamination
  - Transmission of infections
    - Hepatitis B,C
    - HIV
    - CMV
    - Epstein-Barr virus
    - Parvovirus
    - Syphilis
    - Malaria
    - Trypanosomiasis

Surgical and Radiological Control of Bleeding

Damage control surgery was originally described in reference to laparotomy in the exsanguinating patient who is unresponsive to aggressive resuscitation.[1] The aim is to stop bleeding through targeted vascular control and packing and to control contamination, followed by rapid closure to obtain a period of relative physiological stability during which coagulopathy, acidaemia and hypothermia can be reversed. Subsequently, definitive surgery can be carried out. The remit of damage control surgery has been extended to include orthopaedic procedures, including pelvic stabilisation, and even thoracic and neurosurgical procedures.[1] There are no randomised controlled trials comparing damage control laparotomy with definitive laparotomy, and only one evaluating orthopaedic injuries. There is little research on this topic published in the last decade: historical survival in 1988 was 23.8 per cent. A relatively recent retrospective cohort study conducted by Nicholas et al.[10] looked at rates and survival associated with damage control laparotomy in 250 trauma patients. Forty-five patients underwent damage control laparotomy in this study and 73.3 per cent survived, albeit with significantly greater morbidity and length of stay. The improvement from 1988 is clear but understanding of trauma and haemorrhage pathophysiology, more sophisticated management techniques, the advent of dedicated trauma teams and centres and improvements in intensive care may well explain much of this improvement by way of improved medical care.

The use of interventional radiology to embolise arterial bleeding points has increased dramatically in recent years, particularly in the management of pelvic fracture associated bleeding and splenic bleeding. Currently there are no high quality studies evidencing benefit for the use of radiological intervention in these patients but consensus is that it should be considered as part of haemorrhage control.[1] This is particularly pertinent in patients with ongoing pelvic haemorrhage despite fracture reduction techniques such as binder application as the pelvis is notoriously difficult to pack surgically.

Conclusions and Learning Points

Major traumatic haemorrhage is still a major cause of mortality worldwide. Understanding has moved on dramatically in the last decade and trauma care has improved drastically with the use of protocols and bundles of care. There is still some way to go in terms of defining optimal management.

Key Learning Points

- Severely injured patients are likely to be coagulopathic on arrival in the emergency department.
- TEG®/ROTEM® may guide trauma resuscitation but is unlikely to replace major haemorrhage protocols.
- When resuscitating a severely injured patient, aim for 1:1 red cells to plasma/platelets.
- Give tranexamic acid within 3 hours of injury.
- Repletion of fibrinogen is likely to be important.
- Damage control surgery is a pragmatic approach in a very difficult clinical situation.
- Interventional radiology involvement should be considered in the unstable patient.

References

1. Spahn DR, Bouillon B, Cerny V, et al. Management of bleeding and coagulopathy following major trauma: an updated European guideline. *Crit Care* 2013 Apr 19;17(2):R76.

2. Brohi K, Singh J, Heron M, Coats T. *Acute Traumatic Coagulopathy: J Trauma Inj Infect Crit Care* 2003 Jun;54(6):1127–30.

3. Frith D, Goslings JC, Gaarder C, et al. Definition and drivers of acute traumatic coagulopathy: clinical and experimental investigations. *J Thromb Haemost* 2010 Sep;8(9):1919–25.

4. Tauber H, Innerhofer P, Breitkopf R, et al. Prevalence and impact of abnormal ROTEM(R) assays in severe blunt trauma: results of the 'Diagnosis and Treatment of Trauma-Induced Coagulopathy (DIA-TRE-TIC) study'. *Br J Anaesth* 2011 Sep;107(3):378–87.

5. Tapia NM, Chang A, Norman M, et al. TEG-guided resuscitation is superior to standardized MTP resuscitation in massively transfused penetrating trauma patients. *J Trauma Acute Care Surg.* 2013 Feb;74(2):378–85; discussion 385–6.

6. The importance of early treatment with tranexamic acid in bleeding trauma patients: an exploratory analysis of the CRASH-2 randomised controlled trial. *The Lancet* 2011 Mar;377(9771):1096–101.e2.

7. Rourke C, Curry N, Khan S, et al. Fibrinogen levels during trauma hemorrhage, response to replacement therapy, and association with patient outcomes. *J Thromb Haemost JTH* 2012 Jul;10(7):1342–51.

8. Cotton BA, Gunter OL, Isbell J, et al. Damage control hematology: the impact of a trauma exsanguination protocol on survival and blood product utilization. *J Trauma* 2008 May;64(5):1177–82; discussion 1182–3.

9. Holcomb JB, del Junco DJ, Fox EE, et al. The prospective, observational, multicenter, major trauma transfusion (PROMMTT) study: comparative effectiveness of a time-varying treatment with competing risks. *JAMA Surg* 2013 Feb;148(2):127–36.

10. Nicholas JM, Rix E, Easley KA, et al. Changing patterns in the management of penetrating abdominal trauma: the more things change, the more they stay the same. *J Trauma-Inj Infect* 2003;55(6):1095–110.

Chapter 27

Glucose Emergencies

James Keegan and Gordon Craig

Introduction

Hyperosmolar hyperglycaemic state (HHS) and diabetic ketoacidosis are the most serious acute presentations of diabetes mellitus and represent a significant cause of mortality and morbidity. Although the presentations have much in common, there are a number of important differences in diagnosis and management. This case illustrates a common presentation of a hyperglycaemic emergency and discusses the key management principles.

Case Description

A 42-year-old male computer software engineer of African ethnicity was admitted by ambulance following a seizure at home. He had been unwell for 4 days and had become increasingly drowsy and confused. He was obese (BMI 44), but had no other medical history, and did not smoke.

The ambulance crew terminated the seizure with intravenous benzodiazepines and he was found to be profoundly hyperglycaemic with a blood glucose machine (BM) test greater than 55 mmol/l. On arrival in the Emergency Department he remained drowsy (GCS 8) and disoriented. Examination indicated profound dehydration, tachycardia 115 bpm and hypotension (BP 80/50 mmHg). Arterial blood gas analysis revealed a metabolic acidosis (pH 7.23 PaO$_2$ 13.9, PaCO$_2$ 5.4, HCO$_3^-$ 16) and confirmed severe hyperglycaemia (blood glucose 59 mmol/l). Laboratory blood tests indicated haemoglobin 150 g/l, sodium 155 mmol/l, potassium 5.6 mmol/l, urea 27 mmol/l, creatinine 304 umol/l. ECG demonstrated atrial fibrillation with a fast ventricular response.

The patient received a 500 ml 0.9% saline bolus, followed by 1 litre of saline over the next hour. A urinary catheter was inserted and drained small volumes of concentrated urine. Urinary dipstick testing revealed 4+ glucose and a trace of ketones. Capillary ketone measurement was not immediately available. He was subsequently anaesthetised and intubated for airway protection, and admitted to the intensive care unit with a diagnosis of hyperosmolar hyperglycaemic syndrome secondary to undiagnosed type 2 diabetes mellitus.

Invasive arterial blood pressure monitoring and central venous access were established. The patient was started on a titrated fluid replacement regime with 0.9 percent saline and plasma glucose, sodium and potassium concentrations were monitored hourly. Plasma osmolality was calculated at 396 mOsm/kg.

Shortly after admission, T-wave inversion in lead II & III of the ECG was demonstrated, with a significantly raised troponin level. A non-ST elevation myocardial infarction was diagnosed and he was treated with a loading dose of 300 mg Aspirin and therapeutic low-molecular weight heparin.

201

After 6 hours of fluid replacement, an insulin infusion was started at 5 units/hr (0.5 units/kg/hr) and glucose concentrations decreased gradually to 16 mmol/l by day four of admission. The acute kidney injury improved without the need for haemofiltration. He was successfully extubated on day five but required high flow nasal oxygen therapy for a further two days due to bi-basal atelectasis and obese body habitus.

Over the following two weeks, the patient continued to require on-going insulin infusion and was therefore started on a basal-bolus insulin regime. He was discharged for outpatient rehabilitation after three weeks.

Discussion

The importance of DKA has been recognised for some time and management guidelines have become widespread. It is often difficult to differentiate between HHS and DKA, but despite this there are several important diagnostic and management differences.

Presentation & Diagnosis

Patients with both DKA and HHS commonly present with a history of polydipsia, polyuria, dehydration, weight loss and altered mental state. Generalised abdominal pain, nausea & vomiting are uncommon in HHS but occur frequently (greater than 50 percent) in DKA.[1] Abdominal pain may be secondary to the DKA or result from a primary surgical problem and an acute abdomen should be considered in any patient with a relevant history, particularly those with severe DKA.[2]

Examination findings include tachycardia, hypotension, tachypnoea (or Kussmaul respiration in DKA) decreased skin turgor, lethargy or coma. HHS is more frequently associated with coma, focal neurological signs and seizures (as in this case), although these do not normally occur until the serum osmolality is greater than 320mOsm/kg.[1] For this reason, the previous term hyperglycaemic non-ketotic (HONK) coma was modified to HHS.[3]

The diagnostic criteria for DKA are well established (Box 27.1). In contrast precise diagnostic criteria for HHS do not exist, and it is sometimes difficult to differentiate it from DKA. However this differentiation is important as there are some fundamental management differences and complications. Consequently the Joint Diabetes Societies Inpatient Care Group defined characteristic features of HHS (Box 27.2). Importantly significant

---

Box 27.1 DKA Criteria[2]

- Ketonaemia ≥3.0 mmol/l or significant ketonuria (>2+ on standard urine sticks)
- Blood glucose >11.0 mmol/l or known diabetes mellitus
- Bicarbonate <15.0 mmol/l and/or venous pH <7.3

Box 27.2 Characteristic Features of HHS[3]

- Hypovolaemia – severely dehydrated and unwell
- Marked hyperglycaemia (>30 mmol/l) without significant ketonuria (<3 mmol/l) or acidosis (pH >7.3, bicarbonate >15 mmol/l)
- Osmolality usually 320 mosm/kg or more

ketonaemia is rare in HHS, although mild acidosis may still occur due to pre-renal failure,[3] as seen in this case study. Profound dehydration and hypovolaemia are key to the diagnosis of HHS.

HHS patients are classically an older patient group, although the condition is increasingly being diagnosed in younger people as here, and it is often the first presentation of type 2 diabetes in these patients.[3,4] DKA is more common in type 1 diabetics.

Infection is the most common precipitant in both DKA and HHS. Others include inadequate or missed insulin doses, pancreatitis, myocardial infarction, cerebrovascular accident and drugs (e.g. corticosteroids, thiazides, sympathomimetics).[1]

Pathophysiology

In DKA insulin deficiency combined with an increase in counter regulatory hormones (glucagon, cortisol, growth hormone, catecholamines) facilitates increased hepatic glucogneogenesis and glycogenolysis, with impaired peripheral glucose utilisation, and consequent hyperglycaemia. Lipolysis is up-regulated, resulting in an increase in hepatic oxidation of free fatty acids and uncontrolled production of the ketoacids acetone, 3-beta-hydroxybutyrate and acetoacetate. Hyperglycaemia produces an osmotic diuresis and this results in dehydration, with associated extracellular electrolyte shifts (potassium, phosphate) and subsequent electrolyte depletion.[1,2] This is an acute process and patients typically present within hours of onset.

In contrast HHS develops over several days, and consequently the dehydration and metabolic abnormalities are more severe. A relative insulin deficiency again results in hyperglycaemia and subsequent osmotic diuresis. However, insulin levels are adequate to prevent lipolysis and hepatic ketogenesis. Due to the longer natural history, and older patient cohort (with associated co-morbidities, altered thirst response and delayed recognition of symptoms) the level of dehydration and electrolyte disturbance is often severe.

Management

In all patients the initial actions should include immediate assessment of airway, breathing, and circulation and intravenous access. Initial examination and investigations are directed at confirming the diagnosis and establishing the severity. Investigations should include blood ketones, capillary blood glucose, venous blood gases, urea & electrolytes, full blood count, blood cultures, ECG, Chest x-ray and urinalysis. It is often at this stage that a critical care physician is involved.

Detailed protocols for DKA and HHS are available from the Joint British Diabetes Societies.[2,3]

Table 27.1 Typical fluid and electrolyte deficits in DKA & HHS[1–3]

	DKA	HHS
Water	100 ml/kg	100–220 ml/kg
Sodium	7–10 mmol/kg	5–13 mmol/kg
Chloride	3–5 mmol/kg	5–15 mmol/kg
Potassium	3–5 mmol/kg	4–6 mmol/kg

DKA

The key targets in management of DKA are: 1. Restoration of circulating volume, 2. Replacement of potassium, 3. Abolition of ketogenesis and control of hyperglycaemia.

Indications for Critical Care Admission

The presence of one or more of the following criteria are defined by the Joint Diabetes Societies as indicating severe DKA and should prompt consideration for High Dependency (level 2) care:[2]

- Blood ketones >6 mmol/l
- Bicarbonate level <5 mmol/l
- Venous/arterial pH <7.0
- Hypokalaemia on admission (under 3.5 mmol/l)
- GCS less than 12
- Oxygen saturation below 92 percent on air (assuming normal baseline respiratory function)
- Systolic BP below 90 mmHg
- Pulse over 100 or below 60 bpm
- Anion gap above 16 [Anion Gap = $(Na + K) - (Cl + HCO^3)$]

Restoration of Circulating Volume

In severe DKA presenting with systolic BP less than 90 mmHg fluid boluses of 500 ml 0.9 percent saline are recommended over 10 to 15 mins. If there is no improvement after 1L of fluid the cause of hypotension should be urgently re-evaluated.

Once a systolic blood pressure greater than 90 mmHg is established, a standard fluid regime is recommended (Table 27.2), but this should be guided by frequent reassessment of the clinical picture, fluid balance and laboratory results. Caution with aggressive fluid resuscitation should be exercised in young (less than 25 years) or older patients (who are at greater risk of cerebral oedema), those with cardiac or renal dysfunction and in pregnancy.

There is debate regarding the recommendation to use 0.9 percent saline instead of a more balanced fluid such as Hartmann's solution, as the former contributes to a hyperchloraemic metabolic acidosis. The reason for recommending 0.9 percent saline is that it is readily available pre-mixed with potassium chloride. However, in a critical care environment it is acceptable to use other balanced solutions if attention is also given to potassium

Table 27.2 Typical fluid regimen for a 70 kg adult (reproduced with kind permission of The Joint British Diabetes Societies[2])

Fluid	Volume
0.9% sodium chloride 1l	1000 ml over 1 hour
0.9% sodium chloride 1l with potassium chloride	1000 ml over next 2 hours
0.9% sodium chloride 1l with potassium chloride	1000 ml over next 2 hours
0.9% sodium chloride 1l with potassium chloride	1000 ml over next 4 hours
0.9% sodium chloride 1l with potassium chloride	1000 ml over next 4 hours
0.9% sodium chloride 1l with potassium chloride	1000 ml over next 6 hours

replacement, as addition of extra potassium can be more safely managed. A recent study failed to demonstrate superiority of Ringer's lactate solution in DKA.[5] The aim of fluid administration is to restore circulating volume, clear ketones and correct electrolyte disturbance.[2] It is important to note that addition of 40 mmol of potassium chloride increases the calculated osmolality of 1L 0.9 percent saline by 80 mosmol/l to 388 mosmol/l.

Replacement of Potassium

In hyperglycaemic states, there is a shift of potassium into the extracellular space due to acidosis. If this is combined with pre-renal dysfunction from dehydration the patient may present with hyperkalaemia. Therefore, potassium replacement is not recommended in the initial fluid replacement if serum potassium is greater than 5.5 mmol/l. Nevertheless, there is normally a total body deficit of potassium, and this becomes apparent after initial fluid resuscitation and insulin administration, which prompts an intracellular shift of potassium and consequently hypokalaemia may develop. Therefore serum potassium should be measured 1 to 2 hourly (via venous blood gas), and replacement should be routinely provided if serum potassium is 3.5 to 5.5 mmol/l. If the patient is significantly hypokalaemic on presentation, potassium should be replaced before insulin administration.

Insulin Administration

Insulin should be provided via a weight-based fixed-rate intravenous insulin infusion (FRIII). Previous variable rate regimens ('sliding scale') do not adequately adapt to the obese or pregnant patient. Insulin at 0.1 units/kg should be started as soon as fluid resuscitation is commenced. If the patient is already taking long-acting subcutaneous insulins, these should be continued to prevent rebound hyperglycaemia.[2]

Modern bedside monitors are now able to measure blood ketone (3-beta-hydroxy-butarate) levels. This represents the best practice in monitoring resolution of ketonaemia, and a rate of fall of more than 0.5 mmol/l/hr should be targeted. If it is not available, a venous glucose fall of 3 mmol/l/hr and not greater and bicarbonate rise of more than 3 mmol/l/hr should be used as alternative markers. More rapid decreases in blood glucose should be avoided. If these targets are not met, the insulin infusion should be increased by 1 unit per hour every hour until the targets are achieved.

Once the serum glucose is less than 14 mmol/l, a 10 percent glucose infusion should be started at 125 ml/hr, in addition to the 0.9 percent saline fluid replacement (as long as there is no evidence of fluid overload), to prevent hypoglycaemia. The insulin infusion should be changed to a subcutaneous regime once blood ketone levels are less than 0.6 mmol/l and the patient is able to eat and drink. Urinary ketones should not be used to guide treatment as they will remain positive even after the DKA has resolved.[2]

HHS

In HHS the biochemical derangement has normally developed over a longer period. Hyperglycaemia increases serum osmolality and the resultant shift of water from the intracellular to the extracellular space causes a dilutional hyponatraemia. An osmotic diuresis occurs causing the patient to become dehydrated and this exacerbates the hyper-osmolar state, with associated pre-renal failure. Hypernatraemia occurs as a late sign, with on-going contraction of the intravascular space.[1]

The key to management of HHS is therefore the appreciation and close monitoring of the serum osmolality. Rapid reduction of glucose or sodium with insulin or hypotonic fluid will cause a precipitous fall in osmolality and risks uncontrolled excessive fluid and electrolyte shifts that may result in cardiovascular collapse, cerebral oedema and electrolyte disturbance. High serum osmolality combined with immobility also increases the risk of arterial and venous thromboembolic disease.

Assessment of Severity

The Joint Diabetes Societies define the following criteria as signs of severe HHS that warrant High Dependency (level 2) care:[3]

- Osmolality greater than 350 mosmol/kg
- Sodium above 160 mmol/l
- Venous / arterial pH below 7.1
- Hypokalaemia (less than 3.5 mmol/l) or hyperkalaemia (greater than 6 mmol/l) on admission
- Glasgow Coma Scale (GCS) less than 12
- Oxygen saturation below 92 percent on air (assuming normal baseline respiratory function)
- Systolic blood pressure below 90 mmHg
- Pulse over 100 or below 60 bpm
- Urine output less than 0.5 ml/kg/hr
- Serum creatinine above 200 μmol/l
- Hypothermia
- Macrovascular event such as myocardial infarction or stroke

The key principles of management of HHS are:[3]

1. Replace fluid and electrolyte losses, 2. Slowly restore osmolality and glucose to normal levels and 3. Prevent secondary complications

Replacement of Fluid and Electrolyte Losses

Initial fluid resuscitation with 1L 0.9 percent sodium chloride over 1 hour is recommended.

This will cause a fall in blood glucose even without concurrent insulin infusion. As blood glucose falls serum sodium will inevitably rise due to the movement of water back into the intracellular space. A sodium rise of 2.4 mmol/l occurs for each 5.5 mmol/l fall in glucose.[6] If serum osmolality is falling, this rising sodium is not an indication for hypotonic 0.45 percent saline.

On-going fluid resuscitation should be based upon regular patient re-assessment, with a target to achieve 2 to 3 l positive fluid balance over 6 hours. Serum sodium should not fall by greater than 10 mmol/l in 24 hours.[3] If serum sodium is rising and serum osmolality is not falling at the appropriate rate this suggests under-resuscitation and the rate of fluid should be increased. Hypotonic 0.45 percent saline should only be used if the osmolality is increasing despite a positive fluid balance.

As with DKA, serum potassium should be maintained in the range 3.5 to 5.5 mmol/l.

In the case presented above, the patient was managed with carefully titrated 0.9 percent saline and Hartmann's solution and serum electrolytes were monitored with arterial blood gas analysis hourly. Serum potassium was maintained with concentrated potassium given via a central venous catheter. However, it is important to note that these techniques for electrolyte replacement should only be performed in an intensive care environment with regular blood gas monitoring.

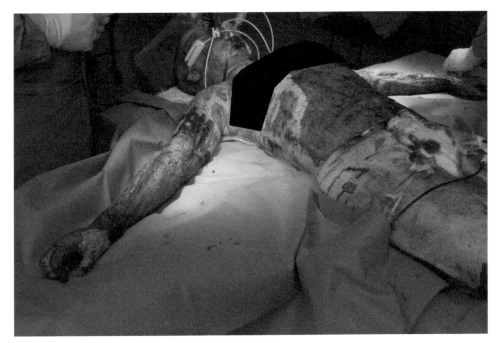

Figure 3.1 Image: intra-op wound debridement and grafting.

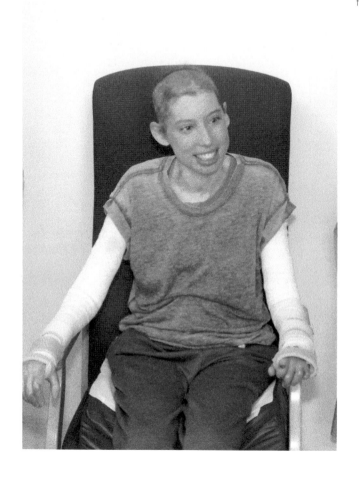

Figure 3.3 Image: patient attending for outpatient follow up.

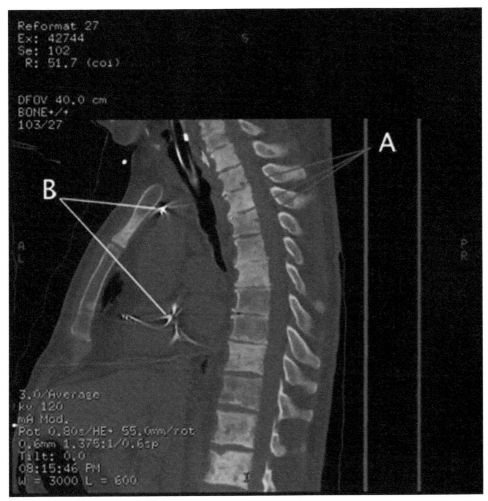

Figure 20.1 Computed tomography of the chest, sagittal section. The red-lines marked with the letter 'A' highlight some of the multiple sclerotic lesions demonstrated by the scan felt to be in keeping with metastatic prostate disease. The yellow lines from letter 'B' point to the ICD device, seen entering the heart. The endotracheal tube can also be seen in situ.

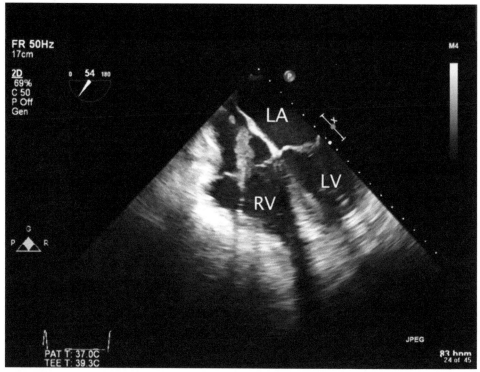

Figure 20.2 A transoesophageal echocardiogram showing the mid-oesophageal four chamber view. The ICD can be seen entering the right atrium, passing through the tricuspid valve and continuing into the right ventricle. A large vegetation can clearly be seen attached to the ICD contained within the right atrium. The tricuspid valve was clear of vegetation as were the other remaining valves, There were no atrial or ventricular septal defects and biventricular function was normal. RV – right ventricle, LA left atrium, LV – left ventricle.

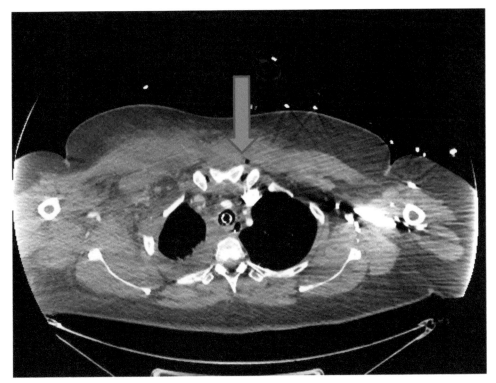

Figure 23.1 CT scan demonstrating free air in the soft tissue.

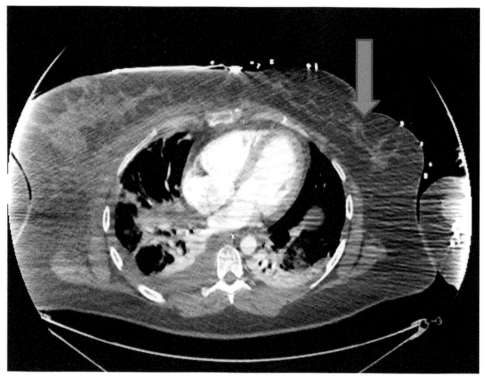

Figure 23.2 CT scan demonstrating soft tissue inflammation.

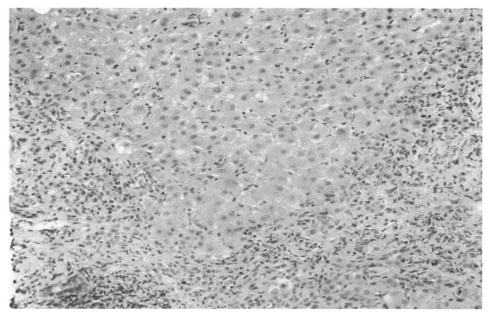

Figure 25.1 Liver biopsy showing interface hepatitis (inflammation of hepatocytes at the junction of the portal tract and hepatic parenchyma).

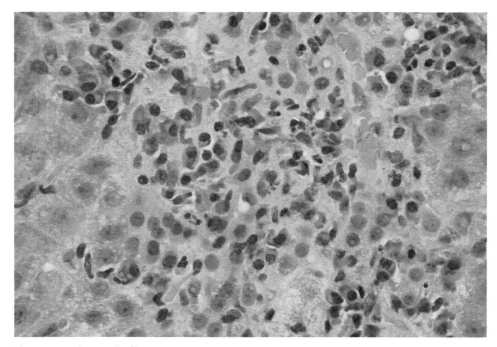

Figure 25.2 Plasma cell infiltrate.

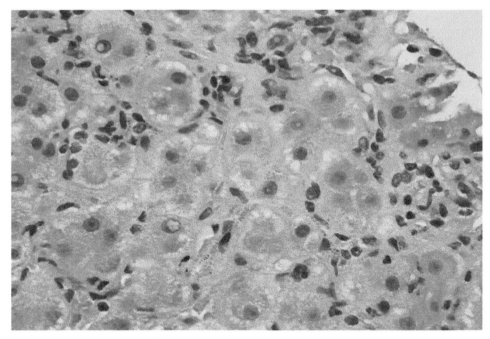

Figure 25.3 Rosettes (clusters of reactive hepatocytes surrounded by inflammatory cells).

Normalise the Osmolality

Serum osmolality should be calculated unless laboratory measurement of osmolality is easily available. This forms an important aspect of diagnosis and monitoring, and should be repeated hourly.

Calculated osmolality $= 2Na^+ + glucose + urea$

Osmolality will decline with fluid resuscitation and insulin infusion. Excessively rapid correction places the patient at risk of neurological complications such as central pontine myelinolysis and cerebral oedema. The target rate of fall in osmolarity is 3 to 8 mosm/l/hr[3].

Normalise Blood Glucose

In HHS, the serum glucose level will often fall with initial fluid resuscitation, and patients are normally highly insulin sensitive. Therefore there is a risk of a precipitous initial fall in blood glucose and serum osmolality. Consequently, the presence of relative hypo-insulinaemia should be identified by testing for significant ketonaemia (blood 3-beta- hydroxybutarate greater than 1 mmol/l). Only if this is present should insulin be started. For all other patients, insulin is only introduced when the rate of fall of glucose from fluid resuscitation has reached a plateau.

Where insulin is started, the dose is reduced in HHS to 0.05 units/kg as a fixed rate insulin infusion. A maximum decrease in blood glucose of 5 mmol/l/hr should be targeted.

Biochemical normalisation is more gradual in HHS and may take up to 72 hours. Once blood glucose of 10 to 15 mmol/l has been achieved, transfer to subcutaneous insulin should be considered.

All patients should have specialist diabetic team input during their hospitalisation and follow up. This gives an opportunity to optimise diabetic control and improve patient education, both of which are vital in preventing recurrence complications.

Complications

Thromboembolic Disease

All diabetic patients are at increased risk of venous and arterial thromboembolic disease, particularly in hyperglycaemic states. The risk is highest in HHS as demonstrated in this case, where the patient suffered an associated myocardial infarction. Hypernatraemia and associated activation of pro-coagulant factors induces a hyper-coagulable state.[7] Prophylactic low molecular weight heparin is recommended for all HHS and DKA patients. Full anticoagulation should be used on an individual patient basis where acute coronary syndrome or venous thromboembolic disease is suspected,[3] although some advocate full anticoagulation for all HHS patients.[8]

Cerebral Complications

Confusion, decreased conscious level and seizures are all relatively common in HHS. The causes are probably multi-factorial: electrolyte disturbance, hyper-osmolality (confusion is more common if serum osmolality greater than 320 mosm/l)[1] dehydration, sepsis, renal dysfunction and hypoglycaemia during treatment may all be implicated.

Cerebral oedema and central pontine myelinolysis are rare but potentially devastating complications. HHS patients are particularly prone to these problems especially if excessive fluid and insulin administration cause precipitous shifts of glucose, sodium and water. Cerebral hypoperfusion with subsequent reperfusion injury may also be implicated.[9]

Young adults and children with DKA are also particularly at risk of cerebral oedema, and separate paediatric guidelines are available for these cases.

Foot Protection

All patients are at risk of peripheral neuropathy and foot ulceration. Appropriate heel care and careful monitoring should be instituted early.

Conclusion

DKA and HHS are both important complications of diabetes. This case illustrates that although there are some similarities such as an elevated blood glucose on presentation, differentiation between them is vital as the treatment pathways are different. National and local guidelines for the management of these conditions are widely available.

Key Learning Points

- The aim of treatment in DKA is controlled correction of fluid losses, ketoacidosis and glucose over 12 to 48 hours, depending on severity.
- Treatment of HHS should be more gradual over 48 to 72 hours.
- Normal saline is the recommended fluid in a ward environment though balanced salt solutions are used in critical care as potassium replacement can be safely managed.
- Extra caution should be taken in children and young adults with DKA as they are more at risk of developing cerebral oedema.
- Fixed rate insulin infusions should be used in preference to a 'sliding scale', at a rate of 0.1 units/kg in DKA. In HHS 0.05 units/kg insulin should be started only after adequate fluid replacement.
- DKA patients should be monitored with regular venous blood gas and blood ketone levels.
- HHS patients should be monitored with regular calculation of the serum osmolality.
- Careful management of serum potassium is important in DKA and HHS.
- Flow charts should be used to document and track changes in ketones, acid-base, electrolytes, glucose and osmolality along with accurate fluid balance.
- Thromboembolic disease, leg ulceration and cerebral complications should be considered in patients with HHS.

References

1. Kitabchi AE, Umpierrez GE, Miles JM, Fisher JN. Hyperglycemic crises in adult patients with diabetes. *Diabetes Care* 2009; 32(7):1335–43.

2. Dhatariya K, Savage M. Joint British Diabetes Societies guideline for the management of diabetic ketoacidosis. 2013. www.diabetes.org.uk/Documents/About%20Us/What%20we%20say/Management-of-DKA-241013.pdf (Accessed 21 July, 2014)

3. Scott A, Claydon A. The management of the hyperosmolar hyperglycaemic state (HHS) in adults with diabetes. 2012. www.diabetes.org.uk/Documents/Position%20statements/JBDS-IP-HHS-Adults.pdf (Accessed 21 July, 2014)

4. Rosenbloom AL. Hyperglycemic hyperosmolar state: an emerging pediatric problem. *J Pediatr* 2010; 156(2):180–4.

5. Van Zyl DG, Rheeder P, Delport E. Fluid management in diabetic-acidosis–Ringer's

lactate versus normal saline: a randomized controlled trial. *QJM* 2012;105(4): 337–43.

6. Katz MA. Hyperglycemia-induced hyponatremia: calculation of expected serum sodium depression. *N Engl J Med* 1973;289(16):843–4.

7. Carr ME. Diabetes mellitus: a hypercoagulable state. *J Diabetes Complicat* 2001;15(1):44–54.

8. Gouveia CF, Chowdhury TA. Managing hyperglycaemic emergencies: an illustrative case and review of recent British guidelines. *Clin Med* 2013;13(2):160–2.

9. Glaser N, Barnett P, McCaslin I, et al. Risk factors for cerebral edema in children with diabetic ketoacidosis. The Pediatric Emergency Medicine Collaborative Research Committee of the American Academy of Pediatrics. *N Engl J Med* 2001;344(4):264–9.

Chapter 28

Endocrine Emergencies

Aylwin J. Chick

Introduction

Endocrine disorders, particularly syndromes of thyroid overactivity or adrenal deficiency, may be important differential diagnoses in adults with critical illness. Although the initial symptoms of such conditions may be non-specific and gradual in onset, once the patient becomes critically unwell they require immediate recognition and management in order to achieve a successful outcome.

Case Presentation

A 40-year-old man presented to the Emergency Room overnight and was referred to Critical Care with a clinical impression of septic shock. The Emergency Room physicians were concerned that despite giving 20 ml/kg of intravenous crystalloid, his blood pressure had remained low at 70/46 mmHg. Other vital signs were reported as respiratory rate 38 breaths/minute, oxygen saturation 92 per cent on air, heart rate 120 bpm, temperature 37.7 °C. The receiving team had already taken blood for culture and administered a broad-spectrum antibiotic.

The man was of African ethnicity and appeared breathless at rest and agitated on initial assessment. Breath sounds were clear and oxygen saturations rose to 98 per cent with supplementary nasal oxygen.

His skin was hot and dry, pulse regular and a further intravenous fluid bolus of 500 ml 0.9 per cent saline (<10 ml/kg was administered). Although opening eyes to voice, he was restless and disorientated, with a random blood sugar of 5.4 mmol/litre. There was no meningism or focal neurological deficit, and no skin lesions (oral or cutaneous) or rashes were evident.

Further history was obtained from the patient's sister who explained that he had collapsed overnight while vomiting, after being lethargic and vomiting intermittently for the preceding 3 days. For 6 weeks he had complained of abdominal pains, loss of appetite and weight loss of 7 kg associated with occasional fevers. Two days earlier his general practitioner (GP) had sent basic biochemical blood tests for investigation.

Further social history revealed that although originally from South Africa, he had been working in the United Kingdom as a schoolteacher for some years. He had recently visited family in South Africa although there were no known tuberculosis contacts and no family history of note. He had no known allergies, took no medications and had been previously well.

Initial Investigations

Table 28.1 indicates the initial biochemistry results and the GP's blood tests, sent two days previously. Initial ECG showed a sinus tachycardia and portable chest radiograph (CXR) indicated evenly distributed, diffuse 'miliary' opacifications across both lung fields.

Table 28.1 Biochemistry results from admission & during treatment

	Initial patient result at GP practice	8 hours after treatment commenced	Reference range & units
Sodium / Na+	127	131	133–146 mmol/litre
Potassium / K+	5.9	5.4	3.5–5.3 mmol/litre
Urea	24	14	2.5–7.8 mmol/litre
Creatinine	125	105	64–104 µmol/litre
Chloride	95	99	95–108 mmol/litre
Venous glucose (random)	5.7	6.8	3.5–7.7 mmol/litre

	Initial arterial blood gas sample on air (Emergency Room)	8 hours after treatment commenced, on 2 litres/ minute nasal O2	Reference range & units
pH	7.20	7.31	7.35–7.45
pO2	9.9	14.0	>8.0 kpa
pCO2	3.8	3.9	4.0–6.0 kpa
Base excess	−10	−7	+/− 2 mmol/L
Bicarbonate	18	20	22–29 mmol/L
O2 saturations	92	96	>93%

Despite two further 500 ml fluid challenges, the patient remained restless and hypotensive.

Subsequent Intensive Care Unit Progress

Further baseline blood samples for urea, electrolytes and bicarbonate were taken in addition to a random cortisol measurement and an ACTH (adrenocorticotrophic hormone) level. 100 mg intravenous hydrocortisone was given as a bolus and prescribed to continue at 100 mg every six hours in addition to intravenous antiemetics.

The patient was transferred to an isolation room on the intensive care unit and given a further 1000 ml 0.9 per cent saline over the next hour. Despite this his blood pressure remained less than 80 mmHg systolic and he was oliguric with an initial hourly urine output of just 10 ml.

With invasive blood pressure monitoring and central venous access, vasopressors were commenced with a target mean arterial pressure (MAP) of 70 mmHg. Further volume depletion was corrected with a combination of Hartmann's crystalloid solution and 0.9 per cent saline, to a total of a further 3 litres over the following 12 hours. The vasopressor requirements improved significantly within 8 hours and a repeat arterial blood gas at 8 hours post-ICU admission showed improvement in all parameters. (see Table 28.1) Vasopressors were discontinued 16 hours after admission to ICU.

Over the following two days, he was reviewed by Infectious Diseases and Endocrinology specialists. After a series of investigations (Table 28.2), he was started on

Table 28.2 Selected investigation results (MTB: mycobacterium tuberculosis)

	Investigation result
Random cortisol at admission	<6 (reference range 180–620 nmol/l at 6am)
ACTH (adrenocorticotropic hormone) at admission	44 (reference range 2.2–13.3 pmol/l at 8am)
Blood cultures at admission	Negative after five days
HIV antigen & antibody tests	Negative
Sputum: acid-fast bacilli smears	Positive
Sputum: Xpert MTB/RIF test	Mycobacterium TB detected, no Rifampicin resistance detected
Lumbar puncture	normal – no evidence of TB meningitis
Chest X-ray report	"reticulonodular infiltrate distributed uniformly throughout both lung fields, 3 mm diameter. Bilateral hilar lymphadenopathy noted. Differential would include miliary TB, lymphangitic spread of malignancy."
CT chest and abdomen	"numerous 3 mm nodules throughout lung fields. Bilateral hilar lymphadenopathy. No pericardial effusion. Multiple foci of low attenuation in liver and spleen, without contrast enhancement. Both adrenal glands are enlarged. Findings consistent with disseminated TB."

anti-tuberculous treatment and public health authorities notified. Steroid treatment was continued as an oral preparation prescribed by the endocrinology team, who also arranged education for the patient and his family regarding the importance of continued steroid treatment.

After four days in critical care, the patient regained appetite and was mobilising with the physiotherapists. After a four further days in the regional Infectious Diseases unit, he was discharged home to continue steroid replacement and anti-tuberculous treatment under close follow-up.

Case Discussion

Clinical Features of Adrenal Insufficiency

This man presented with clinical features consistent with septic shock. However, the biochemical picture of elevated potassium and low sodium, coupled with the history of progressive lethargy, vomiting, weight loss, weakness and fever, were all in keeping with a 'classical' presentation of an adrenal crisis.

Adrenal crisis refers to overwhelming and life-threatening adrenal insufficiency. Most cases presenting in the United Kingdom and Europe are due to autoimmune adrenalitis;[1] however, this patient was at risk for TB given his travel history. Although the typical clinical features of chronic adrenal insufficiency may be non-specific, the Critical Care physician should be alert to these in the background history of patients presenting with shock (Table 28.3). Adrenal crisis should be suspected if there is volume depletion, dehydration or shock that seems out of proportion to the severity of the apparent illness.

Table 28.3 Clinical features of chronic adrenal insufficiency / features raising suspicion of acute adrenal crisis (source: Burke CW, *Clin Endocrinol Metab.* 1985;14(4):947)

	Symptoms	Signs	Laboratory findings
Clinical features of chronic adrenal insufficiency (present in ≥30% of cases)	Lethargy, tiredness, weakness	Hypotension (systolic BP <110mmHg)	Hyponatremia
	Nausea, vomiting	Hyperpigmentation	Hyperkalaemia
	Loss of appetite	Weight loss	Raised urea (azotemia)
	Abdominal pain, constipation		Anaemia
Clinical features raising suspicion of an adrenal crisis	Nausea / vomiting on a background of weight loss, loss of appetite	Hypotension, dehydration	As above, plus:
	Abdominal pain, may present as "acute abdomen"	Shock out of proportion to severity of current illness	Other autoimmune endocrine disorders such as hypogonadism, hypothyroidism
	Fever (otherwise unexplained)	Hyperpigmentation or vitiligo	Unexplained hypoglycaemia

One 'classical' feature of primary adrenal insufficiency, skin or buccal hyperpigmentation due to chronic excess ACTH stimulating melanocytes is not universally found, as in this case. Similarly, hypoglycaemia is only rarely a presenting feature of adrenal crisis.

Myocardial dysfunction and cardiomyopathy have been described in young patients presenting with adrenal crisis and should be screened for by means of ECG initially and consideration for subsequent echocardiography.[2]

Adrenal crisis still accounts for death in 15 per cent of patients with known adrenal insufficiency[3] and patients and their family members should be educated regarding the features of the condition and 'sick-day' rules for steroid replacement.

There are several major reasons for an underlying adrenal insufficiency, which is more common in women than men:[1]

- Autoimmune adrenalitis, leading to destruction of the adrenal cortex
  - There may be a background of other autoimmune disorders such as pernicious anaemia, diabetes mellitus or thyroid disease.
- Infectious adrenalitis
  - Disseminated TB or invasive fungal infections in patients from countries with a high prevalence of such diseases
- Bilateral adrenal haemorrhagic infarction
  - associated with severe sepsis from meningococcemia (Waterhouse-Friderichsen syndrome) and certain other severe bacterial infections;
  - other risk factors include physical trauma and recent anticoagulation

- Adrenal infiltration by malignancy or systemic disease
  - . lymphoma, disseminated lung or breast cancer may infiltrate adrenals;
  - . sarcoidosis, amyloidosis or haemochromatosis that involves the adrenal glands.

- Drugs
  - . Etomidate, ketoconazole, fluconazole may inhibit cortisol biosynthesis, while rifampicin, phenytoin and barbiturates may accelerate the metabolism of cortisol

- Genetic disorders leading to adrenal insufficiency, e.g. congenital adrenal hyperplasia.

TB as a Cause of Adrenal Insufficiency

Tuberculosis (TB) was the most common cause of primary adrenal insufficiency when first described by Thomas Addison. Although autoimmune adrenalitis is now a more common cause in Europe and in the United Kingdom, TB remains an important cause worldwide. The adrenals are involved in 40 percent of cases of miliary TB, although actual adrenal dysfunction may be present in only 3 percent of cases.[6] The incidence of TB continues to be high in the United Kingdom compared to other western European countries.

If TB is suspected as a cause, appropriate hospital infection control measures should be observed to reduce the potential for cross-infection. Specific advice is required from Infectious Diseases or other TB specialists regarding investigations and possible treatment.

Secondary adrenal insufficiency is also crucial to appreciate, although frequently overlooked by doctors.[3,4] Patients who regularly receive physiologically significant doses of exogenous corticosteroids are at risk when their steroid intake is abruptly reduced, or when significant physiological stress is encountered. Importantly, inhaled corticosteroids (ICS), such as fluticasone, are a significant independent risk factor for hospitalisation due to adrenal insufficiency.[5]

The electrolyte disturbances in primary adrenal insufficiency usually include hyponatremia and hyperkalaemia (Table 28.3). Hyponatremia occurs because of both mineralocorticoid deficiency and inappropriate secretion of antidiuretic hormone (vasopressin), caused by cortisol (not aldosterone) deficiency.[1]

Aldosterone plays a significant role in maintaining acid-base balance, inducing the secretion of H+ ions in the renal collecting ducts and tubules. A deficiency of mineralocorticoids such as in this case would thus be expected to produce a metabolic acidosis with a normal anion gap. The persistent vomiting, which is such a common feature at presentation, may result in an atypical hypochloremic acidosis with a raised anion gap.[7]

In terms of specific imaging, abdominal CT scanning is not indicated if autoimmune adrenalitis is confirmed as the diagnosis, but may be helpful in distinguishing between adrenal infection, haemorrhage or malignant disease.[1]

Adrenal Crisis

This may develop in several distinct clinical scenarios (1 & 2 being the most commonly encountered):

1. When a patient with previously undiagnosed Addison's disease is exposed to a new insult, such as trauma or severe infection as in this case;
2. If a patient with known adrenal insufficiency fails to absorb an adequate dose of his or her usual glucocorticoid (due to lack of medication, vomiting or physiological stress);

Approximately 8 per cent of patients with known adrenal insufficiency will develop an adrenal crisis each year by this means;[3]

3. After a vascular event affecting the adrenals (see adrenal haemorrhagic infarction, below);

4. In pituitary apoplexy due to infarction (which may result in sudden, severe loss of cortisol production and excretion);

5. Rarely, those with underlying pituitary disease may develop secondary or tertiary adrenal insufficiency due to acute physiological stress or severe illness.

Regardless of the aetiology, if an adrenal crisis is suspected it will require immediate treatment. A proposed management strategy is detailed below, but the crucial specific aspects are to obtain timely venous blood samples for biochemistry, giving immediate intravenous steroid replacement and addressing volume depletion with IV 0.9 per cent saline. The diagnosis of adrenal crisis often cannot be immediately confirmed in the acute setting as cortisol level results are not usually available. Therefore it is also important to consider and treat any other possible triggers or differential diagnoses, such as acute bacterial infection. Blood cultures and broad spectrum antibiotics should be administered pending definitive diagnosis.

Specific reasons for critical care admission would include shock that fails to respond to IV fluid boluses as in this case, severe electrolyte derangements with a risk of arrhythmias, or an altered conscious level with potential for airway compromise.

Diagnosis and Investigations in Adrenal Crisis

The most important aspects in recognition of adrenal crisis are history and clinical examination, coupled with a high index of suspicion. The key to confirming adrenal insufficiency is to demonstrate inappropriately low cortisol production. Cortisol results will not be available immediately and treatment must not be delayed for the sake of these tests. Patients with suspected adrenal crisis should have blood drawn immediately for random cortisol level (and ideally ACTH as here) prior to receiving intravenous bolus glucocorticoid. A brief discussion with the biochemistry laboratory will ensure the sampling method is correct.

In primary adrenal insufficiency, cortisol production is deficient despite continued secretion of ACTH (which should stimulate cortisol production at the adrenal cortex). The 'short ACTH stimulation test' may be performed within a few days of commencing glucocorticoid replacement, but only if dexamethasone is being given. (hydrocortisone will be measured in the cortisol assay so invalidates the results). A synthetic ACTH analogue is given and baseline and 1-hour cortisol and ACTH levels are checked to detect if there is indeed a primary adrenal problem, or if adrenal insufficiency is secondary to a lack of ACTH secretion.

Emergency Treatment of Suspected Adrenal Crisis

Immediate treatment is essential in suspected cases:

1. Establish intravenous access, check bedside glucometer reading and obtain blood samples.

2. Send blood for urgent serum electrolytes and glucose; request routine measurement of plasma cortisol and ACTH.

3. Begin treatment before obtaining laboratory results, by infusing 1 litre of 0.9 per cent saline as quickly as possible. Correct any hypoglycaemia.
4. Give 100 mg hydrocortisone as an intravenous bolus or 4 mg dexamethasone. (Dexamethasone does not interfere with the measurement of plasma cortisol, and is given over 1 to 5 minutes as a slow injection.)
5. Look for a precipitant (e.g. sepsis, trauma, medications etc.) and treat as indicated.
6. Repeated fluid boluses (e.g. up to 3000 ml) may be required. Repeated measurement of serum electrolytes and assessment of haemodynamic and volume status should prevent iatrogenic fluid overload and electrolyte problems.
7. If shock persists, admit the patient to the critical care unit and begin vasopressor therapy as per unit protocols. Consider avoiding use of etomidate if anaesthesia is required due to its effects on adrenal function (see below).
8. Ensure steroid replacement is prescribed to continue. Intravenous hydrocortisone 100 mg is given every 6 hours, dexamethasone every 12 hours. Specific mineralocorticoid replacement, e.g., fludrocortisone, is not usually recommended or necessary in the emergency management of an adrenal crisis.
9. Seek specialist advice promptly from endocrinology colleagues.

Other Important Aspects of Adrenal Insufficiency in the Critically Ill

In critical illness there may be sub-optimal corticosteroid production (in the absence of a specific structural abnormality in the adreno-cortical axis).[8] There is no agreed diagnostic definition of this 'relative adrenal insufficiency'. Current evidence does not support routine use of supplementary corticosteroids in patients with shock, although some centres advocate intravenous steroids in severe septic shock (defined as a systolic blood pressure less than 90 mmHg for more than one hour despite both adequate fluid resuscitation and vasopressor administration).

The carboxylated imidazole induction agent, etomidate, causes less pronounced haemodynamic effects compared with other IV induction agents, and therefore may seem ideal as an induction agent in the context of critically ill patients. However, etomidate suppresses the adreno-cortical axis (inhibiting 11-ß-hydroxylase) and significantly reduces the cortisol response to stimulation in critically ill patients for up to 24 hours.[8] There is current controversy regarding its use in critical illness.

It is vital from both a clinical and a medico-legal perspective not to overlook the need for steroid replacement therapy in the perioperative or critical illness management of patients with known adrenal insufficiency, or in those at risk due to regular steroid use.[3,9] Management guidelines for these patients are readily available, as is a wealth of information regarding endocrine disorders for healthcare professionals, patients and their relatives.[10]

Conclusion

Acute adrenal crisis is a hormone deficiency syndrome that is rapidly fatal if untreated, but can be treated with relatively simple measures of fluid, electrolyte and steroid replacement once the condition is suspected. This case example highlights the need for the Critical Care doctor to be alert to the possibility of adrenal crisis as a differential for shock unresponsive to fluid resuscitation. Urgent action to correct steroid deficiency is needed along with prompt investigations and endocrinology specialist opinion.

Key Learning Points

- The major clinical features of adrenal crisis are hypotension and volume depletion. There may be profound shock necessitating vasopressor support, in addition to glucocorticoid replacement and fluid resuscitation.
- It is necessary to treat suspected life-threatening adrenal insufficiency immediately rather than wait for any laboratory confirmation.
- IV hydrocortisone 100 mg is appropriate initial steroid replacement therapy.
- The preceding symptoms of adrenal insufficiency may be non-specific and insidious in onset, and may be overlooked or mistaken for an eating disorder or intentional overdose.[7]
- Hyponatremia, hyperkalaemia and a metabolic acidosis with a normal anion-gap are typical biochemical findings.
- Autoimmune adrenal inflammation is the most common cause of primary adrenal insufficiency in the United Kingdom & Europe. Other causes include infectious diseases (including TB), adrenal haemorrhage/infarction, metastatic cancer or lymphoma.
- In any critical illness and in the perioperative period, patients will need steroid replacement if they have known adrenal insufficiency or are – at risk due to regular oral or inhaled steroid use.

References

1. Allolio B, Arlt W. Seminar: Adrenal insufficiency. *Lancet* 2003;361: 1881–93.

2. Wolff B, Machill K, Schulzki I, Schumacher D, Werner D. Acute reversible cardiomyopathy with cardiogenic shock in a patient with Addisonian crisis: A case report. *Int J Cardiol*. 2007 Mar 20;116(2): e71–3. Epub 2006 Oct 31.

3. Wass J A H, Arlt W. How to avoid precipitating an acute adrenal crisis. *BMJ* 2012;345:e6333.

4. Society for Endocrinology. Position statement of the Society for Endocrinology on the endocrine effects of inhaled corticosteroids in respiratory disease. 2011. www.endocrinology.org/policy/docs/ 1107_endocrine%20effects%20of% 20inhaled%20steroids%20in%20respiratory %20disease.pdf (accessed 15 October, 2014.)

5. Lapi F, Kezouh A, Suissa S, Ernst P. The use of inhaled corticosteroids and the risk of adrenal insufficiency. *Eur Respir J* 2013;42:79–86.

6. Lam K Y, Lo C Y. A critical examination of adrenal tuberculosis and a 28-year autopsy experience of active tuberculosis. *Clin Endocrinol* 2001;54:633.

7. Sinha N, Rahman F, Shin M, Burbridge P. An endocrinological emergency masquerading as an overdose. *BMJ Case Reports* 2012; 10.1136/bcr.12.2011.5328, Published 11 July 2012.

8. Baudouin S V, Ball S. The endocrine response to critical illness. In: G M Hall, J M Hunter, M S Cooper, editors, *Core Topics in Endocrinology in Anaesthesia and Critical Care*. 1st ed. Cambridge University Press; 2010.

9. Martin C, Steinke T, Bucher M, Raspé C. Perioperative Addisonian crisis. *Der Anaesthesist* 2012;61:503–11.

10. Addison's Clinical Advisory Panel. Glucocorticoid medication requirements for surgery and dentistry. 2011. www.addisons.org.uk/topics/2005/10/ 0021.html (accessed 15 October, 2014).

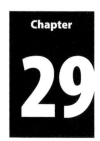

Acid Base Abnormalities

Alastair Glossop

Introduction

Ethylene glycol (EG) toxicity is an uncommon but potentially serious form of poisoning, accounting for less than 100 deaths per year in the United States. Data registry figures from the United States in 2007 report 5,731 cases of known EG poisoning, although as reporting of cases by medical professionals is not mandatory this is likely to be an underestimate. It usually occurs as a result of deliberate self-harm, attempted inebriation or unintentional poisoning. There have also been reported cluster outbreaks following contamination of foodstuffs. EG is found in domestic products such as antifreeze and some cleaning solutions, and also in a variety of industrial solvents. Ingestion of as little as 1.4 ml/kg of undiluted EG may be fatal, although larger volumes than this are frequently ingested in deliberate self-harm attempts. The clinical presentation of EG toxicity is variable and depends upon many factors, including time from ingestion to presentation, volume of EG ingested and presence of other alcohols or poisons at the time of ingestion.

Case Description

A 42-year-old man was referred to critical care with a complicated clinical picture. He had been admitted to hospital nine days earlier with renal failure, retention of urine, hypertension and a severe headache. His serum creatinine at the time was 1026 mmol/l, he had a residual volume following urethral catheterisation of 2.1l of urine and a blood pressure of 190/100 mmHg. He was initially admitted to the Renal Unit for haemodialysis. Admission blood tests revealed deranged liver function tests (AST 1234 mmol/l, ALT 1272 mmol/l), a low platelet count (94 x 10^9/l) and a prolonged bleeding time (244 seconds). An arterial blood gas performed on admission was abnormal with an acidosis (pH 7.13), high lactate (9.7 mmol/l), raised anion gap (28 mmol/l) and attempted respiratory compensation demonstrated by a $PaCO_2$ of 1.9 kPa. His PaO_2 was normal on air (13.2 kPa).

Over the following 8 days he received intermittent haemodialysis with some improvement in his acidosis and biochemistry. However on day nine he developed an acute, painful ascending motor and sensory neuropathy. Despite being awake and oriented he was noted to have fixed, dilated pupils. He began to develop subjective difficulty breathing and was noted to have saturations on room air of 92 per cent. His tidal volume at this stage was measured at 190 mls and arterial blood gas measurement revealed a $PaCO_2$ of 6.8 kPa. At this stage he was transferred to the intensive care unit to be intubated and mechanically ventilated due to the onset of respiratory failure.

A renal biopsy had been taken earlier in his admission and whilst the results were awaited, the rapid onset of ascending motor and sensory paralysis led to concerns that Guillan Barré syndrome might be developing. Following consultation with a neurologist, intravenous (iv) immunoglobulin was started and nerve conduction studies arranged. Ongoing renal replacement was provided in critical care via continuous veno–venous haemofiltration (CVVH).

Following intubation, he was noted to have autonomic instability, with labile blood pressure and heart rate despite adequate sedation. Later during his intensive care admission, cranial nerve neuropathies producing facial weakness, absent cough and gag reflex became evident and the patient was noted to be apnoeic. He suffered profound thrombocytopaenia with a lowest recorded platelet count during his admission of 2 x 10^9/l. On day 14 of his admission a percutaneous tracheostomy was performed, with platelet cover, to aid weaning from mechanical ventilation.

Despite a 5-day course of iv immunoglobulin the patient's neuropathy worsened and nerve conduction tests were expedited to investigate the profound weakness. These revealed features of neuropathy consistent with ethylene glycol toxicity. The results of the renal biopsy became available during this period and showed appearances consistent with acute tubular necrosis (ATN) and oxalate crystal deposition, again suggestive of ethylene glycol induced damage. In light of these findings serum taken and saved at the time of the patient's admission was re-examined, and the presence of breakdown products of ethylene glycol was confirmed.

After 18 days on ITU the patient was awake and oriented and able to answer questions about his illness and recent medical history. The patient had initially strongly denied any deliberate consumption of products containing ethylene glycol and denied any history of psychiatric illness or suicidal ideations. However the clinical picture, findings of nerve conduction studies, and also presence of ethylene glycol breakdown products in serum all provided compelling evidence for the diagnosis of ethylene glycol poisoning, and following a series of interviews with the patient and his close family members, it became evident that he had deliberately consumed antifreeze with suicidal intent approximately 3 days prior to being admitted to hospital.

He made a slow recovery with requirements for ongoing respiratory and renal support gradually reducing over a period of several weeks. Weaning was complicated by an episode of pseudomonas aeruginosa ventilator associated pneumonia. His serum creatinine returned to a baseline of 123 mmol/l and he no longer required renal replacement therapy. His ascending neuropathy and marked weakness also resolved gradually. His total length of critical care stay was 73 days, and he was later discharged from hospital.

Discussion

Making an accurate diagnosis of ethylene glycol toxicity can be difficult in the acute setting. It is confirmed by the laboratory findings of EG or its breakdown products in serum, with the detection of calcium oxalate crystals in urine or on renal biopsy. However the serum tests for EG are not available in all hospitals and thus a delay frequently occurs between patient presentation and the availability of diagnostic information. For this reason this initial diagnosis should be clinical and based on history, clinical features and marked biochemical abnormalities. Treatment should be started on the basis of a high index of clinical suspicion rather than waiting for laboratory confirmation of the diagnosis.[1]

A raised serum anion gap is the most marked biochemical abnormality associated with EG poisoning and should alert clinicians to the diagnosis. The anion gap is an indicator of the presence of unmeasured ions in serum and is calculated using the following equation:

Anion gap $= ([Na^+] + [K^+]) - ([Cl^-] - [HCO_3^-])$

Electrical neutrality is maintained via buffering of unmeasured ions present in serum, such as serum proteins, paraproteins and sulphates and by bicarbonate. In health therefore there are fewer anions than cations measurable in serum. This results in a measured anion gap of 6 to 10 mEq/l. However in the presence of certain disease states the serum concentration of unmeasured ions increases, resulting in depletion of bicarbonate and an increase in this measured gap between cations and anions and hence an increased anion gap acidosis occurs. The following are causes of an increased anion gap acidosis:[2]

Box 29.1   Causes of a raised anion gap acidosis

Ketoacidosis
Diabetic ketoacidosis
Alcoholic ketoacidosis
Starvation ketoacidosis

Lactic acidosis
Renal failure
Uraemia
Acute renal failure with reduced acid excretion

Drugs and toxins
Ethylene glycol
Methanol
Salicylates
Isoniazid
Cyanide
Propylene, Paracetamol

Ingestion of ethylene glycol (EG) becomes a clinically significant problem following the metabolism of EG, via the enzyme alcohol dehydrogenase, into the metabolites glycolic acid, oxalic acid, glycoaldehyde and glycoxylic acid. Whilst EG ingestion per se causes relatively few problems in terms of end organ damage, the toxic metabolites produced by metabolism of ethylene glycol – particularly glycolate and oxalate – are responsible for causing a number of serious pathological processes that affect several different organ systems. Oxalate may combine with ionised serum calcium to form calcium oxalate crystals, which are may then be deposited in several different organs – including the kidneys, liver and myocardium – and exert toxic effects.

The clinical syndrome that follows ingestion of EG begins once this metabolism of EG into its toxic metabolites begins and is commonly described as occurring in three stages.[4]

The first stage of signs and symptoms following EG ingestion is neurological and may frequently mimic the appearance of acute alcohol intoxication. It begins approximately 30 to 60 minutes after the ingestion of ethylene glycol. In some cases, particularly when higher doses of EG have been ingested, the initial excitatory symptoms may progress to cerebral oedema, convulsions, CNS depression and coma.

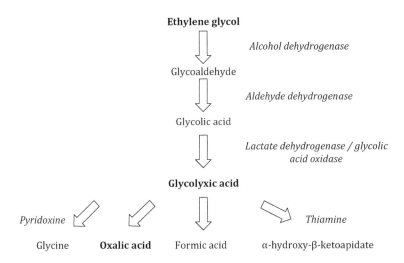

Figure 29.1 Breakdown pathway for ethylene glycol.[3]

The second phase is one of cardiorespiratory symptoms and usually begins 12 to 18 hours following ingestion of EG. Breakdown of EG into its constituent organic acids and also an increase in serum lactate following ingestion may result in the development of a marked metabolic acidosis, which in turn promotes cardiovascular instability. Cardiovascular effects during this phase are pronounced and include dysrhythmias, myocardial depression, hypotension and cardiac failure. The acidosis that may be seen results in tachypnoea and Kussmaul respiration in attempted respiratory compensation. Death from acute EG poisoning most frequently occurs during this phase, especially if specific treatment has not been instituted.

The third phase, which tends to be seen two to three days following ingestion of EG, affects renal function via the damaging end organ effects of EG metabolites. Acute tubular necrosis (ATN) occurs due to both the direct toxic effects of glycolate on renal tubules and also due to the deposition of calcium oxalate crystals within renal tubules. Depending on the extent of renal injury, progression to acute renal failure requiring renal replacement therapy may be seen. During this period urine dipstick often shows haematuria and proteinuria, and the diagnosis may be confirmed by a renal biopsy demonstrating the characteristic presence of calcium oxalate crystals. Recovery of renal function is not universal, and in some cases may take several months.

In addition to the three phases described above, a further 'delayed neurologic' phase has also been described as occuring, albeit very infrequently, following EG poisoning. In such cases patients tend to present late following ingestion of large volumes of EG. Neurological effects such as profound limb weakness and cranial nerve palsies are prominent features and tend to occur 5 to 20 days post ingestion of EG. Bulbar, facial and trigeminal cranial nerves are most likely to be affected, as in this case, and resolution of these palsies may take several months.[4,5] The precise mechanism of nerve injury is unclear – one theory is that metabolites of EG are directly neurotoxic, another is that the metabolism of glycolate leads to depletion of thiamine and pyridoxine, which in turn contributes to neuronal dysfunction. It has also been suggested that this delayed neurological phase is more likely to occur in individuals whose consumption of EG is chronic or staggered over several days, resulting in a gradual depletion of thiamine and pyroxidine as glycolate is metabolised, but with less prominent acute toxic effects occurring.

The treatment of ethylene glycol poisoning involves initial supportive measures and resuscitation, use of specific inhibitors of ethylene glycol metabolism and enhanced elimination.[6] Patients may present with varying degrees of cardiorespiratory compromise and neurological depression: an 'ABCDE' approach to assessment and resuscitation should be followed. As in all cases of acute poisoning, consideration should be given to activated charcoal gastric lavage, although it should be remembered that ethylene glycol is rapidly absorbed from the stomach and therefore lavage is unlikely to be helpful unless the patient presents to hospital very rapidly post ingestion.

Given that the pathogenesis of EG toxicity is derived almost entirely from the products of its breakdown, it is logical that use of inhibitors of ethylene glycol metabolism is an important step in management of poisoning. By preventing the production of the toxic metabolites glycolate, oxalate and other acids the harmful effects associated with high serum levels of toxic metabolites can be significantly reduced. It is also vital, once EG metabolism has been inhibited, to promote enhanced excretion of EG in its unchanged form, and given the solubility of EG in serum and its predominant renal excretion this can be achieved using haemodialysis or CVVH.

Historically ethanol was utilised as an inhibitor of EG breakdown, however more recently fomepizole (4 – methylpyrazole), a potent inhibitor of the alcohol dehydrogenase enzyme, has supplanted its use due to its greater efficacy, safer therapeutic index, easier dosing and more favourable side effect profile. Fomepizole is given intravenously at a loading dose of 15 mg/kg and then at 10 mg/kg every 12 hours for the next 48 hours. Following this period the dose is increased again to 15 mg/kg 12 hourly to ensure adequate plasma levels in the face of increased metabolism. It is continued at this dose until plasma EG levels are less than 20 mg/dL. This regime provides stable, predictable and therapeutic levels of fomepizole and appears to be associated with none of the serious side effects seen with intravenous ethanol treatment such as hypoglycaemia, pancreatitis and liver impairment. Minor side effects have been reported with its use, including eosinophilia and skin rashes.

There is evidence from multicentre trials in France and the USA that early use of fomepizole may reduce the incidence of renal injury and prevent progression to dialysis.[7,8] The META study, which included both an EG and methanol poisoning subset, examined the outcome of poisoning patients who were treated with fomepizole and renal replacement therapy (RRT). Of 19 patients presenting with EG poisoning treated with fomepizole and haemodialysis 18 survived. Fomepizole was also demonstrated in the study to be effective in the treatment of methanol poisoning, which may present in a similar clinical manner to EG poisoning.[8,9] The trial did not use controls or provide any comparison to treatment with ethanol, however the overall mortality rates demonstrated were far lower than historical rates of death following EG ingestion which has led to the authors suggesting a potential mortality benefit for the combined use of fomepizole and RRT.[10]

Enhanced elimination of ethylene glycol is achieved via haemodialysis or haemofiltration. As well as removing ethylene glycol and some of the harmful metabolites from the patient's circulation, dialysis is also helpful in the correction of acid base disturbance and treatment of renal failure.[11] There has also been a suggestion that supplementation of thiamine and pyridoxine for the first 72 hours post ingestion may reduce production of oxalate and reduce the onset of prolonged peripheral and cranial nerve damage.

Conclusions

EG poisoning is an uncommon clinical presentation in the United Kingdom, and although the consequences of ingestion and metabolism are potentially very serious, many can be prevented by prompt diagnosis and early institution of specific treatments that reduce the metabolism and enhance the elimination of EG. Despite adequate early treatment EG poisoning may have several long term sequelae that have a major impact on patient morbidity. A high index of clinical suspicion is required in all patients presenting with a severe and unexplained metabolic acidosis to allow effective treatment to begin with the minimum delay.

Key Learning Points

- Calculation of anion gap should be part of the assessment of interpreting blood gases that show a metabolic acidosis.
- An abnormal anion gap should cause consideration of the possible differentials, close scrutiny of blood tests results and measurement of paracetamol, salicylate and blood alcohol levels.
- If possible diagnoses include methanol and EG poisoning, interventions such as fomepizole and renal replacement therapy may prevent the development of severe complications of poisoning and the need for longer term dialysis.
- Suspicion of EG toxicity should be high in any patient presenting with renal impairment, neurological symptoms and an unexplained high anion gap acidosis.
- Although it is only effective whilst unmetabolised EG is present in the circulation, the side effect profile and wide therapeutic index of fomepizole make it a relatively safe drug to be given 'blind' in cases of suspected poisoning until serum EG levels are known.
- Treatment with thiamine and pyridoxine may also play a role in prevention of late neurological problems, to counteract the depletion of these compounds that occurs during EG metabolism, and therefore these vitamins should be given in short courses in all cases of ethylene glycol poisoning.

References

1. Eder AF, McGrath CM, Dowdy YG, et al. Ethylene glycol poisoning: toxicokinetic and analytical factors affecting laboratory diagnosis. *Clinical Chemistry* 1998;44(1):168–77.
2. Mehta AN, Emmett JB, Emmett M. GOLD MARK: an anion gap mnemonic for the 21st century. *Lancet* 2008;372(9642):892.
3. Henderson WR, Brubacher J. Methanol and ethylene glycol poisoning: a case study and review of current literature. *Cjem* 2002;4(1):34–40.
4. Pellegrino B, Parravani A, Cook L, Mackay K. Ethylene glycol intoxication: Disparate findings of immediate versus delayed presentation. *The West Virginia Medical Journal* 2006;102(4):32–4.
5. Lewis LD, Smith BW, Mamourian AC. Delayed sequelae after acute overdoses or poisonings: cranial neuropathy related to ethylene glycol ingestion. *Clinical Pharmacology and Therapeutics* 1997;61(6):692–9.
6. Brent J. Current management of ethylene glycol poisoning. *Drugs* 2001;61(7):979–88.
7. Megarbane B, Borron SW, Baud FJ. Current recommendations for treatment of severe toxic alcohol poisonings. *Intensive Care Medicine* 2005;31(2):189–95.
8. Brent J, McMartin K, Phillips S, et al. Fomepizole for the treatment of ethylene

glycol poisoning. Methylpyrazole for Toxic Alcohols Study Group. *The New England Journal of Medicine* 1999;340(11):832–8.

9. Brent J, McMartin K, Phillips S, Aaron C, Kulig K, Methylpyrazole for Toxic Alcohols Study G. Fomepizole for the treatment of methanol poisoning. *The New England Journal of Medicine* 2001;344(6):424–9.

10. Brent J. Fomepizole for ethylene glycol and methanol poisoning. *The New England Journal of Medicine* 2009;360(21): 2216–23.

11. Goodman JW, Goldfarb DS. The role of continuous renal replacement therapy in the treatment of poisoning. *Seminars in Dialysis* 2006;19(5):402–7.

Chapter 30

Nutrition and Refeeding Syndrome

Sarah Irving

Introduction

Around 30 per cent of all patients at the point of admission to hospital in the United Kingdom are malnourished.[1] Reduced nutritional intake in the days prior to an admission to critical care is common, as are significant co-morbidities. This means that many critical care patients will be undernourished by the time of admission to the intensive care unit (ICU).

Catabolism provoked by critical illness with inflammatory and endocrine stress responses, leads to severe protein loss and muscle weakness which affects outcomes. Nutrition support during this acute period cannot halt the process, but can limit the energy deficit which occurs, allowing muscle mass to be rebuilt during the anabolic recovery phase of illness. Hence, nutrition must be considered promptly in any malnourished patient, or those who may become undernourished. Protocols usually aim to reach a target goal for nutrition in the first 24 to 48 hours after commencement of feed. However, immediately meeting full caloric goals in patients at risk can cause refeeding syndrome.

Refeeding syndrome consists of the metabolic and physiologic processes that occur as a consequence of depletion during starvation and repletion during refeeding. It may result in profound hypophosphatemia, hypokalaemia, hypomagnesaemia as well as sodium retention/fluid overload and thiamine deficiency.[2,3,4,5]

With careful management, refeeding can be mitigated, but in a small subset of at risk patients, it can be life threatening. Signs and symptoms often overlap with others due to critical illness; hence, it can easily be missed.

The case below and discussion following will outline in more detail the pathophysiology of refeeding syndrome and how to identify and manage those at risk.

Case Description

A 28-year-old lady woman referred in extremis to the ICU team 6 days after admission to the gastroenterology ward for investigation and management of weight loss. On review she was drowsy, but oriented and found to be in type 1 respiratory failure, requiring 15 litres of oxygen via a non-rebreathing face mask. She was in uncontrolled atrial fibrillation (AF) with a rate of 140 bpm, profoundly hypotensive with a prolonged capillary refill time of 4 seconds and was oligo-anuric. Further clinical examination revealed normal heart sounds, reduced breath sounds bibasally, pitting oedema peripherally, but no calf tenderness. Abdominal examination was unremarkable.

The ward team had performed a fluid challenge with little improvement in her clinical state and initiated treatment with broad spectrum antibiotics for a possible hospital acquired pneumonia.

Biochemistry and haematology results had been performed two days previously. Full blood count (FBC) had shown a normocytic, normochromic anaemia, with normal white cell count (WCC). Biochemistry had shown sodium, potassium, magnesium and phosphate levels to be at the lower end of the normal range, but renal function was otherwise normal and apart from an albumin level of 30 g/L, her liver function was normal. Blood gas results taken after clinical deterioration showed her to be in type 1 respiratory failure, have a metabolic acidosis with a base deficit of -10, and a lactate of 5 mmol/l.

On admission to the ICU, she required ventilation due to deteriorating gas exchange. Intubation was straightforward and she was sedated with propofol and alfentanil and established in a biphasic positive airway pressure (BIPAP) ventilation mode with lung protective settings. Invasive arterial and central venous access was gained.

Following further unsuccessful fluid challenges, noradrenaline was started and a mean arterial pressure of 65 mmHg achieved on moderate doses. Initial blood gases showed an improvement in oxygenation, but a continued metabolic acidosis. Both sodium and potassium were found to be extremely low on blood gas and laboratory results, as were magnesium and phosphate levels. Lab results also confirmed an acute kidney injury and elevated hepatic transaminases. FBC again revealed a normocytic, normochromic anaemia, but a normal WCC. Clotting showed a mildly raised PT and normal APTT.

On further review of the notes, it was established that her admission body mass index (BMI) was 12 kg/m^2. Gastro-intestinal investigations into the cause of weight loss had been unremarkable. Nursing observations confirmed poor nutritional intake and a possible diagnosis of anorexia nervosa were being explored. Twenty-four hours before the current deterioration, B vitamins had been given and nasogastric feeding started (at 10 kcal/kg/24 hrs). A dextrose infusion which had been begun following an episode of low blood sugar was continued after the enteral feed began.

A diagnosis of refeeding syndrome was made. Malnutrition Universal Screening Test (MUST) confirmed she had been at high risk on admission to hospital. Full dose IV B vitamins (pabrinex) were started and continued for a total of 10 days and aggressive electrolyte replacement was undertaken. Estimated total eventual caloric requirements were 25 kcal/kg/24 hrs. The glucose infusion was stopped and standard feed (Nutrisan) started at 5 kcal/kg/24 hrs and built up slowly over the course of 1 week to 25 kcal/kg/24 hrs. Electrolytes continued to be monitored closely throughout this period and replaced whilst feeding was being established. Other essential minerals and trace elements were also prescribed. In addition, broad spectrum antibiotics were continued as CXR revealed a right lower lobe pneumonia. Sputum samples confirmed the diagnosis of hospital-acquired pneumonia.

Over the subsequent 4 days, the AF resolved, ventilatory and vasopressor requirements reduced, and extubation was performed successfully on day 5 of ICU admission. Renal and hepatic function gradually improved and she was discharged on day 8 on full feed at 25 kcal/kg/24 hrs.

Case Discussion

Pathophysiology of Refeeding Syndrome

Glucose is the body's preferred fuel, coming from the intake of carbohydrates. Insulin release leads to carbohydrate breakdown by glycolysis and pyruvate/ATP is produced.

In the first few days of starvation, plasma glucose and protein levels fall, so insulin levels decrease and glucagon levels rise, stimulating gluconeogenesis and glycogenolysis.

Once glycogen stores are depleted, gluconeogenesis has to take place by proteolysis and lipolysis. Amino acids in muscle are broken down and free fatty acid oxidation leads to ketone production. Ketones are substituted for glucose as energy substrates in brain and other organs. This decreases skeletal muscle protein breakdown and amino acid release by reducing the obligatory demand for glucose. Once fat stores are depleted, muscle bulk diminishes quickly. Insulin secretion reduces further and basal metabolic rate slows by up to 25 per cent.

These processes are exaggerated by critical illness. In addition to metabolic rate, cardiac output and haemoglobin levels, renal concentration capacity will decrease with time. Respiratory and cardiac function declines due to muscular wasting. Fluid and electrolyte imbalances are common, although serum electrolyte concentration may remain normal as they are mainly in the intracellular compartment. It is important to recognise that an overweight or obese patient can also be malnourished.

When a malnourished patient is given aggressive nutritional support, the increase in glucose levels increases insulin release by the pancreas and reduces secretion of glucagon. Insulin stimulates glycogen, fat and protein synthesis. This process requires electrolytes such as phosphate and magnesium and cofactors such as thiamine. Insulin stimulates the absorption of potassium into the cells through the sodium-potassium ATPase symporter, which also transports glucose into the cells. Magnesium and phosphate are also taken up into the cells and water follows by osmosis. These processes result in a decrease in the serum levels of phosphate, potassium and magnesium, all of which are already depleted. The clinical features of the refeeding syndrome occur as a result of the functional deficits of these electrolytes and the rapid change in basal metabolic rate. The result can be a life-threatening depletion of these vital electrolytes.

Hypophosphataemia is central to the causation of refeeding syndrome. It is needed to produce adenosine triphosphate (ATP) and provides energy for almost all cellular functions. Phosphate is an essential part of RNA and DNA, and is needed in red blood cells for 2, 3-diphosphoglycerate production for easier release of oxygen to the tissues.

Refeeding-induced hypophosphatemia can result in respiratory failure due to a decrease in available ATP, which is needed to maintain the diaphragm's normal contractility. In addition, hypophosphatemia can cause red and white blood cell dysfunction, muscle weakness and rhabdomyolysis and seizures.

Mild decreases of potassium and magnesium may cause nausea, vomiting, constipation, diarrhoea, muscle twitching or weakness. Severe depletion of the serum concentrations of potassium and magnesium can cause dysrhythmias, cardiac dysfunction, skeletal muscle weakness, seizures and metabolic acidosis.[2,3,4,5]

Clinical Presentation of Refeeding Syndrome

There are no widely accepted diagnostic criteria for refeeding syndrome, so available published data may not reflect clinically relevant cases. Most definitions adopt hypophosphataemia as a surrogate marker, but many patients are hypophosphataemic without evidence of organ dysfunction. Hypophosphataemia in the general hospital population has been found to be low, at 2 per cent. Another study of (10,197 hospitalised patients) showed the incidence of severe hypophosphataemia was 0.43 per cent, with malnutrition being one of the strongest risk factors.[3,4]

A few studies have analysed the incidence of refeeding syndrome in the ICU, but a prospective cohort study of 62 patients in the intensive care unit refed after being starved for 48 hours showed that 21 patients (34 per cent) experienced refeeding hypophosphatae-mia. However, there are limitations to relying on low serum phosphate within the critical care population, as levels may be normal in patients with multiorgan failure or in the presence of impaired renal function.[3]

Many case reports highlight the potentially fatal nature of the condition. In an observational study of 68 patients admitted to critical care with anorexia nervosa, 5 died due to the effects of refeeding.[6] Anorexic patients are not representative of the general ICU population, so these results cannot be fully extrapolated.

Rio et al. in 2013 used a definition of serum electrolyte shifts plus observed clinical complications of acute circulatory fluid overload and organ dysfunction. In a study of 243 hospital inpatients starting nutritional support, only 3 (2 percent) met this definition, but all 3 survived. There were 13 (5.3 percent) deaths during hospital admission, which were not attributed to refeeding syndrome. The independent predictors for refeeding syndrome were starvation and baseline low serum magnesium concentration. Of note, other described risk factors[7] for refeeding syndrome were not found to be associated. Intravenous carbohydrate infusion prior to artificial nutrition support may have precipitated the onset of the syndrome. Careful electrolyte replacement and initial hypocaloric feed were standard in this study. This may have prevented refeeding deaths.[8]

The clinical manifestations of the symptoms of refeeding syndrome are unpredictable and can occur late and without warning. Changes in serum electrolytes alter the cell membrane potential, hence affect nerve, cardiac and skeletal muscle cells. With mild derangements in these electrolytes, there may be no symptoms. The spectrum of presentation ranges from mild nausea, vomiting and lethargy to multiorgan failure with respiratory insufficiency, cardiac failure, hypotension, arrhythmias, delirium, coma and death. Clinical deterioration may occur rapidly if the diagnosis is not made and appropriate measures taken.[3,4] (See Table 30.1)

Management of Refeeding Syndrome

No randomised controlled trials of treatment are published, hence management is mainly based on consensus guidelines. In 2006 National Institute for Health and Care Excellence (NICE) published Guidelines for Nutritional Support and published updated evidence in 2013. The guidelines emphasise the need to identify those at risk and introduce feeding carefully to prevent the occurrence of the syndrome. In other words, management is largely based on prevention.[7]

Those with little or no intake for more than 10 days, or with a BMI less than 16 kg/m^2 are at high risk. Little intake for 15 days or a BMI less than 14 kg/m^2 leads to very high risk. Alcohol abuse, drugs including insulin, chemotherapy, antacids or diuretics increase the likelihood.[2]

All hospital admissions, including critical care admissions, in the United Kingdom should undergo MUST assessment, which identifies those who are already malnourished or at risk of malnutrition. This forms the basis on which a refeeding risk assessment can be performed.

NICE suggests that nutrition support should be cautiously introduced in all seriously ill patients, at no more than 50 per cent of estimated target energy and protein needs and built

Table 30.1 Manifestations of refeeding syndrome

Derangement	Mechanism	Presentation
Hypophosphatemia Hypokalemia Hypomagnesemia	Insulin release causes intracellular shift of electrolytes	Arrhythmias Weakness Rhabdomyolysis Reduced 2,3 DPG and anaemia, haemolysis and reduced oxygen delivery.
Hyperglycemia	Glucose administration to starved system adapted to fat metabolism.	Osmotic diuresis Dehydration Ketosis, metabolic acidosis Increased CO_2 production
Thiamine deficiency	Depleted through starvation, then required as co-enzyme for increased carbohydrate metabolism	Wernicke's encephalopathy Korsakoff's psychosis
Fluid overload	Introduction of carbohydrate and rapid reduction in renal sodium and water clearance.	Congestive cardiac failure Pulmonary oedema
Steatohepatitis	Lipogenesis	Fatty liver, deranged LFTs

up over 24 to 48 hours. In those who have had negligible intake for over 5 days, the 50 per cent target should be maintained for 2 days and only increased if the clinical and biochemical monitoring reveal no refeeding problems.

Full target needs can be estimated using several methods. The ESPEN (European Society for Clinical Nutrition and Metabolism) guidelines[9] are 25 kcal/kg/24 hrs, while ASPEN[10] (American Society for Parenteral and Enteral Nutrition) suggests either 25 to 30 kcal/kg/24 hrs, predictive equations, or indirect calorimetry. ASPEN advises consideration of hypocaloric feeding in the critically ill obese (BMI greater than 30 kg/m^2) patient, at either 60 to 70 percent of target energy requirements, 11 to 14 kcal/kg actual body weight, or 22 to 25 kcal/kg ideal body weight.

NICE guidance (see Figure 30.1) is that nutritional targets should be between 25 to 35 kcal/kg/day total energy (including that derived from protein), 0.8 to 1.5 g protein (0.13 to 0.24 g nitrogen)/kg/day, 30 to 35 ml fluid/kg (with allowance for extra losses or input), adequate electrolytes, minerals, micronutrients (allowing for any pre-existing deficits, excessive losses or increased demands) and fibre if appropriate.

In those at high risk, feeding should be started at a maximum of 10 kcal/kg/day. In very high risk cases, caloric intake should begin at 5 kcal/kg/day. Enteral feed should be used as first line, although parenteral feed can be used safely. Nutrition should slowly be increased to meet full needs by day 4 to 7. Specialised feed is unnecessary.

NICE also advise cardiac monitoring for those at highest risk, restoration of circulatory volume and careful fluid balance. It is important that B vitamins are replaced prior to commencing nutrition. Potassium, phosphate and magnesium should be measured and corrected at least daily. For patients with electrolyte deficit, nutritional support should be started at the lower rate rather than being delayed until the imbalance is corrected, as this avoids further nutritional deterioration.

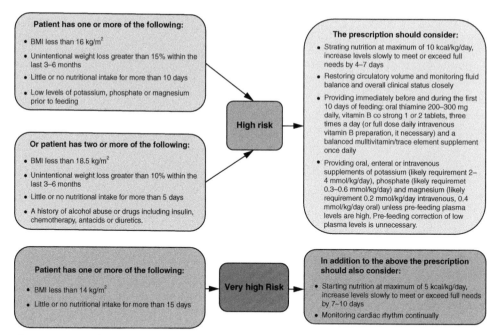

Figure 30.1 Simplified NICE guidance for refeeding risk assessment and prevention.

Conclusion

Clinically relevant refeeding syndrome is very rare but does occur. Good awareness of the condition and a high degree of suspicion is necessary, as the presentation can be similar to other causes of critical illness and multi-organ dysfunction. Careful assessment of the patient and introduction of hypocaloric feed with electrolyte and B vitamin replacement can, in most cases, prevent the worst complications.

Those at highest risk include those who have a BMI of less than 14 kg/m^2, or with negligible intake for over 15 days. Certain groups are at particular risk, including those with a history of alcohol abuse.

Some cases are thought to have been precipitated by glucose infusion without other nutrition and this should be carefully monitored. Management in a critical care area with cardiac monitoring and more careful electrolyte and fluid management should be considered for the highest risk cases and in particular, those who have already had arrhythmias.

More research is needed to identify more clearly who is at highest risk and if the syndrome can be prevented by early, aggressive electrolyte replacement. This may allow extreme caloric restriction to be used only for a smaller number at very high risk.

Key Learning Points

- Refeeding syndrome is due to a switch from lipid and fatty acid metabolism of starvation back to carbohydrate metabolism with increased phosphate and thiamine requirements. Acute thiamine deficiency, release of insulin and intracellular shift of potassium, magnesium and phosphate leads to life threatening multiorgan dysfunction.
- Signs of refeeding syndrome include hypophosphataemia, hypokalaemia and hypomagnesaemia.

- A careful assessment of nutrition on admission using a tool such as MUST should be performed on all patients, to identify those at risk.
- Those at highest risk are those with a history of alcohol abuse, chemotherapy and drugs such as antacids and diuretics.
- Prevention in at-risk groups is key.
- Glucose infusion can increase insulin production and may produce refeeding syndrome.
- Replacing electrolytes should begin in tandem with careful re-introduction of feed at a slower rate.
- Management within a critical care environment should be considered for those at highest risk of refeeding syndrome.

References

1. British Association for Parenteral and Enteral Nutrition (BAPEN) Nutrition Screening Survey in The UK and Republic of Ireland in 2011. Published 2012. www.bapen.org.uk/pdfs/nsw/nsw-2011-report.pdf

2. Byrnes MC, Stangenes J. Refeeding in the ICU: an adult and pediatric problem. *Curr Opin Clin Nutr Metab Care* 2011 Mar; 14(2):186–92.

3. Khan LU, Ahmed J, Khan S, et al. Refeeding syndrome: a literature review. *Gastroenterol Res Pract* 2011;2011: 410971.

4. Mehanna HM, Moledina J, Travis J. Refeeding syndrome: what it is, and how to prevent and treat it. *BMJ* 2008 Jun 28; 336(7659):1495–8.

5. Boateng AA, Sriram K, Meguid MM et al. Refeeding syndrome: Treatment considerations based on collective analysis of literature case reports. *Nutrition* 2010 Feb;26(2):156–67.

6. Vignaud M, Constantin JM, Ruivard M. et al. Refeeding syndrome influences outcome of anorexia nervosa patients in intensive care unit: an observational study. *Crit Care* 2010;14(5):R172.

7. National Institute for Health and Clinical Excellence. Nutrition support in adults: Oral nutrition support, enteral tube feeding and parenteral nutrition. NiCE Guidelines [CG32] Published 2006. www.nice.org.uk/guidance/cg32

8. Rio A, Whelan K, Goff L, et al. Occurrence of refeeding syndrome in adults started on artificial nutrition support: prospective cohort study. *BMJ Open* 2013;3(1):e002173.

9. Kreymann KG, Berger MM, Deutz NE. et al. ESPEN Guidelines on Enteral Nutrition: Intensive care. *Clin Nutr* 2006 Apr;25(2):210–23.

10. McClave SA, Martindale RG, Vanek VW. Guidelines for the Provision and Assessment of Nutrition Support Therapy in the Adult Critically Ill Patient: Society of Critical Care Medicine (SCCM) and American Society for Parenteral and Enteral Nutrition (A.S.P.E.N.). *JPEN J Parenter Enteral Nutr* 2009 May–Jun; 33(3):277–316.

31

Pre-eclampsia and Eclampsia in Critical Care

Martin J Feat

Introduction

Pre-eclampsia remains one of the leading causes of maternal and neonatal morbidity and mortality. It is the commonest medical problem encountered in pregnancy and can complicate up to 15 percent of pregnancies. Up to 5 percent of patients with severe pre-eclampsia or eclampsia may require admission to the intensive care unit (ICU). There are also risks for the foetus, with 5 percent of stillbirths without congenital abnormalities occurring in cases of pre-eclampsia. A significant proportion of women with pre-eclampsia will also give birth before 34 weeks gestation as a result of their disease. This case study discusses the management of pre-eclampsia and eclampsia on the labour ward and ICU.

Case Presentation

A 23-year-old woman, pregnant for the first time and at 26 weeks, presented via ambulance to the accident and emergency department with seizures. On arrival, seizure activity was continuing and she required intubation both to maintain oxygenation and for airway protection. Prior to intubation, her oxygen saturation was 91 per cent and her arterial blood pressure was 190/125 mmHg.

Anaesthesia was induced in the wedged supine position using alfentanil 2 mg, thiopentone 450 mg and suxamethonium 150 mg. Despite this, her systolic blood pressure increased to 240 mmHg at intubation and she was thus commenced on intravenous labetalol. This was initially started at a rate of 50 mg per hour and the dose was increased by 10 mg per hour every 30 minutes until the systolic blood pressure was less than 160 mmHg and the diastolic blood pressure less than 100 mmHg.

As seizure activity in a pregnant woman should be treated as eclampsia until proven otherwise, she was thus also started on intravenous magnesium sulphate (a 4 g loading dose followed by continuous infusion at 1 g/hour). The immediate management issues to be considered were:

1. Stabilisation of blood pressure
2. Prevention of further seizure activity
3. Appropriate investigations, including consideration of other causes of seizures
4. Safe delivery of the baby

Immediate blood tests requested included full blood count, urea and electrolytes, uric acid and coagulation screen. A sample was sent for crossmatching blood in the event that emergency caesarean section was required.

The results obtained were:

Haemoglobin 89 g/l	Sodium 134 mmol/l
White cell count 13 x 10^9/l	Potassium 4.9 mmol/l
Platelets 74 10^9/l	Urea 12.1 mmol/l
Prothrombin time 12.1s	Creatinine 125 mmol/l
APTT 31 seconds	Alkaline phosphatase 156 IU/l
Fibrinogen 2.1 g/l	ALT 41 IU/l
Uric acid 408 umol/l	Albumin 29 g/l
	Total bilirubin 20 umol/l

After catheterisation, urinalysis showed 3+ proteinuria and a urinary protein to creatinine ratio (PCR) of 120 mg/mmol

Foetal heart rate monitoring demonstrated reduced variability with a baseline tachycardia and there were concerns about foetal wellbeing. However, given the woman's prolonged seizure activity, hypertensive response to intubation and low platelet count there were also concerns that she may have suffered an intracerebral haemorrhage. A CT scan of her head was thus urgently performed. This showed no evidence of haemorrhage but did demonstrate a minor degree of cerebral oedema. As her blood pressure was now relatively stable at 160/90 mmHg and with evidence suggesting the development of haemolysis, elevated liver enzymes, low platelets (HELLP) syndrome, a decision was made to proceed to emergency caesarean section. As she remained intubated and ventilated, general anaesthesia was used. Following delivery, she was returned ventilated to the ICU for continued supportive care. She remained oliguric for the next six hours after which her urine output improved spontaneously. She was extubated the following day, although she required continued antihypertensive therapy and transfer to the obstetric high dependency area for ongoing care.

Case Discussion

Causes of death from pre-eclampsia/eclampsia include intracerebral haemorrhage (which reflects a failure of anti-hypertensive treatment), haemorrhage (abruption, hepatic rupture), multi-organ failure and death directly due to seizures (hypoxia, aspiration). Many of these cases will be managed initially in obstetric units but may present through accident and emergency departments, in some cases with undiagnosed or concealed pregnancy. Such patients may have had no routine antenatal care and thus present with severe, untreated disease.

Deaths from pre-eclampsia and eclampsia have been highlighted in the triennial Confidential Enquiries into Maternal Deaths in the United Kingdom. Reduction in deaths has been thought to reflect better use of guidelines and protocols and indeed deaths, including those associated with HELLP syndrome and acute fatty liver of pregnancy, are now at the lowest level ever recorded in the United Kingdom.[1]

In the 2011 'Saving Mothers Lives' report, 22 deaths were included in the chapter on eclampsia/pre-eclampsia.[2] Five of these women died from cardiac arrest associated with eclampsia. Whilst most deaths occurred from other complications of pre-eclampsia, such as intracerebral haemorrhage, it must be remembered that eclampsia carries its own intrinsic risks. Better antenatal management may lead to a reduced incidence of eclamptic seizures, but this also means a relative lack of experience for medical staff in dealing with these patients. Following local and national guidelines therefore becomes even more important and in the United Kingdom, guidance has been produced by The National Institute for Health and Care Excellence (NICE).[3]

Although the diagnosis of severe pre-eclampsia may seem apparent, it is worth remembering that it can be mimicked by other conditions. Phaeochromocytoma presenting in pregnancy may be misdiagnosed as pre-eclampsia and although rare there are numerous case reports in the literature. Failure to make the correct diagnosis is associated with a high mortality.

Airway Management in Eclampsia

Initial airway management should be in the left lateral position in order to reduce both aortocaval compression and the risk of aspiration. A Guedel^{TM} airway may be used if required. Nasopharyngeal airways are generally avoided in the pregnant patient due to the increased risk of bleeding from the nasal mucosa. Whether to intubate or not can be a difficult decision in the emergency department or critical care unit in a case of eclampsia. The majority of eclamptic seizures will be brief and self-limiting. The major risk in this situation will come from an exaggerated hypertensive response to intubation, with the risk of intracerebral haemorrhage. Intubation may be more difficult due to airway oedema and repeated, prolonged attempts at intubation by inexperienced staff may increase the hypertensive response. The failed intubation rate in obstetrics (1 in 224) is higher than in the non-obstetric population.[4] There is also likely to be a higher risk when intubation is performed outside the operating theatre environment in less than ideal circumstances. There is a tendency to gastric reflux due to progesterone mediated reduction in lower oesophageal sphincter tone which, coupled with the potential for a full stomach in the emergency situation, makes rapid sequence induction with cricoid pressure mandatory. Left lateral tilt to avoid aortocaval compression may make it easier for cricoid pressure to distort airway anatomy. Use of an inadequate dose of suxamethonium (recommended dose 1.5 mg/kg) particularly in cases with a raised body mass index, may also increase the risk of failed intubation.

Management of Hypertension

Recent publications have stressed the importance of systolic hypertension in pre-eclampsia. Severe hypertension, with systolic blood pressures of greater than 180 mmHg, needs urgent and effective treatment. Saving Mothers' Lives reports several cases where failure to appreciate the urgency and adequately control severe hypertension led to death from intracerebral haemorrhage.[2]

First line therapy for hypertension should be labetalol and other antihypertensive agents should only be used where the side effect profile of labetalol makes its use inappropriate (such as in asthma). Hydralazine is an alternative but it can produce marked hypotension so may require consideration of concomitant administration of a fluid bolus in the antenatal patient to prevent this. This is potentially problematic as these patients are at significant risk of pulmonary oedema due to low serum albumin and increased vascular permeability. However, rapid lowering of the blood pressure may reduce uteroplacental flow with effects on oxygen delivery to the potentially already compromised foetus.

The other issue in the case described is the possibility that she had already suffered an intracerebral haemorrhage. In this case, raised intracranial pressure would require a higher systolic blood pressure to maintain cerebral blood flow and rapid lowering of the blood pressure might be unwise.

Magnesium

There is level-1 evidence for the use of magnesium to prevent recurrent seizures in eclampsia. This is typically given as per the Collaborative Eclampsia Trial regime (4 g intravenous loading dose over 5 minutes followed by an infusion of 1 g/hr).[5] The infusion should be continued for 24 hours after the last seizure and recurrent seizures may be treated with a further bolus dose of 2 to 4 g given over 5 minutes. There is rarely a role for other anticonvulsant drugs such as benzodiazepines and these should not form part of the initial management.

NICE also recommends considering administration of intravenous magnesium sulphate in severe pre-eclampsia if the patient is in a critical care setting and delivery is planned within 24 hours. This is based on evidence derived from the Magpie trial.[6]

There is some evidence emerging from meta-analyses suggesting a benefit to the neonate from antenatal administration of magnesium sulphate in cases of premature delivery. Greatest benefit is shown where delivery is at 28 weeks or earlier. This may prove to be important as there is an association between pre-eclampsia and the need for early delivery.

Delivery

Ultimately, the treatment for pre-eclampsia will be delivery of the foetus and placenta. However, this is not something to undertake urgently without prior stabilisation of the mother. The exaggerated hypertensive response to intubation in the pre-eclamptic patient with uncontrolled hypertension may lead to death from intracerebral haemorrhage. It is essential that the blood pressure is controlled prior to surgery. This being the case, foetal monitoring during an eclamptic seizure is of no benefit as it is unlikely to be reassuring and will not change the initial management.

The vast majority of patients with eclamptic seizures will not require intubation and ventilation at presentation. They may not even need delivery by caesarean section as they may be amenable to induction of labour instead. This is an obstetric decision that will be influenced by individual circumstances, such as the gestational age and previous obstetric history. Even when the patient with a recent eclamptic seizure does require emergency delivery by caesarean section, it may still be possible to perform a regional anaesthetic (usually spinal anaesthesia) as this will produce greater haemodynamic stability and avoid problems associated with intubation. This will require a knowledge of the patient's platelet count and coagulation results, all of which may be abnormal.

HELLP Syndrome

This patient had some of the features of HELLP syndrome. This is an uncommon but well recognised complication of severe pre-eclampsia. Not all of the features may be present and indeed hypertension and proteinuria may be absent. It may present with epigastric pain, nausea, vomiting, haematuria and jaundice and is easily misdiagnosed in the early stages. The woman is likely to require urgent delivery of the baby and management is then aimed at supporting maternal renal and hepatic function until spontaneous resolution occurs. Platelet transfusions are unlikely to be required unless there is active bleeding, such as may occur during caesarean section.

Corticosteroids do not form part of the management of HELLP syndrome. However, they may be useful to aid foetal lung maturation in the case of premature birth. Two doses of betamethasone 12 mg intramuscularly should be given 12 hours apart where delivery is likely within the next 7 days and gestational age is between 24 and 34 weeks. It may also be useful up to 36 weeks gestation. This should be discussed with the obstetrician in charge of the patient

Prevention of Venous Thromboembolism

A thromboembolism risk assessment must be performed as pregnant patients are at high risk of this complication. Low molecular weight heparins form the mainstay of pharmacological prophylaxis but should not be administered until a plan for delivery has been made. In addition, abnormal coagulation or a low platelet count may make administration unwise. Use of physical methods such as compression stockings would be appropriate for all patients.

Renal Function

This has classically been assessed using automated reagent strips. Whilst this may detect proteinuria, there is a poor correlation with 24 hour protein levels as it may be affected by factors such as the patient's hydration status.[7] A result of 1+ or greater requires quantification using either a spot urinary protein to creatinine ratio (PCR) or a 24-hour urine collection. A urinary PCR greater than 30 mg/mmol or a 24-hour collection containing more than 300 mg of protein represents significant proteinuria.

Fluid restriction forms an essential part of the management of severe pre-eclampsia and eclampsia. Patients are likely to remain oliguric for several hours after delivery, but it is reassuring to note that, unlike other critically ill patients, this is likely to resolve without treatment and a spontaneous diuresis often occurs during the recovery phase. Aggressive fluid boluses are likely to cause pulmonary oedema and are best avoided. Cautious fluid challenges may be required, particularly if intraoperative/delivery losses have been underestimated and not replaced. Careful attention to fluid balance in the perioperative period is essential. Monitoring of central venous pressure is rarely useful as it does not correlate with the development of pulmonary oedema and use of pulmonary artery catheters has also not been shown to improve outcome.

Interpretation of Blood Results

This should be done in the knowledge of the normal ranges in a pregnant woman. In the case described, a creatinine of 125 umol/l represents significant renal impairment. Renal blood flow and glomerular filtration rate are both increased in pregnancy and a creatinine greater than 75 umol/l or a urea greater than 4.5 mmol/l warrants further investigation. The low serum albumin is associated with an increased risk of pulmonary oedema and the raised uric acid is consistent with a diagnosis of pre-eclampsia.

The low haemoglobin level may have multiple causes, including physiological anaemia of pregnancy (relative haemodilution), iron/folic acid deficiency, haemorrhage, sickle cell disease or thalassaemia. More worryingly, it may represent haemolysis as part of HELLP syndrome.

The thrombocytopenia seen in this patient is most likely to represent severe pre-eclampsia with or without HELLP syndrome. Other causes are possible though, including gestational thrombocytopenia (which accounts for 70 to 80 percent of cases) and idiopathic thrombocytopenic purpura. Access to previous blood results may help to identify the acute versus the chronic problem and give an indication of whether the platelet count is stable or falling.

Of equal concern is the mild coagulopathy. While at 2.1 g/l her fibrinogen may appear to be within the normal range, this actually represents a low level for a pregnant woman and 4.5 g/l would be a more normal value. This is important to recognize, as severe pre-eclampsia is associated with placental abruption, a cause of major obstetric haemorrhage and disseminated intravascular coagulation. Early recourse to fibrinogen concentrates or cryoprecipitate may be appropriate in this situation and liaison with a haematologist is advisable.

Early Warning Scoring Systems

All pregnant women who present to hospital should be assessed using an early warning scoring system. This should be a maternity specific one as the physiological changes of pregnancy make some of the parameters used in a normal adult early warning scoring system inappropriate. While this may be of little immediate help in the face of an eclamptic seizure, it may be of use for the non-obstetrically trained when dealing with pre-eclampsia.

Conclusion

Successful management of patients with pre-eclampsia and associated conditions requires a multidisciplinary approach. Obstetricians, anaesthetists, midwives and neonatologists will all be involved in delivery of the baby. Stabilisation of the mother remains the initial priority and safe delivery can only occur once this has happened.

Key Learning Points

- Severe systolic hypertension in pre-eclampsia needs urgent and effective treatment. Blood pressure must be stabilised as a priority before delivery.
- There may be an exaggerated hypertensive response to intubation in these patients that must be attenuated to prevent intracerebral haemorrhage.
- Most eclamptic seizures are self-limiting. Prolonged or recurrent seizures unresponsive to treatment must raise the possibility of alternative diagnoses such as intracerebral haemorrhage or epilepsy.
- Oliguria is common in severe pre-eclampsia and will usually resolve spontaneously. Aggressive fluid therapy may precipitate pulmonary oedema.
- Physiological, haematological and biochemical parameters must be interpreted with reference to the normal values for pregnant patients.

References

1. Knight M, Kenyon S, Brocklehurst P, Neilson J, Shakespeare J, Kurinczuk JJ (Eds.) *on behalf of MBRRACE- UK. Saving Lives, Improving Mothers' Care:Lessons Learned to Inform Future Maternity Care from the UK and Ireland Confidential Enquiries into Maternal Deaths and Morbidity 2009–2012.* Oxford: National Perinatal Epidemiology Unit, University of Oxford 2014.

2. Centre for Maternal and Child Enquiries (CMACE). Saving Mothers' Lives: reviewing maternal deaths to make motherhood safer: 2006–2008. The Eighth Report on Confidential Enquiries into

Maternal Deaths in the United Kingdom. *BJOG* 2011;118(Suppl. 1):1–203.

3. Hypertension in pregnancy: The management of hypertensive disorders during pregnancy. NICE guidelines [CG107] Published date: August 2010.

4. Quinn AC, Milne D, Columb M, Gorton H, Knight M. Failed tracheal intubation in obstetric anaesthesia: 2 yr national case-control study in the UK. *Br J Anaesth* 2013 Jan;110(1):74–80.

5. The Eclampsia Trial Collaborative Group. Which anticonvulsant for women with eclampsia? Evidence from the Collaborative Eclampsia Trial. *The Lancet* 1995;345:1455–63.

6. The Magpie Trial Collaborative Group. Do women with pre-eclampsia, and their babies, benefit from magnesium sulphate? The Magpie Trial: a randomised placebo-controlled trial. *The Lancet* 2002;359: 1877–90.

7. Meyer NL, Mercer BM, Friedman SA, Sibai BM. Urinary dipstick protein: a poor predictor of absent or severe proteinuria. *Am J Obstet Gynecol* 1994;170:137–41.

Airway Management

Timothy Wenham and Aditya Krishan Kapoor

Introduction

Airway management is integral to patient care in the intensive care unit. Although much attention is given to ventilator management, lung protective ventilation and weaning strategies, establishing an artificial airway can be a time of significant risk to the patient. Often this occurs in an emergency time-pressured situation; possibly in a remote area of the hospital and often occurs out of hours when staffing levels and senior support may be limited or not immediately available. The patient may be compromised and respiratory failure makes the development of hypoxaemia a significant risk.

The key to successfully managing these situations is preparation and planning; ensuring consideration is given to the possible complications and knowing in advance what action will be taken should problems be encountered. Guidelines and algorithms can aid this decision-making process and unload some of the cognitive burden. In order to draw upon these aids in the emergency situation, it is also useful to mentally or verbally rehearse the process during all intubations. This case highlights the issues that may be faced with airway management in an emergency.

Case Description

A 67-year-old patient with chronic obstructive pulmonary disease presented acutely to the emergency department (ED) having been brought in by ambulance. He had been found collapsed and unresponsive by his son. His past medical history included obesity (body mass index, BMI, of 47), obstructive sleep apnoea, ischaemic heart disease and tablet controlled diabetes.

Initial assessment revealed a Glasgow Coma Scale (GCS) of 3/15 with chest examination demonstrating widespread wheeze and crepitations throughout both lungs. Initial observations were pulse 110 bpm, BP 115/60 mmHg, SpO_2 82 percent (15 l/min O_2 via face mask with reservoir bag). The initial arterial blood gas measurements were pH 7.21, $PaCO_2$ 16.7 kPa, PaO_2 6.4 kPa, $HCO3^-$ 31 mmol, BE +7, lactate 2.4 mmol/L. The critical care doctor was called for an opinion on critical care admission.

On review, a decision was made to intubate the patient to provide respiratory support and airway protection. He was positioned in a slight head up position on the ED trolley and preoxygenated using a Waters (Mapleson C) breathing circuit with high flow oxygen. Monitoring included ECG, non-invasive blood pressure, pulse oximetry, and capnography. Despite preoxygenation, a SpO_2 of 92 percent was the maximum that could be achieved. Intravenous sodium thiopentone and suxamethonium were administered in appropriate induction doses and the ED nurse applied cricoid pressure. At the initial intubation attempt with a size 3 Macintosh blade, the view was a Cormack and Lehane grade 3 view and so a gum elastic bougie (GEB) was used to pass the endotracheal tube. On attempted ventilation no chest rise or carbon dioxide trace on the capnograph was observed and the tube was removed. A second attempt at laryngoscopy was made; however, despite repositioning and altering cricoid pressure, no improvement in view was possible. The patient began to desaturate therefore manual ventilation with face mask and oropharyngeal airway was commenced. Urgent help was summoned and the on-call anaesthetist was requested to attend urgently for a failed intubation. Manual ventilation proved difficult requiring a two-person technique to provide chest movement and a trace on the capnograph and cricoid pressure was released. Insertion of a laryngeal mask airway (LMA) in the form of an iGel™ was attempted but there was excessive leak and minimal ventilation so facemask ventilation was resumed.

The anaesthetist arrived with an operating department practitioner to provide assistance. The patient had saturations of 88 per cent and was beginning to show some signs of spontaneous respiration. A videolaryngoscope and fibre-optic bronchoscope from theatres were obtained. In addition the availability of surgical airway equipment was ensured. The patient was given intubating doses of midazolam and rocuronium and the videolaryngoscope used. A grade-2 view was obtained and with difficulty a GEB was passed through the cords under vision and the endotracheal tube was railroaded over it. Ventilation of the lungs was confirmed by auscultation and capnography.

The patient's oxygen saturation improved and mechanical ventilation commenced with subsequent transfer to the ICU for on-going management.

Case Discussion

This case of a failed intubation is an uncommon but potentially life-threatening airway emergency. The probability of failing with any procedure must always be considered and this is especially important with airway management in the critically ill. Predicting difficulty, optimising the environment and ensuring the availability of all equipment is important. Training and rehearsing emergency procedures and algorithms should form a key part of critical care team training.

Predicting and Planning

Most important is to be aware of predictors of when difficulty may be encountered. Patient characteristics indicative of difficulty include pregnancy, obesity, rheumatological conditions such as rheumatoid arthritis and ankylosing spondylitis, previous head and neck surgery or radiotherapy. The mode of presentation can also provide information with cervical spine injury or immobilisation, facial or laryngeal trauma, and oral and pharyngeal masses such as tumours or abscesses all being associated with potential difficulty.

It is important to always assess the airway and there are a number of predictive tests for difficult intubation, difficult LMA insertion and difficult mask ventilation which are often used in anaesthetic practice. Their extension into critical care can be difficult as the patient may not be able to comply with assessment; however it remains useful to consider these as markers of potential difficulty (Box 32.1)

It is evident that the patient population will differ in the ICU compared with anaesthetic practice. Patients may be suffering from significant cardio-respiratory compromise and intubation conditions may be suboptimal. Specific tests for use in intensive care may therefore be of more use. The MACOCHA score is a tool that has been described recently[1,2] (Box 32.2). This was developed in a prospective multicentre study of adult non-obstetric patients. Difficult intubation was defined as 3 or more attempts at laryngoscopy or attempts lasting more than 10 minutes. In this case the MACOCHA score would have been 3 and so the possibility of a difficult intubation should have been considered.

Box 32.1 Markers of difficult intubation and difficult mask ventilation

Predictive tests of difficult intubation

Mouth opening / Interincisor gap	<3 cm indicates difficulty
Mandibular advancement / protrusion / Upper lip bite test	Inability to advance lower incisors beyond upper incisors
Mallampati / Modified mallampati (Samsoon & Young)	>Class 3 associated with difficulty
Cervical spine extension	Increasing risk with restriction
Thyro-mental distance (Patil test)	<6 cm associated with difficulty
Sterno-mental distance (Savva test)	<12.5 cm associated with difficulty
Wilson score	Combines 5 risk factors: weight, head & neck movement, jaw movement, receding mandible and buck teeth

Predictive Tests of Difficult Mask Ventilation
Elderly
Edentulous
Raised BMI
Presence of beard

Box 32.2 MACOCHA score calculation

Factors	Points
Patient	5
Mallampati Score III or IV	2
Obstructive Sleep Apnoea	1
Reduced Mobility of Cervical Spine	1
Limited mouth opening <3 cm	
Factors Related to Pathology	1
Coma	1
Severe Hypoxaemia (<80%)	
Factor Related to Operator	1
Non-anaesthetist	
Total	12

MACOCHA: **M**allampati ≥3, Obstructive Sleep **A**pnoea, **C**ervical spine limitation, Limited mouth **o**pening, **C**oma, **H**ypoxia, Non-**a**naesthetist.
    Score from 0–12 with increasing difficulty.
    A score of ≥3 gives a sensitivity of 73% and specificity of 89%. The positive predictive value was 36% but the negative predictive value was 98%.

Given that the MACOCHA score is only relatively recently described it is not known if its routine use or use similar prediction tools of difficulty in intubation can be translated into a reduction in the incidence of difficult intubation and subsequent complications by increasing preparedness regarding equipment and personnel. Despite full assessment of the airway, unexpected difficulty may still arise and so thought must be given prior to all intubations of what steps will be taken if the procedure does not turn out to be straightforward. The Fourth National Audit Project of The Royal College of Anaesthetists and the Difficult Airway Society report on major complications of airway management in the United Kingdom (NAP4) identified poor airway assessment and the failure to plan for failure as important clinical themes associated with complications.[3] The lack of anticipation and planning for difficult cases was a major concern.

Preoxygenation

Preoxygenation is a core component of the intubation of critically ill patients who are likely to be suffering from cardio-respiratory compromise.[4,5] There are risks of aspiration due to a non-starved status, critical illness or intra-abdominal pathology, and rapid sequence induction of anaesthesia is usual UK practice. With apnoea an inevitable consequence of induction of anaesthesia and the administration of neuromuscular blocking agents to facilitate intubation, preoxygenation serves to provide a degree of safety against the development of hypoxaemia.

The aim of preoxygenation is to replace the nitrogen content of the functional residual capacity (FRC) with oxygen – termed denitrogenation. Classical preoxygenation involves 3 minutes of tidal volume breathing of 100 percent oxygen. This serves to maximise the alveolar oxygen content and denitrogenate both the FRC and the bloodstream (minor effect). Attention needs to be directed to ensuring an appropriately sized face mask and the minimisation of leaks which adversely affect the efficacy of preoxygenation. Efficacy can be measured by assessing end tidal oxygen concentration and aiming for a target greater than 90 per cent if facilities are available for this. While administration of oxygen helps fill the FRC with oxygen, the FRC itself can be increased by optimisation of the patient's position and the use of positive end-expiratory pressure or continuous positive airway pressure.

The causes of hypoxaemia in critically ill patients are often multi-factorial with ventilation/perfusion mismatch and shunt, airway or alveolar pathology, anaemia and low cardiac output all playing a role. In these patients the efficacy of preoxygenation may be decreased and it may not be possible to raise the patient's saturations to close to 100 per cent. In these circumstances, as in this case, as the SpO_2 was less than 95 per cent, it may be prudent to provide manual ventilation while awaiting full neuromuscular blockade in order to prevent rapid desaturation. This has to be balanced with the risk that excessive pressures may result in lower oesophageal sphincter incompetence and gastric distension leading to regurgitation and aspiration.

The combination of the above techniques serves to increase the duration of 'safe' apnoea as long as possible to facilitate tracheal intubation while minimising the risks of dangerous hypoxaemia and aspiration.

Management of Failed Intubation

Prior to intubation it is important to ensure that all equipment, personnel and drugs are prepared in advance and that the team present is aware of the plan. In particular, attention must be given to action to take in the case of a difficult or failed intubation and equipment for this must be available. If time permits, additional or senior personnel can be summoned if difficulty is predicted. In this case, additional help could have been called upon early as there were indications that the intubation might be complicated. It is important to consider the urgency of the situation, the patient's clinical state and balance this against the risks of intervention. One option sometimes overlooked is to consider a tracheostomy under local anaesthesia performed by an ENT surgeon.

One of the recommendations of NAP4 is that an intubation checklist should be developed and used for all intubations of critically ill patients in order to ensure adequate preparation of the patient, equipment, drugs and the team.[3] An example is provided in the full report. In addition the checklist should also include the identification of back-up plans should difficulty be encountered. The other recommendations of significance for critical care include the provision of algorithms for management of intubation, extubation and re-intubation; that every ICU should have immediate access to a difficult airway trolley and that a fibrescope should be immediately available for use on ICU.

The management of a difficult or failed intubation is an emergency situation. A number of difficult intubation algorithms exist. An algorithm can be defined as a set of rules for solving a problem in a finite number of steps, in this case the process of achieving an artificial airway in order to provide oxygenation and ventilation. Oxygenation is at the forefront of all difficult airway algorithms and must always remain the primary objective.

The Difficult Airway Society (DAS) published their guidelines for the management of the unanticipated difficult intubation in 2004[6] (Figure 32.1).

These guidelines were developed for use in anaesthesia and the focus of the approach is one of maintaining oxygenation while minimising airway trauma. The American Society of Anaesthesiologists published the most recent update to their Practice Guidelines for Management of the Difficult Airway in 2013.[7] These guidelines have much in common with the DAS guidelines; however, these are again developed for the practise of anaesthesia and give importance to the early consideration of awakening the patient in cases of intubation difficulty which may not be an option in the critically ill. The final common pathway of both guidelines is the use of emergency techniques for direct tracheal access.

Some common themes are important in managing a difficult or failed intubation. The first is to ensure that the initial attempt at intubation is performed under optimal conditions. Important considerations here are optimum patient position, adequate neuro-muscular blockade and the availability of all required equipment (e.g., patient monitoring including pulse oximetry and capnography, at least two laryngoscopes/videolaryngoscopes and an introducer/gum-elastic bougie and equipment for failed intubation). The import-ance of the use of pre-oxygenation, cricoid pressure, optimum external laryngeal manipu-lation (OELM) by the laryngoscopist and the BURP (backwards, upwards and rightwards pressure on the thyroid cartilage) manoeuvre are emphasised. The use of OELM and BURP with an alternative laryngoscope and a bougie may allow success in cases of difficulty, being mindful that cricoid pressure itself can cause airway obstruction and worsen the view at laryngoscopy. It is important to ensure adequate oxygenation between attempts at intub-ation. It is also important to emphasise the limitation of intubation attempts to prevent trauma causing laryngeal oedema which could lead to a 'can't intubate can ventilate' scenario deteriorating into a 'can't intubate can't ventilate' scenario.

Once it becomes apparent that intubation has failed, this should be announced to the team present. If awakening the patient is an option, then this should be considered. If this is

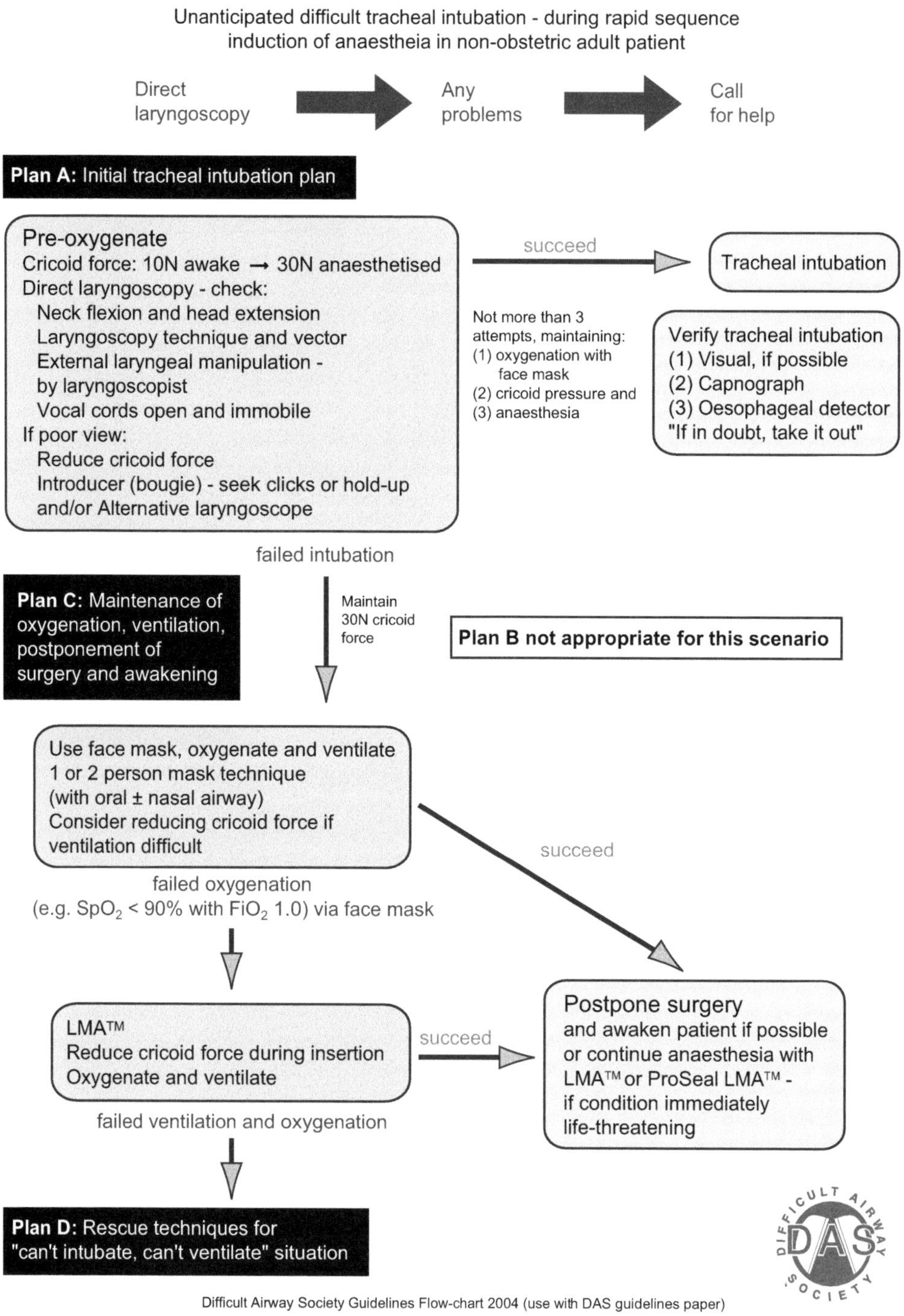

Unanticipated difficult tracheal intubation - during rapid sequence
induction of anaestheia in non-obstetric adult patient

Direct laryngoscopy ➡ Any problems ➡ Call for help

Plan A: Initial tracheal intubation plan

Pre-oxygenate
Cricoid force: 10N awake → 30N anaesthetised
Direct laryngoscopy - check:
  Neck flexion and head extension
  Laryngoscopy technique and vector
  External laryngeal manipulation -
  by laryngoscopist
  Vocal cords open and immobile
If poor view:
  Reduce cricoid force
  Introducer (bougie) - seek clicks or hold-up
  and/or Alternative laryngoscope

succeed → Tracheal intubation

Not more than 3 attempts, maintaining:
(1) oxygenation with face mask
(2) cricoid pressure and
(3) anaesthesia

Verify tracheal intubation
(1) Visual, if possible
(2) Capnograph
(3) Oesophageal detector
"If in doubt, take it out"

failed intubation

Plan C: Maintenance of oxygenation, ventilation, postponement of surgery and awakening

Maintain 30N cricoid force

Plan B not appropriate for this scenario

Use face mask, oxygenate and ventilate
1 or 2 person mask technique
(with oral ± nasal airway)
Consider reducing cricoid force if
ventilation difficult

succeed

failed oxygenation
(e.g. SpO$_2$ < 90% with FiO$_2$ 1.0) via face mask

LMA™
Reduce cricoid force during insertion
Oxygenate and ventilate

succeed →

failed ventilation and oxygenation

Postpone surgery
and awaken patient if possible
or continue anaesthesia with
LMA™ or ProSeal LMA™ -
if condition immediately
life-threatening

Plan D: Rescue techniques for
"can't intubate, can't ventilate" situation

Difficult Airway Society Guidelines Flow-chart 2004 (use with DAS guidelines paper)

Figure 32.1 Reproduced from Henderson JJ, Popat MT, Latto IP, Pearce AC. Difficult Airway Society guidelines for management of the unanticipated difficult intubation. *Anaesthesia* 2004; 59: 675–94, with permission from Blackwell Publishing Ltd.

not a possibility then the focus must be on maintaining oxygenation. Initial attempts at maintaining oxygenation can be via face mask and oral airway as these are readily available. If these prove difficult or fail, a supraglottic airway device can be tried. Although the classic LMA^{TM} has been suggested, second generation supraglottic airway devices (e.g., ProSeal LMA^{TM}, iGel^{TM}, LMA Supreme^{TM}) are now in common use and may offer advantages of improved seal pressure and the incorporation of a gastric port to allow the stomach to be decompressed. Supraglottic airway device insertion may be hampered by cricoid pressure which may need to be reduced to facilitate insertion. It is possible that these devices may allow a sufficiently secure airway to allow patient stabilisation but it is likely that more a more definitive airway will be required. This may take a number of forms including the use of a video or fibre-optic laryngoscope to achieve intubation or use of a percutaneous tracheostomy.

If all attempts at achieving oxygenation and ventilation discussed above have failed, rescue techniques for the 'can't intubate, can't ventilate' situation will be required. Although these techniques carry risks, they must be balanced against the risk of hypoxic brain injury and death if the situation goes uncorrected. The choice of techniques here are needle/cannula versus surgical cricothroidotomy. Although both are advocated, the cannula technique could require equipment that may not be readily to hand such as a kink resistant cannula and mechanism to deliver percutaneous transtracheal jet ventilation (e.g., Manujet; ENK Flow Modulator). The surgical technique can be performed rapidly and will allow connection to conventional ventilation equipment and circuits. The NAP4 report highlighted a high failure rate of cannula techniques of the order of 60 per cent which were often rescued by surgical cricothroidotomy or tracheostomy. The ideal method for achieving direct tracheal access is still not known with certainty.

Video-laryngoscopes and equipment for indirect laryngoscopy have become increasingly common, as have intubating optical stylets. In this case successful intubation was facilitated by the use of a video-laryngoscope. These devices may be effective in reducing complications from difficult intubation in critically ill patients but large multicentre studies are required before they will feature in published guidelines. Ensuring their availability in areas such as the emergency department and intensive care will also need to be addressed. It is important that no matter what equipment is used the practitioner is fully trained in its use and aware of its limitations.

Simulation is increasingly being recognised as an important tool in training in all aspects of medical practise. In particular its value in understanding the non-technical and human factor influences is invaluable and these often are difficult to learn with conventional teaching. Multi-disciplinary training within critical care teams is important to ensure that everyone is aware of the failure to intubate algorithms and the actions that should be undertaken.

Conclusion

This case is one of a failed intubation, an uncommon but potentially life-threatening airway emergency in a critically ill patient. There were several predictors that intubation might prove to be difficult and perhaps if they had been identified, the problems encountered could have been avoided and the initial intubation attempt optimised. The risks are increased in the emergency situation when the environment is unfamiliar, where trained assistance may be absent and when a full range of equipment may be lacking. Knowledge of difficult and failed intubation algorithms is essential and the key principles are anticipating difficulty, optimising the environment, prioritising oxygenation and where necessary undertaking emergency tracheal access without delay.

Key Learning Points

- Always assess the patient and the situation when performing airway management.
- Always assess the patient's airway for markers of potential difficulty and consider using tools developed for use in the ICU / critically ill population. (e.g., the MACOCHA score)
- Anticipate difficulty and plan in advance what actions to take.
- Optimise the environment by ensuring that all personnel and equipment are present and checked.
- Ensure familiarity with the equipment present in areas where airway management will be undertaken.
- Optimise patient positioning, undertake effective pre-oxygenation and ensure adequate neuromuscular blockade to provide ideal conditions for the first intubation attempt. The usefulness of OELM by the laryngoscopist and the BURP manoeuvre should never be overlooked.
- Ensure familiarity with failed / difficult intubation drills and algorithms and undertake regular team training to ensure retention of knowledge and skills.
- Always prioritise oxygenation over ventilation.
- Undertake rapid emergency tracheal access to achieve oxygenation in a 'can't intubate, can't ventilate' situation.

References

1. De Jong, Molinari, Terzi, et al. Development and Validation of the MACOCHA Intubation Score in a Multicenter Cohort Study. *Am J Respir Crit Care Med* 2013;187(8):832–39.

2. De Jong A, Jung B, Jaber S. Intubation in the ICU: we could improve our practice. *Critical Care* 2014;18:209.

3. Cook T, Woodall N, Frerk C. 4th National Project of The Royal College of Anaesthetists and The Difficult Airway Society. Major complications of airway management in the United Kingdom 2011.

4. Sirian R, Wills J. Physiology of apnoea and the benefits of preoxygenation. *Continuing Education in Anaesthesia, Critical Care and Pain* 2009;9(4):105–8.

5. Weingart SD, Levitan RM. Preoxygenation and prevention of desaturation during emergency airway management. *Annals of Emergency Medicine* 2012;59(3):165–75.

6. Henderson JJ, Popat MT, Latto IP, Pearce AC. Difficult airway society guidelines for management of the unanticipated difficult intubation. *Anaesthesia* 2004;59:675–94.

7. Apfelbaum J, Hagberg C, Caplan R, et al. Practice guidelines for management of the difficult airway: an updated report by the American Society of Anesthesiologists task force on management of the difficult airway. *Anaesthesiology* 2013;118(2): 251–70.

Bronchoscopy and Tracheostomy

Steve Cantellow and Victoria Banks

Introduction

Indications for a tracheostomy include long-term ventilation, airway protection, the management of secretions and to bypass an upper airway obstruction. The TracMan trial revealed that performing an early tracheostomy did not reduce 30-day mortality. Despite this, tracheostomy may be associated with improved comfort, reduced sedation requirements, better oral hygiene, a reduced rate of ventilator associated pneumonia (VAP) and improved weaning success rates.[1,2]

There are risks involved in tracheostomy insertion, some of which may be fatal and so an understanding of the anatomy and potential complications is crucial.

Case Description

A 47-year-old obese man with severe pancreatitis secondary to gallstones was admitted to the intensive care unit for circulatory and ventilatory support. During the second week of his admission, percutaneous dilatational tracheostomy (PDT) was felt to be appropriate on the grounds that he was likely to require prolonged mechanical ventilation.

Family assent for the procedure was obtained. The patient had a normal coagulation profile and the previous laryngoscopy grade was noted. Appropriate staffing and equipment were assembled, his nasogastric feed was stopped and the stomach aspirated. A pillow was positioned under his shoulders to fully extend the neck. He was fully sedated, given an opioid analgesic and a muscle relaxant and was ventilated on 100 per cent oxygen. Fibreoptic bronchoscopy (FB) was used to guide the procedure.

The tracheal rings, thyroid and cricoid cartilages were palpated. The skin and subcutaneous tissues were injected with a lignocaine-adrenaline solution and a 1.5 cm horizontal skin incision made below the cricoid cartilage. Blunt dissection was used to identify the anterior tracheal wall. The trachea was noted to be rather deep. The endotracheal tube was withdrawn until there was a 'give' below the operator's finger and the bronchoscope was pulled back into the endotracheal tube. A needle mounted on a syringe was inserted under direct vision into the trachea between the first and second rings and air successfully aspirated. Correct placement of the J-wire (12 o' clock position, between rings 1 and 2) was confirmed by FB. Dilatation was achieved using a single stage dilator tracheostomy kit. A pre-mounted 8.0 mm internal diameter tracheostomy tube was railroaded over an 8-French 'wire stiffener'. The cuff was inflated and cuff pressure checked. Direct fibreoptic visualisation confirmed its position within the trachea. The ventilator circuit with capnography monitoring was attached and a chest X-ray was requested. Four corner sutures and a soft tie held the tube in place. It was noted that the tracheostomy tube looked a little short as the flange was indenting the neck.

After repositioning the patient, the monitoring began to alarm, indicating low oxygen saturations, a flat capnography trace and high airway pressures. The patient's neck, face and thorax had dramatically swollen. It wasn't possible to ventilate via the tracheostomy or pass a suction catheter past the end of the tracheostomy tube, even after removal of the inner tube. It was felt that the tracheostomy had become displaced and was no longer in the trachea. The tracheostomy was removed and the neck incision covered. Attempts to hand ventilate were challenging so the patient was urgently re-intubated with a cuffed oral endotracheal tube. His oxygenation quickly improved.

Over the course of the next five days, the surgical emphysema and mediastinal air reduced significantly. A surgical tracheostomy was performed and a longer tracheostomy tube with an adjustable flange was inserted. The patient had a protracted stay within critical care but was eventually decannulated after sixty days.

Case Discussion

Tracheal Anatomy[3]

It is normally possible to palpate the thyroid and cricoid cartilages in the neck, and a number of tracheal rings above the sternal notch.

There are two main fascial planes, the investing fascia and the deeper pretracheal fascia. The strap muscles are in the midline, deep to the investing fascia.

The thyroid isthmus covers the trachea between rings two and four. Depending on the percutaneous tracheostomy technique, the isthmus may be encountered during dilation but this is usually without consequence, probably due to a tamponading effect.

The lateral relations of the trachea include the lateral lobes of the thyroid and the carotid sheath containing the carotid artery, jugular vein, and vagus nerve. The recurrent laryngeal nerve runs along the tracheo-oesophageal groove. Posterior to the trachea is the oesophagus.

The trachea is lined with a respiratory mucosa whose capillary pressure ranges from 20–30 mmHg. Increasing the cuff pressure can impair blood flow which increases the risk of tracheal complications including stenosis, tracheomalacia and fistulation between trachea and oesophagus or blood vessels. Cuff pressure should ideally be 15 to 20 mmHg and never above 35 mmHg.[4]

An important vessel to mention is the innominate artery (brachiocephalic trunk), a branch of the aorta which ascends and crosses the trachea from left to right (Figure 33.1).

It is occasionally high riding and is associated with massive haemorrhage both at the time of tracheostomy or subsequently if the tracheostomy tube erodes into the vessel. Fistula formation between the artery and trachea can also occur.

The anterior jugular veins are superficial, and often have communications that cross the midline. Other vessels in the region include the thyroid arteries (sometimes including an aberrant thyroid ima artery) and veins.

Tracheostomy Technique

Tracheostomy can be either surgical or percutaneous.

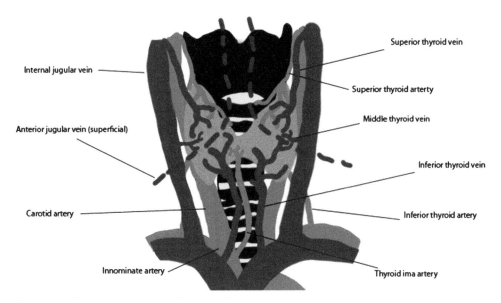

Internal jugular vein

Anterior jugular vein (superficial)

Carotid artery

Innominate artery

Superior thyroid vein

Superior thyroid artery

Middle thyroid vein

Inferior thyroid vein

Inferior thyroid artery

Thyroid ima artery

Figure 33.1 Tracheostomy anatomy: blood vessels.

Percutaneous

The three main percutaneous techniques are:

1. Ciaglia:[5] dilatation with a series of tapered dilators, now usually modified to use a single stage dilator. This technique is described in the case above, and is the commonest PDT technique in the UK
2. Griggs:[6] dilatation with modified Kelly forceps
3. Fantoni:[7] translaryngeal technique with balloon dilatation

Surgical

After skin incision, the investing fascia is opened vertically and the strap muscles split in the midline. Retractors are used to hold the tissues apart and the isthmus is either moved out of the way or divided. A tracheal hook is inserted below the cricoid to pull the trachea upward and forward. Bleeding is controlled and the trachea opened. In children, a vertical incision suffices, whereas in adults it is common to make a window by removing the anterior parts of the third and fourth rings. Traction sutures are inserted so that the trachea can be accessed should the tracheostomy tube become displaced before a tract has formed.[8] In the case of accidental decannulation, it is relevant to know whether the patient had a surgical tracheostomy or PDT. A permanent tract may take between 7–10 days in the case of PDT but occurs much sooner with a surgical tracheostomy.

Choice of Technique

PDT does not require transfer of the critically ill patient to theatre (with its related complications) and is associated with a lower infection rate, cost savings and a complication rate similar to surgical technique. Nevertheless, a surgical technique should be considered when there are anatomical concerns such as

- midline mass
- previous radiotherapy
- scar tissue
- trachea not midline
- fixed neck/unstable neck
- inability to palpate cricoid/short neck/obesity
- head and neck trauma
- high innominate artery
- large overlying midline vessels
- burns

A percutaneous technique should not be performed in the unintubated patient, the paediatric patient nor used for airway rescue (cricothyroidotomy is more appropriate).

Tracheostomy Safety

The Fourth National Audit Project (NAP4) of the Royal College of Anaesthetists found that half of all airway-related deaths and cases of brain damage in critical care were related to tracheostomy complications (see Box 33.1). Tracheostomised patients are also cared for on the wards and so complications can occur outside monitored environments. Both the NCEPOD report 'On the Right Trach?' and the National Tracheostomy Safety Project (NTSP) make some key recommendations which are essential reading.[2,4] The principal themes are:

- Patients with tracheostomy should be cared for in an appropriate risk-assessed environment;
- Equipment for the management of tracheostomy should be immediately available and checked regularly;
- Staff should trained and competent;
- There should be clinical leadership for tracheostomy care in hospitals, along with appropriate policies and guidance on issues such as humidification, cuff pressure, cleaning of the inner tube and resuscitation;
- Tracheostomy tubes should be appropriate for the patient's anatomy;
- Multidisciplinary care should be the standard for all patients with tracheostomy, especially with regard to decannulation and discharge planning;
- Unplanned nighttime discharge from critical care is not recommended;
- Tracheostomy should be recorded and coded as an operative procedure and tracheostomy-related data should be collected and analysed

Planning for Tracheostomy

It is inappropriate to perform this elective procedure 'out of hours' and the patient's relatives should be fully informed of the proposed procedure and assent should be obtained. Printed information leaflets can aid this discussion. Full consideration needs to be given regarding specific patient factors (e.g: anatomy/ coagulation/ PEEP should be less than 10 cmH_2O/ FiO_2 less than 60 percent), staffing and equipment requirements. Before 'knife-to-skin,' it is crucial to have a 'time out' and run through a pre-procedure checklist (**Box 33.2**). The insertion of an inappropriately sized tracheostomy tube in the case described above might have been averted if a safety checklist had been used.

Box 33.1 Complications of tracheostomy

Intraoperative
Loss of PEEP (hypoxia)
Bleeding (see text)
False passage
Right endobronchial placement
Tracheal injury: ring fracture, tears, perforation
Laryngeal injury: cricothyroid muscle, vocal cords

Delayed
Bleeding (see text)
Pneumonthorax, pneumomediastinum, surgical emphysema
Displacement & accidental decannulation
Obstruction: mucus, blood clot, herniated cuff, tube abutting tracheal wall or carina
Cuff leak/aspiration
Fistulae: Trache-oesophageal, Trache-arterial
Infection: local, mediastinitis, VAP
Discomfort, impaired communication

Late
Tracheomalacia and stenosis
Persistent sinus
Permanent tracheostomy
Psychological problems (anxiety, altered body image)

Tube Choice and Long Term Care

Obese patients are better suited to tubes with a longer proximal length, while patients with tracheomalacia may require tubes with a longer distal length. Patients with fixed flexion abnormalities may not tolerate tubes with fixed angulation.[4] Tube diameter is also relevant to patient size and also if flexible bronchoscopy is required (see below). It is recommended that tracheostomy tubes with a removable inner-tube are used.[4]

If there is a requirement for ongoing ventilation or an aspiration risk, a cuffed tube is mandatory; however, uncuffed smaller tubes may be more comfortable during the latter stages of weaning. Fenestrated tubes permit phonation when used in conjunction with a speaking valve. The benefits of using uncuffed tubes need to be balanced against the risk of their limited ability to protect against aspiration or to provide the application of PEEP/high ventilator pressures. The timing of this step (and subsequent decannulation) must be carefully considered seeking input from speech and language therapists, physiotherapists, dieticians and outreach nurses.[2,4]

Drying out of secretions can cause tube obstruction and so humidification is vital, as is the immediate availability of suction. Best practice suggests that removable inner tubes should be removed and cleaned at least every eight hours. Patients should have all equipment concerned with the management of a tracheostomy, including a change of tube, at their bedside.[4]

Anyone caring for patients with tracheostomies should remain vigilant for so-called 'red flags' which the NTSP classifies into airway flags, breathing flags, general flags and tracheostomy specific flags. The tracheostomy specific flags are:

1. a visibly displaced tube
2. blood around the tube

> **Box 33.2** Pre-procedure check list
>
> # Percutaneous Tracheostomy
> ### *Critical Care Time-outs*
>
> *Time-out 1: Pre-Procedure (before operator scrubs)*
>
> | | |
> |---|---|
> | Assent? | (Form 4 signed twice with assent documented and filed in patient notes) |
> | Contra-indications considered? | (e.g C-spine, coagulopathy, anatomy and drug allergies) |
> | Feed? **STOP INSULIN?** | (Plans regarding enteral feeding and risk of hypoglycaemia understood) |
> | Roles? | (Operator, anaesthetist, nurse and runner roles delegated) |
> | Trache tube? | (Trache type and size considered and available) |
> | Kit? | (Tracheostomy trolley complete and airway equipment to hand) |
>
> **The Team Agree Tracheostomy in Patient's Best Interest and it is Safe to Proceed**
>
> *Time-out 2: Prior to Incision (operator scrubbed)*
> **The team agree**:
>
> - The patient is anaesthetised, paralysed and appropriately ventilated
> - The patient is optimally positioned, the neck is clean and local anaesthetic has been infiltrated
> - No one has any unvoiced concerns
>
> *Time-out 3: Post procedure (operator happy airway secure)*
> **The team agree**:
>
> - Chest X-ray and audit form responsibility delegated
> - Scope decontamination and documentation responsibility delegated
> - Feed (with or without insulin) restarted
> - No one has any unvoiced concerns
>
> Reproduced with kind permission from Dr. G Gibbon, Nottingham University Hospitals NHS Trust.

3. increased pain/discomfort
4. difficulties keeping the cuff inflated despite large volumes or air (could indicate cuff damage or tube displacement).

In a tracheostomy emergency, it is essential to rapidly establish whether the patient has a tracheostomy (manage according to the 'Green Algorithm') or a laryngectomy (Red Algorithm).[4] Key elements include the need to call for expert help, an assessment of whether the patient is breathing and an assessment of tracheostomy patency. If the patient is not improving, it is necessary to remove the tracheostomy and prioritise oxygenation. Oxygenation can be achieved by simple primary techniques such as hand ventilating via the stoma or oro-nasal route. It can also involve specialist secondary techniques such as oral intubation, re-siting a tracheostomy, or fibreoptic bronchoscopy (e.g. to place an Aintree™ catheter or to 'railroad' a tracheostomy tube).

The use of bed head labeling can be helpful to indicate the presence of a tracheostomy, whether it was surgical or percutaneous, the tube size and who to call in an emergency.[4]

Fibreoptic Bronchoscopy

Fibreoptic bronchoscopy (FB) is used to assist percutaneous dilatational tracheostomy (PDT) in 85 per cent of patients undergoing the procedure in the United Kingdom.[2] FB is an important skill to acquire and a firm grasp of bronchial anatomy is necessary (see section below). The reader also is referred to online video tutorials that demonstrate bronchoscopic anatomy in real time.

A good resource is www.bronchoscopy.nl/teaching-files.html

The operator can stand at the head of the patient, where the patient's orientation is essentially aligned with the operator's, or facing the patient where the orientation is reversed. If a camera and monitor are used, the bronchoscope's orientation and movements must be aligned with the monitor prior to use.

Anatomy of the Flexible Bronchoscope[9]

Flexible bronchoscopes are delicate and expensive and need to be handled with utmost care. They comprise:

1. **Control handle:** with eyepiece, body, control lever, suction valve, and access port to the working channel. It is conveniently held in the left hand because the universal cord comes off to the left.
2. **Insertion cord:** outer diameter usually around 6 mm and length 55 to 60 cm. It contains two light bundles to transmit light, a working channel, a viewing bundle and wires to control movement at the tip.
3. **Universal cord:** goes between the light source and the side of control handle to transmit light down insertion cord.

Considerations and Complications

The internal diameter of an endotracheal tube should be around 1.5 mm greater than the external diameter of the scope. There is frequently an imperfect seal (with a gas leak and loss of PEEP) or the opposite situation where the physical obstruction caused by the scope results in gas trapping. It is essential that a second person is available at all times throughout bronchoscopy to respond to changes in patient physiology. Bronchoscopy can exacerbate haemodynamic instability and cause a significant increase in intracranial pressure. Pneumothorax and pneumomediastinum are also described, especially in the context of transbronchial biopsy.

Flexible Bronchoscopy for PDT

The use of the FB to guide PDT was first described by Marelli et al.[10] While evidence is lacking, many value the reassurance it confers, namely that wire placement is in the midline, the posterior tracheal wall has not been breached and that cartilage rings remain intact. The scope can be used to immediately reintubate the patient or remove blood clots which can occlude bronchi.

Anatomy of the Tracheobronchial Tree[3]

The tracheal cartilages form arches anteriorly, while the trachealis muscle runs longitudinally along its flat posterior wall. Trachealis divides and enters both main bronchi, usually continuing into the right and left lower lobes.

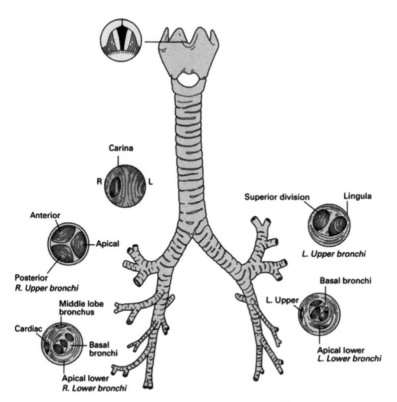

Figure 33.2 The bronchoscopic anatomy of the bronchial tree.[3]

As the scope is advanced into the **right main bronchus** after only 1.5 cm the **right upper lobe bronchus** (Figure 33.2) appears on the lateral wall in the 3 o' clock position. It has a characteristic trifurcation into **anterior, apical** and **posterior** segments. As the scope advances further, the right main bronchus becomes the **bronchus intermedius** for about 2.5 cm. Anteriorly (12 o' clock position) the origin of the **right middle lobe bronchus** is seen. Posteriorly the **right lower lobe bronchus** is seen. As the scope advances into the lower lobe, the first segment to arise is the **apical segment** which is posteriorly positioned (at about the 6 o' clock position). Continuing deeper into the right lower lobe one finds the basal trunk which divides into four segments directly ahead: on the medial side is the **medial basal ('cardiac')** segment and on the lateral side are the vertically arranged **anterior basal, lateral basal** and **posterior basal** segments.

The longer (approximately 4.5 cm) **left main bronchus** has no early branches and divides into **left upper lobe** and **left lower lobe** bronchi. Upon the scope's entry into the upper lobe, the opening to the **lingula** is seen and the trifurcation of the left upper lobe into **apical, posterior** and **anterior** segments. Withdrawing the scope and then continuing down into the **left lower lobe bronchus**, the origin of the **apical segmental bronchus** may be seen posteriorly (at about the 6 o' clock position). Advancing further, the basal segmental bronchi are seen as a cluster of three (**anteromedial*, lateral, posterior basal**).

*The anterior and medial segments are commonly fused.

Conclusion

Tracheostomy insertion, whether surgical or percutaneous, has considerable risk of morbidity and may be fatal. Safety and appropriate planning of the procedure are vital to minimise complications and the patient's relatives should be fully informed of the indications for the procedure and the associated risks and benefits. An understanding of the anatomy and potential complications is necessary for anyone performing the tracheostomy or associated bronchsocopy.

Key Learning Points

- Percutaneous tracheostomy may be associated with early or late complications, the most serious of which involve loss of airway and major haemorrhage.
- An awareness of relevant anatomy is critical in minimising risk during tracheostomy procedures.
- Pre-procedural check-lists have an important role in promoting tracheostomy safety.
- The NTSP has valuable learning resources and emergency algorithms.
- Most intensive care units in the United Kingdom use flexible bronchoscopy to guide percutaneous tracheostomy.

References

1. Young D, Harrison DA, Cuthbertson BH, Rowan K. Effect of early vs late tracheostomy placement on survival in patients receiving mechanical ventilation: the TracMan randomized trial. *Jama* 2013;309(20):2121–9.

2. Wilson KA, Martin IC. On the Right Trach? A review of care received by patients who underwent a tracheostomy. A report by the the National Confidential Enquiry into Patient Outcome and Death.: NCEPOD, 2014.

3. Ellis H, Lawson A. *Anatomy for Anaesthetists*. 9th ed, Wiley, 2014.

4. McGrath B. *Comprehensive Tracheostomy Care: The National Tracheostomy Safety Project Manual*. Wiley Blackwell, 2014.

5. Ciaglia P, Firsching R, Syniec C. Elective percutaneous dilatational tracheostomy. A new simple bedside procedure; preliminary report. *Chest* 1985;87(6):715–19.

6. Griggs WM, Myburgh JA, Worthley LI. A prospective comparison of a percutaneous tracheostomy technique with standard surgical tracheostomy. *Intensive Care Medicine* 1991;17(5):261–3.

7. Fantoni A, Ripamonti D. A non-derivative, non-surgical tracheostomy: the translaryngeal method. *Intensive Care Medicine* 1997;23(4):386–92.

8. Kost KMM, Myers EN. Tracheostomy. In Myers E, editor. *Operative Otolaryngology: Head and Neck Surgery*. Elsevier, 2008:577–94.

9. Garland R. Anatomy and Care of the Bronchoscope. In: Ernst A, editor. *Introduction to Bronchoscopy*. Cambridge University Press, 2009.

10. Marelli D, Paul A, Manolidis S, et al. Endoscopic guided percutaneous tracheostomy: early results of a consecutive trial. *The Journal of Trauma* 1990;30(4):433–5.

Chapter 34

Central Venous Catheter Infections

Andrew Leeson and Stephen Webber

Introduction

A central line is defined as an intravascular catheter that terminates at or close to the heart, or in one of the great vessels which is used for infusion, withdrawal of blood or haemodynamic monitoring.

Central line infection may be local (at the site of insertion) or systemic and is an example of a health care associated infection (HCAI); it is one of the most serious complications of vascular access device use. A central line associated bloodstream infection (CLA-BSI) is defined as the presence of a bloodstream infection that cannot be attributed to another source in a patient with a central line in place for at least 48 hours.[1,2] A catheter-related blood stream infection (CR-BSI) is a more rigorous definition of catheter-related infection, requiring bloodstream infection plus quantitative microbiological evidence of catheter infection.[3] These definitions will be explained in greater detail later in the text.

In 2011, a point prevalence survey of English hospitals that included 52,443 patients from 103 trusts showed an incidence of bloodstream infections (BSIs) of 0.5 percent for all hospital admissions, accounting for 7.3 percent of all HCAIs. Sixty-four percent of all BSIs occurred in patients with, or who had previously had, vascular access devices. Use of central venous access catheters (CVCs) is responsible for 86 percent of CR-BSIs.[4] North American data suggest a CR-BSI incidence of 1.3 to 5.6 per 1000 catheter days depending on the patient population, leading to around 80,000 BSIs and 28,000 deaths in intensive care unit (ICU) patients per annum.[1,5] In the year 2000, the United Kingdom National Audit Office estimated the financial burden of CR-BSI to be £6209 per patient.[6]

Case Report

A 75-year-old woman with a three-month history of weight loss was admitted to the emergency department with acute abdominal pain, vomiting and fever. Physical examination revealed a peritonitic abdomen. A computerised tomography (CT) scan of the abdomen demonstrated a mass in the sigmoid colon and free intra-abdominal fluid. The patient underwent an emergency laparotomy and Hartmann's procedure for bowel perforation secondary to a sigmoid tumour. Pre-operatively a radial arterial line and a multi-lumen CVC in the right internal jugular vein were sited. Despite the patient receiving four litres of crystalloid fluid resuscitation, vasopressor therapy with a noradrenaline infusion via the CVC was necessary to maintain the blood pressure. A 5-day course of intravenous piperacillin-tazobactam was started.

Postoperatively, the patient was admitted to critical care for ongoing respiratory support, fluid resuscitation and vasopressor therapy. Nasogastric feeding was begun the following day; however a paralytic ileus with high volume nasogastric aspirates prevented escalation of feed volume. Given the history of pre-morbid weight loss, parenteral nutrition was started via the CVC. Over the next 5 days, the patient was gradually weaned off the noradrenaline and the ventilatory parameters progressively improved.

On the 6th postoperative day, following discontinuation of the antibiotics, the patient developed a fever of 38.7 °C but remained systemically well. Blood cultures were taken from a peripheral vein and the arterial and central lines. Sputum, urine and drain fluid were sent for microbiological culture. The following day, the white blood cell count increased to 23×10^9/l and peripheral and CVC blood cultures were positive for *enterococcus*, with the CVC culture becoming positive two hours earlier than the peripheral. A repeat abdominal CT scan was unremarkable.

A diagnosis of a CR-BSI was made, the patient was started on intravenous vancomycin and the infected line was removed. Following this, the inflammatory markers improved and there were no further episodes of pyrexia. After 24 hours of normothermia, a peripherally inserted central catheter (PICC) was sited, allowing continued administration of parenteral nutrition. The patient was subsequently extubated and discharged to the surgical ward with a plan to complete a 5-day course of vancomycin.

Discussion

Pathogenesis of Central Line Infection

Central venous catheter colonisation and infection is thought to occur by one of four possible routes, listed in order of decreasing incidence:

1. Migration of skin flora from the insertion site, either at the time of insertion or subsequent translocation along the catheter tract.
2. Contamination of the catheter or catheter hub, usually by the person accessing the line.
3. Haematogenous spread from a distant site of infection (e.g., respiratory tract).
4. Infusion of contaminated fluid.[3,7]

The most common causative pathogens of CR-BSI are skin flora such as coagulase negative staphylococcus (e.g., *Staph. epidermidis*), *Staphylococcus aureus*, *Enterococci spp.* and *Candida spp.*[7] Gram negative bacteria comprise approximately 20 per cent of CR-BSIs.[3]
Other factors that contribute to the development of CR-BSI include:

- Device factors: polytetrafluroethylene (Teflon[TM]) and polyurethane catheters are associated with fewer infections than polyvinyl chloride or polyethylene.[2,8] Multilumen catheters may be a greater risk of infection than single lumen. Devices impregnated with antimicrobial substances may be a lower risk of infection than non-impregnated devices.
- Host factors: increasing severity of illness, neutropenia and parenteral nutrition can all increase the likelihood of line infection.[3]
- Pathogen factors: Coagulase negative staphylococcus, *Staph. aureus*, *Pseudomonas aeruginosa* and Candida spp. produce exopolysaccharide rich extracellular polymeric substance (EPS), which forms a biofilm capable of promoting bacterial binding. Furthermore, this biofilm layer provides protection from the host's cellular immune system and limits antimicrobial agent penetration.[3]
- Institutional factors: lapses in infection control processes during catheter insertion and maintenance.[2,3]

Definition of Central Line Infection

The terminology used to describe central line infections can be confusing: a colonised line may show microbial growth without bloodstream infection or the clinical manifestations of infection. Colonisation may progress to bloodstream infection, which can be defined as either a CLA-BSI or a CR-BSI. The criteria for these definitions are shown in Box 34.1.

CR-BSI is a clinical definition often used in research studies with limitations restricting its application to routine practice; in some settings a potentially infected CVC may not be removed (tip not available for culture) and moreover many laboratories are unable to perform quantitative culture analysis. Therefore, a different set of diagnostic criteria is required for 'real world' CVC infection surveillance purposes. The CLA-BSI definition does not require quantitative microbiological data and is used as a surrogate measure of CR-BSI, but because the CLA-BSI definition is less stringent and secondary sources of BSI may not be certain, this can result in false positives for CVC infection, thus overestimating the true CVC infection rate.[3,10]

Treatment of Central Line Infection

It is usually necessary to remove an infected CVC. An exception to this may be when vascular access is difficult: in this circumstance it may be more appropriate to leave the line in situ and treat with systemic antibiotics and line locks. However, should the patient become unwell, the line should be removed.[2]

Box 34.1   Definitions of central line infection

Central line associated bloodstream infection (CLA-BSI)
BSI occurring at least 48 hours after CVC insertion or within 24 hours of a CVC being removed.[9,10] Additionally one of three criteria must be present:

- Identification of a recognised pathogen, cultured from one or more blood cultures and the organism is not related to an infection at another site.
- The patient demonstrates at least one of the following: fever (>38°C), chills or hypotension AND any organism cultured is not related to an infection at another site AND any skin commensal cultured is from two or more cultures taken on separate occasions.
- A child of ≤1 yr of age demonstrating at least one of the following: fever (>38°C), hypothermia (<36°C), apnoea or bradycardia AND any organism cultured is not related to an infection at another site AND any skin commensal cultured is from two or more cultures taken on separate occasions.

Catheter-related bloodstream infection (CR-BSI)
BSI with no other apparent source PLUS one of the following quantitative microbiological cultures:[1,10]

- Simultaneous samples from the catheter lumen and peripheral venepuncture grow the same pathogen, with the catheter sample becoming positive first by at least two hours.
- Simultaneous samples from the catheter lumen and peripheral venepuncture grow the same pathogen, with the catheter sample showing significantly more growth by quantitative culture.
- Peripheral culture and removed catheter tip grow the same pathogen with pre-specified growth by quantitative or semi-quantitative culture methods.

Empiric antimicrobial treatment of a suspected CVC infection requires broad-spectrum intravenous antibiotics covering gram positive and negative bacteria pending microbiological results, e.g., dual therapy with a glycopeptide and a carbapenem. If the patient is at high risk of fungal infection, e.g. the immunocompromised patient, antifungal treatment should be added. Antimicrobial choice and treatment duration should be adjusted based on culture results. If the infecting organism is a skin commensal line removal alone may suffice, but infection with a recognised pathogen requires additional treatment with an appropriate antimicrobial agent. In addition to this, an echocardiogram is required to exclude endocarditis following BSI from *Staph. aureus* and Candida. When central venous access is still required following a CR-BSI, a new line should be inserted rather than exchanging over a guidewire.[2]

Prevention of Central Line Infection

Until relatively recently, CR-BSI was considered an almost inevitable consequence of central venous access. However, in the last decade it has become apparent that catheter-related infection is largely preventable.

In 2006, Pronovost et al. published a landmark paper examining the effect of implementing a care bundle for CVC insertion and management in 108 ICUs throughout the state of Michigan. The care bundle consisted of five elements:

- Hand hygiene
- Use of full barrier precautions during catheter insertion
- Use of chlorhexidine for skin preparation
- Avoiding use of femoral lines
- Removing unnecessary catheters

Other measures introduced comprised the education of staff on infection control practices, the production of dedicated catheter insertion carts and the empowerment of nursing staff to ensure these processes were correctly followed.

The median baseline rate of infection fell from 2.7 per 1000 catheter days to 0 in the first 3 months following implementation of the care bundle and was sustained for the remainder of the study period. A persistent reduction in the incidence rate ratios (IRR) for CR-BSI was also observed over the study period, resulting in an IRR of 0.34 compared with baseline (p of less than 0.001) at 18 months following implementation. The authors concluded that this intervention was coincident with a reduction in CR-BSI but due to lack of blinding and randomisation could not associate a causal relationship between the two.[5]

The Matching Michigan study group implemented a similar care bundle in English hospitals, with participating hospitals grouped into clusters and enrolled in four phases.[10] The premise of the study remained the same, to reduce infection rates using evidence-based changes in clinical practice and non-technical skills. A similar pattern of results was demonstrated, with mean baseline CR-BSI rates falling from 3.7 to 1.48 per 1000 catheter days (p less than 0.0001) for the adult population. Infection rates in the paediatric population fell non-significantly from 5.65 to 2.89 per 1000 catheter days (p = 0.625) by the end of the study period. Interestingly, subsequent clusters entering the study had baseline incidence rates close to the post intervention rate for the preceding group, possibly representing a widespread shift in practice as a result of the Michigan study. The study was also performed at time of intense national pressure to reduce HCAI rates, which may have contributed to the observed results.[10]

A number of organisations have produced guidance on strategies to reduce the risk of catheter infection. The EPIC guidelines – national evidence based guidelines for the prevention of healthcare-associated infections in National Health Service (NHS) hospitals in England – first published in 2001 provide guidance on reducing HCAI as a whole, with particular emphasis on CR-BSI.[2] In 2006, this document along with guidelines produced by the Centres for Disease Control (CDC) in America, formed the basis for the Department of Health's High Impact Intervention Number 1: central venous catheter care bundle. (Box 34.2)[3,11]

The EPIC guidance is currently in a third edition. However, the underlying principles remain the same. Based on the systematic review of available evidence, it divides the recommendations into nine distinct interventions:[2]

Education: the incidence of infection is reduced when infection control measures are in place, whilst infection rates increase when catheters are managed by inexperienced staff. The effects of education appear to be greatest when baseline compliance with best practice is low.

General asepsis: Hands should be decontaminated with alcohol hand gel or soap and water when soiled or potentially soiled and before contact with the catheter or insertion site. Aseptic technique should be used when inserting or accessing the catheter.

Selection of catheter type: Antimicrobial impregnated catheters should be considered when they are expected to remain *in situ* for more than five days, in high-risk patients (e.g. severe burns) and in populations where other efforts to reduce infection rates have failed. The number of lumens should be the minimum required, though the evidence for infection rates increasing as the number of lumens increases is controversial and may simply represent an association rather than causality. Parenteral nutrition should be administered via a dedicated lumen. Long-term access (greater than 6 months) requires the line to be tunneled whereas peripherally inserted central catheters (PICC) can be used for medium term access (6 weeks to 6 months).

Selection of insertion site: the subclavian approach to central venous access has traditionally been viewed as having the lowest rate of infection, but at the expense of other complications, particularly pneumothorax, whereas the femoral route carries the highest risk of catheter colonisation and venous thrombosis. However, a systematic review has cast doubt on these beliefs finding no significant differences in the rate of infection and thrombosis between catheter sites in recent studies.[12] When inserting a CVC, a pragmatic approach to site selection should be taken, weighing the risk of infection against the risk of other complications. Pending further evidence it may be prudent to avoid the femoral route where possible.

Maximum sterile barrier (MSB) precautions during catheter insertion: Use of a surgical cap, mask, sterile gown, gloves and drape reduce the incidence of CR-BSI when siting a catheter.

Cutaneous antisepsis: Skin should be prepared with 2 per cent chlorhexidine gluconate in 70 per cent isopropyl alcohol and allowed to dry. If chlorhexidine is contraindicated (e.g., patient allergy) then povidone iodine in alcohol should be used.

Catheter and catheter site care: Sterile, semipermeable dressings should be used to cover the catheter to allow regular inspection of the insertion site. Dressings should be changed at least every 7 days, or sooner when moisture collects under the dressing. A chlorhexidine impregnated sponge can be used to cover the insertion site as a

Box 34.2 Central line care bundle (adapted from Department of Health High Impact Intervention No.1[11])

Insertion actions

Catheter type
- Single lumen unless indicated otherwise.
- Consider antimicrobial impregnated catheter if duration 1 to 3 weeks and risk of CR-BSI high.

Insertion site
- Subclavian or internal jugular.

Skin preparation
- Preferably use 2 per cent chlorhexidine gluconate in 70 per cent isopropyl alcohol and allow to dry.
- If patient has a sensitivity use a single patient use povidone-iodine application.

Personal protective equipment
- Gloves are single-use items and should be removed and discarded immediately after the care activity.
- Eye/face protection is indicated if there is a risk of splashing with blood or body fluids.

Hand hygiene
- Decontaminate hands before and after each patient contact.
- Use correct hand hygiene procedure.

Aseptic technique
- Gown, gloves and drapes as indicated should be used for the insertion of invasive devices.

Dressing
- Use a sterile, transparent, semi-permeable dressing to allow observation of insertion site.

Safe disposal of sharps
- Sharps container should be available at point of use and should not be overfilled; do not disassemble needle and syringe; do not pass sharps from hand to hand.

Documentation
- Date of insertion should be recorded in notes.

Ongoing care actions

Hand hygiene
- Decontaminate hands before and after each patient contact. • Use correct hand hygiene procedure.

Catheter site inspection
- Regular observation for signs of infection, at least daily.

Dressing
- An intact, dry, adherent transparent dressing should be present.

Box 34.2 *(cont.)*

Catheter access
- Use aseptic technique and swab ports or hub with 2 per cent chlorhexidine gluconate in 70 per cent isopropyl alcohol prior to accessing the line for administering fluids or injections.

Administration set replacement
- Following administration of blood, blood products - immediately.
- Following total parenteral nutrition – after 24 hours (72 hours if no lipid).
- With other fluid sets – after 96 hours.
- No routine catheter replacement

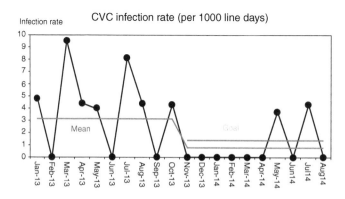

Figure 34.1 Central line infection rate plotted on a run chart.

strategy for reducing CR-BSI. The entry site should be cleaned with 2 per cent chlorhexidine in 70 per cent isopropyl alcohol when performing dressing changes.

Replacement strategies: Routine catheter replacement as a strategy to reduce CR-BSI is not recommended.

General principles for catheter care: needleless connectors may reduce the incidence of infection and should be decontaminated with 2 per cent chlorhexidine in 70 per cent isopropyl alcohol prior to accessing. Routine use of antimicrobial locks and prophylactic systemic antibiotics prior to insertion are not recommended. Although catheter thrombosis is associated with increased infection, routine use of anticoagulation is not recommended. The frequency at which the intravenous giving sets should be changed is dependent on the type of fluid being administered. (Box 34.2)[2]

The Matching Michigan study was one part of the larger, National Patient Safety Agency (NPSA) led, Patient Safety First campaign. Launched in 2008, this campaign aimed to improve the safety culture within the NHS by engaging staff and enabling change.[13] The reduction of CR-BSI rate using the Michigan care bundle, incorporating 'plan do study act' (PDSA) improvement methodology, was one component of the program to reduce harm in critical care. The PDSA methodology introduces, analyses and modifies interventions cyclically on a small scale before implementing the interventions on a larger scale. Improvements are monitored by assessing compliance with the care bundle and tracking infection rates, which can be plotted graphically on a run chart (Figure 34.1).

Conclusions

Infection is a serious complication of central venous catheterisation, carrying high rates of morbidity, mortality and a significant financial burden. Colonisation of the CVC usually occurs during insertion or manipulation of the catheter and may subsequently lead to infection. Diagnosis of central line infection is complex but requires microbiological evidence of the presence of a pathogen or signs of infection unrelated to another source. Treatment usually involves line removal, and depending on the infecting organism, supplemental antimicrobial therapy. Implementation of a central line care bundle has been shown to significantly reduce central line infection rates, requires little financial expenditure and is recommended by a number of healthcare organisations.

Key Learning Points

- Catheter-related bloodstream infection is one of the most serious complications of vascular access device use, with significant associated morbidity, mortality and healthcare costs.
- Common causative pathogens of CR-BSI are skin flora such as coagulase negative Staphylococci (e.g., *Staph. epidermidis*), *Staphylococcus aureus, enterococci spp.* and *candida spp.* Gram negative pathogens account for 20 per cent of CR-BSIs.
- Diagnosis of CR-BSI requires specific diagnostic criteria based on clinical signs and blood culture results.
- Consideration can be given to retaining the catheter in specific situations, though removal of the infected line and systemic antimicrobial therapy are the mainstays of treatment of CR-BSI.
- Implementation of a central line care bundle has been shown to significantly reduce the incidence of CR-BSI and has been incorporated in the Patient Safety First campaign.
- Systems should be in place to monitor the incidence of CR-BSI.

References

1. O'Grady NP, Chertow DS. Managing bloodstream infections in patients who have short-term central venous catheters. *Cleve Clin J Med* 2011;78:10–17.

2. Loveday HP, Wilson JA, Pratt RJ et al. UK Department of Health. Epic 3: national evidence-based guidelines for preventing healthcare-associated infections in NHS hospitals in England. *J Hosp Infect* 2014;86 Suppl 1:S1–70.

3. O'Grady NP, Alexander M, Burns LA, et al. Healthcare Infection Control Practices Advisory Committee (HICPAC). Guidelines for the prevention of intravascular catheter-related infections. *Clin Infect Dis* 2011;52:162–93.

4. Health Protection Agency. *English National Point Prevalence Survey on Healthcare Associated Infections and Antimicrobial Use, 2011: Preliminary data.* Health Protection Agency: London, 2012.

5. Pronovost P, Needham D, Berenholtz S et al. An intervention to decrease catheter-related bloodstream infections in the ICU. *N Engl J Med.* 2006; 355:2725–32.

6. National Audit Office. The management and control of hospital acquired infection in Acute NHS Trusts in England. London: The Stationery Office. 2000. Available at www.nao.org.uk/publications/nao_reports/9900230.pdf (accessed 15 August 2014).

7. Safdar N, Maki DG. The pathogenesis of catheter-related bloodstream infection with noncuffed short-term central venous catheters. *Intensive Care Med.* 2004;30:62–7.

8. Sheth NK, Franson TR, Rose HD, et al. Colonization of bacteria on polyvinyl chloride and Teflon intravascular catheters in hospitalized patients. *J Clin Microbiol.* 1983;18:1061–3.

9. Mermel LA, Allon M, Bouza E et al. Clinical practice guidelines for the diagnosis and management of intravascular catheter-related infection: 2009 Update by the Infectious Diseases Society of America. *Clin Infect Dis.* 2009;49:1–45.

10. Bion J, Richardson A, Hibbert P et al. 'Matching Michigan': a two-year stepped interventional programme to minimise central venous catheter-bloodstream infections in intensive care units in England. *BMJ Qual Saf.* 2013;22:110–23.

11. Saving Lives: delivering clean and safe care. High Impact Intervention No.1 – Central venous catheter care bundle. Department of Health, 2007.

12. Marik PE, Flemmer M, Harrison W. The risk of catheter-related bloodstream infection with femoral venous catheters as compared to subclavian and internal jugular venous catheters: a systematic review of the literature and meta-analysis. *Crit Care Med* 40:2479–85.

13. National Patient Safety Agency. Patient Safety First. The campaign review. Available at www.patientsafetyfirst.nhs.uk/ashx/Asset.ashx?path=/Patient%20Safety%20First%20-%20the%20campaign%20review.pdf (accessed 29 August 2014).

Chapter 35

Ventilator Associated Pneumonia

Alastair Jame Morgan

Introduction

Ventilator associated pneumonia (VAP) is the most common nosocomial infection acquired in the intensive care unit (ICU). It is defined as an inflammation of the lung parenchyma occurring 48 to 72 hours or more following endotracheal intubation, and is characterised by the presence of either new or progressive infiltrates, signs of systemic infection, changes in sputum characteristics and detection of an organism not present at the time mechanical ventilation (MV) was begun.[1]

VAP is estimated to occur in 9 to 28 per cent of all patients who are mechanically ventilated for more than 24 hours, but this incidence depends on case mix and diagnostic criteria used. It accounts for almost 50 per cent of ICU acquired infection.[1,2] More severely ill patients and those with significant co-morbidities have a higher mortality and are especially prone to VAP, making it difficult to determine the independent contribution VAP makes to mortality. Recent studies suggest that the attributable mortality is estimated at 4.4 to 9 percent.[3] It is associated with a prolonged duration of mechanical ventilation, increased ICU, hospital length of stay and healthcare costs.

Risk for VAP is greatest during the first 5 days of mechanical ventilation. Early-onset VAP occurs within the first 4 days post-intubation and is usually due to antibiotic sensitive bacteria. Late-onset VAP develops five or more days after intubation and is commonly caused by opportunistic and multidrug resistant (MDR) organisms. The exact prevalence of MDR organisms is variable between institutions.

Case Description

A 73-year-old woman suddenly develops shortness of breath and haemoptysis. She has a past medical history of hypertension, for which she takes amlodipine and ramipril. She is a smoker of 20 cigarettes per day. She had recently been treated in hospital for lower limb cellulitis and remains on oral flucloxacillin. It is evident from initial assessment that she is in respiratory distress with oxygen saturations of 84 percent on 15 litres of oxygen. An arterial blood gas shows a PaO_2 of 6.5 kPa and a $PaCO_2$ of 3.8 kPa. Her chest x-ray shows cardiomegaly and there is a tachycardia of 120 bpm with poor R wave progression on her ECG. Respiratory distress and hypoxaemia necessitate emergent intubation and ventilatory support. She becomes severely hypotensive post-induction, requiring fluid boluses and commencement of a peripheral adrenaline infusion. A transthoracic echocardiogram shows a profoundly dilated right ventricle containing an echogenic mass, with bowing of the intra-ventricular septum. She is thrombolysed for suspected pulmonary embolus, started on a heparin infusion and transferred to the ICU.

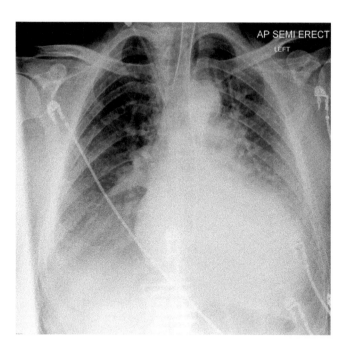

AP SEMI ERECT

LEFT

Figure 35.1 Chest radiology after 3 days of mechanical ventilation. *The nasogastric tube was noted to be in the distal oesphagus and was advanced into the stomach.

Over the ensuing 48 hours, clinical parameters improve and the level of ventilatory support is decreased. On day three post-admission, she develops a tachypnoea and hypoxaemia with a reduced PF ratio, requiring escalation of PEEP to 10 cmH_2O and FiO_2 to 0.6. Purulent secretions are aspirated via the endotracheal tube. Her anterior chest is resonant to percussion but crepitations are auscultated bilaterally. A portable chest radiograph shows diffuse bilateral lower zone opacities (Figure 35.1). The white blood count is 14,200 cells/mm.[3] She is started on cefuroxime but oxygenation continues to deteriorate over the ensuing 24 hours, necessitating turning her to the prone position. Tracheal aspirates taken at the time of deterioration grow Pseudomonas aeruginosa. Antibiotics are changed to piperacillin/tazobactam pending sensitivities.

After 16 hours prone, her PaO_2 is 16.3 kPa and $PaCO_2$ 6.2 on FiO_2 0.45. She is turned back to supine in a semi recumbent position and is re-established onto a spontaneous ventilatory mode. After a further 3 days of treatment with piperacillin/tazobactam, she is felt to be ready for a trial of extubation following a successful sedation hold and spontaneous breathing trial. On day twopost-extubation, she is deemed to be well enough for discharge to the general respiratory ward where she continues to make a good recovery.

Case Discussion

Aetiology

During critical illness, the oropharynx becomes colonised with enteric aerobic gram-negative bacilli (AGNB). Critically ill patients have increased levels of proteases in their oral secretions, which cause a depletion of fibronectin, a glycoprotein that interferes with binding of gram-negative bacteria to the epithelial cells in the oropharynx. As a result, organisms such as Pseudomonas aeruginosa easily attach to buccal and pharyngeal epithelial cell receptors. The presence of an endotracheal tube plays a significant role through its interference with the normal protective upper airway reflexes, inhibiting swallowing and encouraging microaspiration. As a result, accumulation of secretions in the oropharynx creates a suitable environment for colonisation with pathogenic organisms.

Infectious bacteria obtain direct access to the lower respiratory tract via microaspiration along the folds in the wall of the endotracheal tube cuff, or through the formation of a biofilm within the endotracheal tube. Its inner surface acts as a nadir for biofilm formation and a protective layer for the bacteria. The application of positive pressure ventilation and intermittent catheter suction may embolise bacteria into the distal lower airway, where they can proliferate and cause an inflammatory reaction. It is the host's immune response that ultimately determines whether parenchymal infection and VAP will develop. Mechanically ventilated patients have neutrophil dysfunction and impaired phagocytosis, increasing their susceptibility to VAP.

Pathogens

Time of onset of pneumonia is an important epidemiologic variable and risk factor for specific pathogens. Early-onset VAP is usually caused by antibiotic sensitive community pathogens, although MDR organisms are increasingly responsible. Late-onset VAP is usually caused by MDR pathogens and associated with increased mortality and morbidity. Patients with a history of hospital admission for more than 2 days in the previous 3 months, patients receiving chemotherapy or antibiotics in the previous 30 days and patients undergoing chronic haemodialysis are increasingly susceptible to MDR pathogens.[1] The pathogens associated with VAP also depend on the case mix, underlying co-morbidities and duration of hospital stay. The patient in this case-study was at an increased risk of developing an MDR related VAP due to her recent hospital admission and treatment with antibiotics. This may explain why she deteriorated despite treatment with cefuroxime.

Common causative pathogens are listed in Box 35.1. Increasingly VAP is due to polymicrobial infection, particularly in patients with adult respiratory distress syndrome (ARDS). It is rarely caused by anaerobic, viral or fungal pathogens except in the immunocompromised patient.

Box 35.1 Common causative pathogens. * Infections due to gram-positive cocci such as *Staphylococcus aureus*, particularly MRSA, have been rapidly emerging

Early-onset VAP	Late-onset
Haemophilus spp	Methicillin resistant *S. aureus*
Streptococcus pneumoniae	*Acinetobacter*
Methicillin sensitive *S. aureus*	*Pseudomonas aeruginosa*
Escherichia coli	Extended-spectrum beta-lactamases
Klebsiella pneumonia	*Stenotrophomonas maltophilia*
Enterobacter species	
Proteus species	
Serratia marcescens	
Coagulase negative *Staphylococci*	

Box 35.2 Independent risk factors for the development of VAP

Host-Related	Intervention Related
male sex	supine position
advanced age	presence of an endotracheal tube
trauma related admission	presence of a tracheostomy
pre-existing pulmonary disease	failed extubation
Hypoalbuminaemia	stress ulcer prophylaxis
underlying disease severity	excessive sedation
	duration of mechanical ventilation

Risk Factors

There are several risk factors for the development of VAP (Box 35.2). Although multivariate analysis has identified enteral feeding as a risk factor, most clinicians recognise the importance of early enteral feeding. Post-pyloric feeding may reduce this risk.

Diagnosis

Critically ill patients are subject to a multitude of pathologic insults that create overlapping systemic and pulmonary signs of inflammation, meaning that diagnosis of VAP can be complex. Traditional VAP definitions are subjective, lacking sensitivity and specificity. Competing diagnostic criteria have been developed to improve the accuracy of diagnosis and allow comparability of VAP rates (Box 35.3).

The Johanson Criteria use clinical and radiological parameters.[4] This definition has a sensitivity and specificity of 69 percent and 75 percent respectively, which is insufficient to be used alone to diagnose VAP.[5] It is, however, the most accurate of the combinations of clinical and radiological criteria.

The Healthcare Associated Infections in intensive care units (HAI-ICU) criteria, formerly known as HELICS, is widely used for surveillance of VAP rates in Europe. These rely on a combination of clinical, radiological and microbiological scores to diagnose VAP. Five different categories of VAP are assigned depending on the microbiological criteria used. This allows for a diagnosis of VAP to be made with non-quantitative endotracheal aspirate culture, other indirect cultures or without any positive microbiology.

The Clinical Pulmonary Infection (CPIS) score is calculated on the basis of points assigned for various signs and symptoms of VAP. Scores can range between 0 and 12 with a score greater than 6 suggestive of a diagnosis of VAP. It is poorly predictive in trauma and burns patients. A meta-analysis of 13 studies concluded that the CPIS score has a 65 percent and 64 percent sensitivity and specificity respectively.[6] Inter-observer variability remains substantial but the CPIS score may be useful for monitoring response to treatment.

The Centers for Disease Control and Prevention (CDC) diagnostic criteria are predominantly intended to allow reporting of rates of nosocomial pneumonia, and do not specifically apply to VAP.[7] This tool has a sensitivity of 84 percent and specificity of 69 percent.

Investigations

Confirmation of infection depends on culture of an appropriate specimen. Although an aetiological diagnosis can be made from a respiratory tract culture, colonisation of the

Box 35.3 Diagnostic criteria for VAP. Johanson Score,[4] Clinical Pulmonary Infection Score and The Centers for Disease Control and Prevention Criteria.[7]

Johanson Criteria
- Presence of a new or progressive radiographic infiltrate
- Plus at least two of three clinical features:
  - temperature >38 °C
  - leucocytosis (WCC $\geq$12000 cells/mm)[3] or leucopenia (WCC <4000 cells/mm)[3]
  - presence of purulent tracheal secretions

Clinical Pulmonary Infection Score (CPIS)

	0	1	2
Temperature	36.5 – 38.4	38.5 – 38.9	$\leq$ 36 or $\geq$39
Leucocyte count (cells/mm)[3]	4000–11000	<4000 or >11000	band forms $\geq$ 50%
Tracheal Secretions	None	Mild/non-purulent	Purulent
Radiographic findings	No infiltrate	Diffuse/patchy infiltrate	Localised infiltrate
Culture results	None or mild growth	Moderate or florid growth	Moderate or florid growth and pathogen consistent with gram stain
PaO$_2$:FiO$_2$ ratio	>240 or ARDS		$\leq$240 and absence of ARDS

The Centers for Disease Control and Prevention (CDC) Criteria

Radiology	Two or more serial chest radiographs with at least one of: • New or progressive and persistent infiltrate • Consolidation • Cavitation
Clinical Signs	At least one of the following: • Fever (temperature >38 °C with no other recognised cause • Leucopenia (<4000 cells/mm[3]) or leucocytosis ($\geq$12000 cells/mm[3]) • Altered mental status with no other recognised cause in adults 70 years or older Plus at least two of the following: • New onset of purulent sputum, change in character of sputum, increased respiratory secretions or increased suctioning requirements • New onset of worsening cough, dyspnoea or tachypnoea • Rales or bronchial breath sounds • Worsening gas exchange (PaO$_2$/FiO$_2$ $\leq$240)
Microbiology	At least one of the following (optional): • Positive growth in blood culture not related to another source of infection • Positive growth in culture of pleural fluid • Positive quantitative culture from BAL or protected specimen • Five percent or more of cells with intracellular bacteria on direct examination of Gram-stained BAL fluid • Histopathological evidence of pneumonia

trachea precedes development of pneumonia in almost all cases of VAP. Indeed, much of VAP misdiagnosis stems from bacterial colonisation superimposed upon non-infectious pulmonary processes. A sterile culture in the absence of a recent change in antibiotic therapy is strong evidence that VAP is not present.

The relative benefits of non-invasive and invasive techniques for obtaining samples and differentiating between airway colonisation and infection are unclear. However, it does appear that neither invasive nor non-invasive microbiological sampling confers an advantage in terms of survival, length of ICU stay or duration of MV.[8] There is a high likelihood of false positives and false negatives with all techniques, and none is totally reliable.

The least invasive, simplest and cheapest method of obtaining a sample is to pass a sterile suction catheter into the trachea and aspirate any secretions. Tracheal aspirates have a reported sensitivity of 56 to 69 percent and a specificity of 75 to 95 percent, due to contamination of the samples with bacteria from the inner surface of the endotracheal tube. Treatment based solely on non-quantitative cultures of tracheal aspirates may result in over diagnosis of VAP and excessive use of antibiotics. Quantitative cultures significantly improve specificity. The number of colony forming units (CFU) present in a specimen should be greater than or equal to $10^{[5]}$ CFU/ml to be positive for VAP, rather than due to contamination.

Bronchoalveolar lavage (BAL) allows for sampling of secretions from the distal airways. The risk of contamination by upper airway secretions can be minimised by using a dual catheter that prevents the sampling catheter from coming into contact with the bronchoscope, a technique called protected BAL. Increasingly, mini-BAL or non-bronchoscopic BAL is being performed. This procedure uses specially designed catheters that allow sampling of the distal airways via the tracheal tube. This is a quick and technically simple technique, with culture results that are comparable to other lavage methods. A quantitative diagnostic threshold of greater than of equal to 104 CFU/ml is used. The reported sensitivity and specificity for BAL are 42 to 93 percent and 45 to 100 percent respectively. False negatives arise from the failure to sample the correct lung segment, insufficient bacterial growth to cross the quantitative threshold, and damping of bacterial growth by prior antibiotic exposure.

Protected Specimen Brush (PSB) sampling is designed to minimise microbiological contamination from the inside of the endotracheal tube. PSB has a sensitivity and specificity of 33 to 100 percent and 50 to 100 percent respectively. A diagnostic threshold of $10^{[3]}$ CFU/ml is usually used for PSB cultures.

Several biomarkers including procalcitonin, CRP and soluble triggering receptor expressed on myeloid cells type 1 (sTREM-1) have been investigated. Currently, the discriminatory value of these tests is low, but serial measurements may be useful in assessing appropriateness of antibiotic treatment. sTREM-1 levels, when coupled with clinical criteria and results of microbiological cultures, may increase specificity and maintain sensitivity of VAP diagnosis.

Management

Appropriate antimicrobial treatment of patients with VAP significantly improves outcome. Empirical antibiotic therapy should rapidly be commenced after appropriate samples have been obtained, as long as this does not seriously delay treatment. Knowledge of the likely organisms, local microbial epidemiology and their sensitivities, the results of surveillance cultures from the patient, previous antibiotic exposure and duration of MV usually guide initial antibiotic therapy.

The British Society for Antimicrobial Chemotherapy has produced guidelines for the empirical treatment of VAP.[9] The use of cefuroxime or co-amoxiclav is recommended for early-onset VAP in the absence of prior antibiotic therapy or risk factors. For patients recently treated with antibiotics or those with risk factors, a third generation cephalosporin, flouroquinolone or piperacillin/tazobactam is recommended. Patients with late onset VAP or risk factors for MDR pathogens should receive antibiotics with activity against Pseudomonas aeruginosa, such as ceftazidime, ciprofloxacin, meropenem or piperacillin/ tazobactam. The risk of MRSA pneumonia should be considered, particularly in late-onset VAP. Vancomycin and teicoplanin remains the mainstay of treatment, although there is evidence to suggest that linezolid results in improved survival rates.

A de-escalation strategy should be used once the results of antimicrobial susceptibility tests are available. Antibiotics can be safely discontinued when an adequate clinical response is suggested by a resolution in signs and symptoms of active infection. Where patients respond to therapy, routine duration should be no longer than 8 days.[9]

Prevention

Prevention of VAP uses an evidence-based bundle approach, containing a small number of key interventions. Despite reducing VAP rates, several of these interventions have failed to show a significant benefit in clinical outcomes including mortality, length of MV and length of ICU stay. The necessary components of the VAP bundle and how best to implement them remain unanswered, with individual critical care units developing their own set of interventions.

Strategies aimed at reducing the duration of MV may reduce the incidence of VAP. The use of non-invasive ventilation has been shown to reduce the need for MV in certain patient groups with respiratory failure. Its use significantly lowers VAP risk and also demonstrates a mortality reduction since NIV either avoids or minimises duration of MV (please refer to Chapter 19).

Daily sedation breaks and weaning protocols are effective in reducing the duration of MV. Since VAP risk is related to duration of MV, these strategies should be implemented although a reduction in VAP rates has yet to be proven. Although tracheostomy is often advocated to aid weaning from respiratory support, recent evidence suggests that early tracheostomy does not reduce duration of MV or incidence of VAP.

Selective decontamination of the digestive tract (SDD) and selective oral decontamin-ation (SOD) consist of eradicating potentially pathogenic microorganisms in oral, gastric and intestinal flora. Several SDD regimens exist but most frequently consist of the oral and gastric administration of non-absorbable antimicrobials (usually polymyxin E, tobramycin and amphotericin B) to eradicate AGNB, in conjunction with intravenous administration of a broad-spectrum antibiotic. Although there is conflicting evidence, studies have shown that SDD reduces VAP incidence, length of stay and mortality in mechanically ventilated ICU patients, with a reduction in unit-acquired bloodstream infection if the intravenous component is used.[10] SDD is not widely practiced (5.2% of UK general critical care units) since data does not yet exist to promote confidence in long-term safety and emergence of resistant organisms.

There is substantial evidence to support an association between poor oral health and development of VAP. Oral decontamination with topical oral antiseptics appears to reduce the incidence of VAP, especially when combined with thorough mechanical cleaning of the oral cavity. The National Institute for Health and Care Excellence (NICE) recommends that all mechanically ventilated patients should receive oral antiseptics, although as yet no impact on mortality or length of ICU stay has been demonstrated.[11] A recent meta-analysis has challenged this recommendation. VAP risk was not shown to be significantly reduced in ventilated non-cardiac surgery patients receiving routine oral care with chlorhexidine.[12]

Preventative measures targeting the endotracheal tube aim to either minimise tube colonisation and formation of a biofilm, or to avoid microaspiration of oropharyngeal secretions and gastric content.

Silver coated endotracheal tubes are thought to reduce bacterial colonisation and biofilm formation: a prospective randomised single-blind multicentre trial showed a significant risk reduction of 35.9 percent in the occurrence of VAP and a delayed time to VAP occurrence through the use of silver coated endotracheal tubes.[13] Subglottic suction channels allow the continuous aspiration of subglottic secretions and may reduce the risk of aspiration. A recent meta-analysis inclusive of 2242 patients concluded that subglottic suction was effective for the prevention of VAP (RR 0.55; 95 percent CI 0.46 to 0.66), reduced ICU length of stay (-1.52 days; 95% CI -2.94 to 0.11) and decreased duration of MV (-1.08 days; 95 percent CI -2.04 to -0.12).[14] There was no effect on mortality or adverse events. Certain endotracheal tubes also have wrinkle-free cuffs that may reduce the channeling of subglottic secretions.

All patients without specific contraindications should be nursed in the semi recumbent position with the head raised at 30 to 45 degrees. Randomised trials have produced conflicting results. Despite the lack of evidence, this low-cost practical intervention has been recommended by NICE and the NHS Commissioning Board Special Health Authority.[11]

Conclusion

VAP is the most common nosocomial acquired infection within ventilated critically ill patients. It is associated with prolonged mechanical ventilation and attributable mortality may be up to 10 per cent. Diagnosis should be supported by microbiological evidence, although no single technique currently offers a reliability advantage. If a diagnosis of VAP is suspected, an appropriate antibiotic should be rapidly commenced, guided by duration of MV, patient risk-factors for MDR organisms and local microbial epidemiology. Care bundles reduce VAP rates but are yet to significantly reduce length of MV, ICU length of stay and mortality.

Due to the economic and clinical burden, VAP rates are proposed as a quality indicator for patient safety. In the continuing absence of a universal definition and microbiological investigation, this remains a contentious and controversial issue.

Key Learning Points

- VAP is associated with prolonged mechanical ventilation, ICU and hospital length of stay, and increased healthcare costs.
- Accurate diagnosis remains a challenge and should be guided by microbiological sampling.
- Length of ventilation and risk factors for MDR organisms are important factors to consider when commencing antibiotics.
- There is strong evidence that care bundles reduce incidence of VAP but this has not translated into a mortality reduction.

References

1. American Thoracic Society, Infectious Diseases Society of America. Guidelines for the management of adults with hospital-acquired, ventilator-associated, and healthcare-associated pneumonia. *Am J Respir Crit Care Med* 2005;171: 388–416.

2. Vincent JL, Bihari DJ, Suter PM, et al. The prevalence of nosocomial infection in intensive care units in Europe. *JAMA* 1995;274:639–44.

3. Melsen WG, Rovers MM, Koeman M, et al. Estimating the attributable mortality of ventilator-associated pneumonia from randomized prevention studies. *Crit Care Med* 2011;39:1–7.

4. Johanson WG, Pierce AK, Sandford JP, et al. Nosocomial respiratory infections with gram-negative bacilli. The significance of colonization of the respiratory tract. *Ann Intern Med* 1972;77:701–6.

5. Fabregas N, Ewig S, Torres A, et al. Clinical diagnosis of ventilator-associated pneumonia revisited: comparative validation using immediate post-mortem lung biopsies. *Thorax* 1999;54: 867–73.

6. Shan J, Chen HL, Zhu JH. Diagnostic accuracy of clinical pulmonary infection score for ventilator-associated pneumonia: a meta-analysis. *Respir Care* 2011;56: 1087–94.

7. Horan T, Gaynes R. Surveillance of nosocomial infections. In: Mayhall C, ed. *Hospital Epidemiology and Infection Control*, 3rd ed. Philadelphia, Pa: Lippincott Williams & Wilkins; 2004: 1659–1702.

8. Berton DC, Kalil AC, Cavalcanti M, et al. Quantitative versus qualitative cultures of respiratory secretions for clinical outcomes in patients with ventilator-associated pneumonia. *Cochrane Database Syst Rev* 2012;CD006482.

9. Masterton RG, Galloway A, French G, et al. Guidelines for the management of hospital-acquired pneumonia in the UK: report of the working party of hospital-acquired pneumonia of the British Society of Antimicrobial Chemotherapy. *J Antimicrob Chemother* 2008;62:5–34.

10. Liberati A, D'Amico R, Pifferi S, et al. Antibiotic prophylaxis to reduce respiratory tract infections and mortality in adults receiving intensive care. Cochrane Database Syst Rev 2009;CD000022.

11. Campbell F, Cooper K, Czoski-Murray C, et al. Technical patient safety solutions for prevention of ventilator-associated pneumonia in adults. Health Services Research Unit. April 2008. www.nice.org.uk/nicemedia/pdf/ VAPConsultation2SystematicReview.pdf.

12. Klompas M, Speck K, Howell D, et al. Reappraisal of routine oral care with chlorhexidine gluconate for patients receiving mechanical ventilation. *JAMA Intern Med* 2014;174:751–61.

13. Kollef MH, Afessa B, Anzueto A, et al. Silver-coated endotracheal tubes and incidence of ventilator-associated pneumonia: the NASCENT randomized trial. *JAMA* 2008;300:805–13.

14. Muscedere J, Rewa O, McKechnie K, et al. Subglottic secretion drainage for the prevention of ventilator-associated pneumonia: a systematic review and meta-analysis. *Crit Care Med* 2011;39:1985–91.

Abbreviations

AGNB	Aerobic Gram Negative Bacilli
BAL	Bronchoalveolar Lavage
CFU	Colony Forming Units
CPIS	Clinical Pulmonary Infection Score
ECG	Electrocardiogram
PaO$_2$/FiO$_2$	Partial Pressure of Oxygen / Fixed Inspired Oxygen Concentration
ICU	Intensive Care Unit
MDR	Multi-drug Resistant
MRSA	Methicillin Resistant *Staphylococcus Aureus*
MV	Mechanical Ventilation
NICE	National Institute for Health and Care Excellence
NPSA	National Patient Safety Agency
PEEP	Positive End Expiratory Pressure
PSB	Protected Specimen Brush
SDD	Selective Decontamination of the Digestive Tract
SOD	Selective Oral Decontamination
VAP	Ventilator Associated Pneumonia

Chapter 36

Neuromonitoring

Martin Smith

Introduction

In addition to the continuous monitoring of cardiorespiratory functions common to all critically ill patients, several techniques are available for global and regional brain monitoring which provide assessment of cerebral perfusion and oxygenation, and early warning of impending brain hypoxia/ischaemia. Neuromonitors can be used to guide the management of acute brain injury (ABI) and to identify cerebral complications arising as a consequence of critical illness.

Case Description

A 65-year-old male sustained a large right-sided acute subdural haematoma during a road traffic accident whilst riding a bicycle. He had no other significant injuries. On arrival in the emergency department his Glasgow Coma Scale (GCS) was 5 (E1, V1, M3) and both pupils were 3 mm and reactive to light. He underwent emergency craniotomy for evacuation of the haematoma and was admitted to the ICU for postoperative ventilation, and sedation with propofol and fentanyl. A right frontal parenchymal intracranial pressure (ICP) monitor was placed at the end of surgery and ICP was 15 mmHg on arrival to the ICU. He was nursed in a 30° head-up position, ventilation was adjusted to maintain $PaCO_2$ between 4.5 and 5.0 kPa and PaO_2 greater than 13.0 kPa, and standard measures were instituted to maintain cerebral perfusion pressure (CPP) between 50 and 70 mmHg and ICP less than 20 mmHg.

On the following morning the ICP rose to 25 mmHg despite maximum propofol sedation and the addition of midazolam. A repeat CT scan showed no rebleeding but extensive cerebral oedema. A brain tissue PO_2 ($PtiO_2$) monitor was inserted adjacent to the ICP monitor and $PtiO_2$ was 2.5 kPa. In view of the adequate $PtiO_2$ and CPP of 65 mmHg, it was decided to continue current treatment and accept a higher ICP threshold of 25 mmHg.

Over the next 24 hours the ICP rose to 28 to 30 mmHg and increasing vasopressor doses were required to maintain CPP. $PtiO_2$ gradually reduced to 1.2 kPa. An urgent CT scan demonstrated worsened cerebral oedema so the bone flap was removed and craniotomy extended to decompress the cranium. Postoperatively ICP was 17 mmHg and $PtiO_2$ increased above 2.0 kPa over the ensuing hours. Sedation was continued at a reduced dose and ICP and $PtiO_2$ remained stable over the next 48 hours. A CT scan showed resolving cerebral oedema so sedation was reduced and, 48 hours after discontinuation of sedation, the patient's GCS was 4T (E1, VT(intubated), M3). He was flexing his right arm to pain but not moving other limbs. A CT scan confirmed continued resolution of the cerebral oedema. An EEG showed diffuse encephalopathy but no evidence of seizures. Over the next few days the patient made some neurological improvement so a tracheostomy was performed to facilitate weaning from mechanical ventilation and acute neurorehabilitation. He was discharged from the ICU 18 days after admission with a GCS of 8T (E3, VT, M5). He was localising with his right arm, movement was returning in the right leg but the left hemiparesis persisted.

On review at 18 months after the initial injury, and following extensive rehabilitation, the patient was independent with a residual left-sided weakness.

Case Discussion

This case demonstrates how neuromonitoring can be used to guide patient-specific approaches to the management of ABI. Some monitoring modalities are well established whereas others are relatively new to the clinical arena and their indications are still being evaluated (Table 36.1).

Clinical Examination

Fundamental to neuromonitoring is serial clinical assessment of neurological status. The Glasgow Coma Scale (GCS) score provides a standardised, internationally recognised method for evaluating global neurological status by recording best eye opening, motor and verbal responses to physical and verbal stimuli (Table 36.2). In association with identification and documentation of localising signs, including pupil responses and limb weaknesses, the GCS remains the mainstay of clinical assessment forty years since its first description.[1] Clinical assessment is limited in sedated patients or those with decreased conscious level and neuro-monitoring offers assessment of cerebral perfusion and oxygenation in such circumstances.

Intracranial and Cerebral Perfusion Pressures

ICP monitoring allows direct measurement of ICP and calculation of CPP as the difference between mean arterial pressure and ICP.[2] It also allows identification and analysis of pathological ICP waveforms and derivation of indices of cerebrovascular pressure reactivity (see below).

ICP monitoring and management is a standard of care after severe traumatic brain injury (TBI) because intracranial hypertension is associated with deleterious outcome.[3] Consensus guidelines from the Brain Trauma Foundation recommend that ICP should be treated if sustained above 20 mmHg, and CPP maintained between 50 to 70 mmHg. A 2010 meta-analysis suggested that ICP monitoring and management is associated with improved outcome after severe TBI but a recent randomised controlled trial found no difference in three- or six-month outcomes when treatment was guided by ICP monitoring compared to care based on imaging and clinical examination in the absence of ICP monitoring.[4] Whether the findings of this study, conducted in Bolivia and Ecuador, are applicable to wealthier nations with superior pre-hospital care and rehabilitation services remains to be seen. It is important to recognise that this study does not support the abandonment of ICP monitoring after TBI, but it does remind us that ICP monitoring cannot provide a comprehensive picture of cerebral physiology and pathophysiology.[2] Brain hypoxia can occur despite ICP and CPP being within accepted thresholds for normality.

Cerebral Oxygenation

Measurement of ICP and CPP in association with monitors of the adequacy of cerebral perfusion, such as cerebral oxygenation, provides a more complete picture of the injured

Table 36.1 Advantages and disadvantages of current bedside monitoring techniques

Technique	Advantage	Disadvantages
Intracranial pressure	- measurement of absolute ICP - calculation of CPP - analysis of pathological ICP waveforms - derivation of indices of cerebrovascular pressure reactivity	- no assessment of the adequacy of cerebral perfusion
Jugular venous oximetry	- global measure of cerebral oxygenation - assessment of the balance between oxygen supply and demand	- may miss regional ischaemia
Brain tissue PO_2	- complex and highly dynamic variable representing interaction between cerebral oxygen delivery and demand - allows rapid detection of cerebral ischaemia - bedside 'gold standard' monitor of cerebral oxygenation	- focal measurement - knowledge of probe location crucial when interpreting PtiO2 values
Near infrared spectroscopy (cerebral oximetry)	- continuous measure of the balance between cerebral oxygen delivery and utilisation - measurement of cerebral saturation - non-invasive, multi-site	- little evidence for utility in ABI - optical complexity of the injured brain complicates its use
Transcranial Doppler	- non-invasive assessment of CBF velocity - diagnosis and management of cerebral vasospasm - identification of cerebral hypoperfusion/hyperperfusion - assessment of autoregulatory reserve	- does not measure absolute CBF - operator dependent
Cerebral autoregulation	- continuous assessment of autoregulatory reserve - identification of optimal CPP	- several methods described
Cerebral microdialysis	- measurement of local brain tissue biochemistry - assessment of glucose metabolism - identification of hypoxia/ischaemia and cellular energy failure	- labour intensive - thresholds for abnormality uncertain - use currently limited to research centres
EEG	- diagnosis of seizures - confirms/excludes non-convulsive seizures as the cause of continued unconsciousness/delayed awakening	- requires skilled interpretation - affected by sedative agents

ABI, acute brain injury; CBF, cerebral blood flow; CPP, cerebral perfusion pressure; EEG, electroencephalography; ICP, intracranial pressure; $PtiO_2$, brain tissue PO_2.

brain and its response to treatment. Several methods are available to monitor cerebral oxygenation at the bedside, but brain tissue pO_2 ($PtiO_2$) is widely considered the 'gold standard.'

Table 36.2 The Glasgow Coma Score

	Response	Score
Eye opening	Spontaneous	4
	To voice	3
	To pain	2
	None	1
Verbal response	Orientated	5
	Confused, disorientated	4
	Inappropriate words	3
	Incomprehensible sounds	2
	None	1
Motor response	Obeys commands	6
	Localises to pain	5
	Flexion or withdraws to pain	4
	Abnormal flexion to pain	3
	Extension to pain	2
	None	1

Table 36.3 Interpretation of changes in jugular venous oxygen saturation

SjvO2	Relative changes in cerebral blood flow and metabolism	Causes
Normal (55% – 75%)	CBF and $CMRO_2$ balanced	
Low (<50%)	↓ CBF or ↑ CMRO2	- ↓ blood pressure - ↓ PaCO2 - ↓ PaO2 - ↑ ICP or ↓ CPP - Seizures
High (>80%)	↑ CBF or ↓ CMRO2	- cerebral hyperaemia - failure of oxygen utilisation (mitochondrial failure) - arterio-venous shunting - brainstem death - seizures

$SjvO_2$, jugular venous oxygen saturation; CBF, cerebral blood flow; $CMRO_2$, cerebral metabolic rate for oxygen; PaO_2, arterial oxygen tension; $PaCO_2$, arterial carbon dioxide tension; ICP, intracranial pressure; CPP, cerebral perfusion pressure.

Jugular Venous Oximetry

Measurement of jugular venous oxygen saturation ($SjvO_2$) was the first bedside measure of cerebral oxygenation. It is a flow-weighted, global measure and therefore unable to detect regional ischaemia. Normal $SjvO_2$ is 55 to 75 per cent and interpretation of changes is relatively straightforward (Table 36.3). Prolonged or multiple desaturation less than 50 percent has been associated with poor neurological outcome after TBI. Although widely used for decades, $SjvO_2$ monitoring has been superseded by newer modalities.

Brain Tissue Oxygen Tension

$PtiO_2$ is a complex and dynamic variable representing the interaction between cerebral oxygen delivery (including cerebral blood flow) and demand (oxygen metabolism), as well as tissue oxygen diffusion gradients. It provides a highly focal measure of cerebral oxygenation. The probe can be located in peri-contusional tissue to monitor 'at risk' brain regions although this can be technically difficult. In many instances, and especially after diffuse cerebral injury, $PtiO_2$ is measured in normal appearing frontal sub-cortical white matter. Knowledge of probe location is crucial when interpreting $PtiO_2$ values and should be confirmed by CT scan.

There are no large randomised controlled trials assessing the efficacy of $PtiO_2$-guided treatment after TBI but a systematic review of small studies demonstrated that $PtiO_2$-directed therapy supplementing ICP and CPP management is associated with superior outcome compared to standard ICP and CPP-guided therapy.[5] Current guidelines recommend incorporating the monitoring and management of $PtiO_2$ as a complement to ICP and CPP guided care in patients with severe TBI.[3] The treatment threshold for critical brain hypoxia is usually defined as less than 2 kPa (less than 15 mmHg), although the burden of cerebral hypoxia (severity, duration and chronological trend), as opposed to absolute $PtiO_2$ values in isolation, determines clinical outcome.

$PtiO_2$ is strongly influenced by systemic blood pressure and CPP but also by several other factors including PaO_2, $PaCO_2$ and haemoglobin concentration. Optimisation of which of these variables (or combination of variables) in the correction of brain hypoxia to improve outcome remains unclear. Further, it is the responsiveness of the hypoxic brain to a given intervention that appears to be of prognostic significance, with reversal of hypoxia being associated with reduced mortality

As illustrated by the case described in this chapter, $PtiO_2$ monitoring can be used to guide medical and surgical therapies after TBI. It is most widely used to guide ICP and CPP management, including the identification of patients with refractory intracranial hypertension who might benefit from second and third tier ICP-reducing therapies.[3] A suggested approach to $PtiO_2$–guided management of TBI is shown in Figure 36.1.

Cerebral Oximetry

Near infrared spectroscopy (NIRS) based cerebral oximetry provides a continuous measure of the balance between cerebral oxygen delivery and utilisation. It is used relatively widely to monitor the brain during cardiac surgery as there is some evidence of an association between intraoperative cerebral desaturation and an increased risk of perioperative cognitive decline.

There has been limited study of the utility of NIRS after ABI. Small observational studies investigating cerebral desaturation during changes in CPP, impending brain herniation, cerebral vasospasm and pharmacological interventions have produced conflicting results.[6] In particular, there is no evidence that therapy guided by changes in NIRS-derived variables influences outcome after ABI.[3] The use of NIRS is confounded by the optical complexity of the injured brain as well as by the potential for extracranial contribution to the signals. Modern technology is able to overcome some of these issues and it is likely that a single NIRS device will in the future be able to provide continuous assessment of cerebral oxygenation, haemodynamics and metabolism over multiple regions of interest.[6]

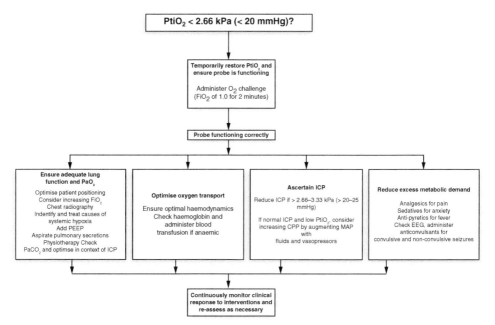

Figure 36.1 Management protocol for a patient with low brain tissue oxygen tension after traumatic brain injury. *CPP, cerebral perfusion pressure; EEG, electroencephalography; ICP, intracranial pressure; MAP, mean arterial pressure; PaCO$_2$, arterial partial pressure of carbon dioxide; PEEP, positive end-expiratory pressure; PtiO$_2$, brain tissue oxygen tension.*

Cerebral Blood Flow

Transcranial Doppler ultrasonography (TCD) is a non-invasive technique for assessing cerebral haemodynamics in realtime. It uses a low-frequency pulsed wave ultrasound probe to measure blood flow velocity (FV) through basal cerebral vessels from the Doppler shift caused by red blood cells moving through the field of view. It measures relative blood flow changes rather than actual cerebral blood flow (CBF). The TCD FV waveform resembles an arterial pulse wave (Figure 36.2) and may be quantified into peak systolic, end diastolic and mean FVs and pulsatility index (PI). PI provides an assessment of distal cerebrovascular resistance.

TCD is most commonly used in the diagnosis and management of cerebral vasospasm after subarachnoid haemorrhage, but in addition has a role in the identification of patients at high risk of critically low brain perfusion and to direct therapy, assess autoregulation and identify the need for brain imaging and invasive neuromonitoring after TBI.[7]

Autoregulation

Cerebral pressure autoregulation (CA) is an important mechanism that protects the brain against fluctuations in CBF in the face of changing CPP. It is impaired in various intracranial pathologies including TBI and SAH, as well as by administration of sedative agents. This may lead to pathophysiological derangements of regional blood flow and increased susceptibility to secondary ischaemic insults.

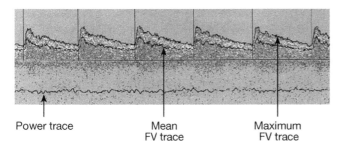

Figure 36.2 Transcranial Doppler.
A typical blood flow velocity (FV) display from transcranial Doppler ultrasound of the middle cerebral artery. Each waveform is 'enveloped' in the outer black line that is drawn electronically to represent the maximum velocity profile of each cardiac cycle; the inner black line represents the mean velocity profile. Systolic, diastolic and mean FV are calculated from the maximum velocity profile. The lower black trace represents the power of the reflected Doppler signal.
Reproduced with permission from Oxford University Press - Moppet and Mahajan, Brit J Anish 2004; 93; 710–24.

Increased arterial blood pressure (ABP) normally leads to cerebral vasoconstriction within 5 to 15 seconds, and a secondary reduction in cerebral blood volume (CBV) and ICP. When CA is impaired, CBV and ICP increase passively with ABP with opposite effects when ABP is reduced. A pressure reactivity index (PRx) can be derived from continuous monitoring and analysis of slow waves in ABP and ICP as a continuous, bedside assessment of CA.[2] A negative value for PRx when ABP is inversely correlated with ICP indicates normal CA, and a positive value a non-reactive cerebrovascular circulation. PRx may be used to guide therapy after TBI and identify optimal CPP, which is the CPP at which autoregulatory reserve is maximal. There is evidence of better outcome when actual CPP is maintained close to optimal CPP.[8] Although continuous monitoring of CA is most often performed using PRx, other approaches using oxygenation, TCD and NIRS variables are described and may be superior.[3]

Cerebral Microdialysis

Cerebral microdialysis (MD) allows bedside analysis of biochemical substances in brain tissue extracellular fluid. Glucose, lactate, pyruvate, glycerol and glutamate are the most commonly measured substances in the clinical setting, and each is a marker of a particular cellular process associated with glucose metabolism, hypoxia/ischaemia or cellular energy failure. Because lactate can be an energy substrate for the brain as well as an indicator of anaerobic metabolism, it is usual to monitor the lactate:pyruvate ratio rather than lactate alone. Cerebral MD monitoring can be considered in patients at risk of cerebral hypoxia/ischaemia, cellular energy failure and glucose deprivation,[3] but its use is currently limited to a few research centres.

Electrophysiology

Non-convulsive seizures and non-convulsive status epilepticus occur in up to one third of patients after ABI and are best detected by continuous electroencephalography (cEEG). It is increasingly recognised that non-convulsive seizures can occur in critically ill patients without a primary brain injury, and current guidelines recommend cEEG monitoring to rule out non-convulsive seizures in all comatose patients with unexplained and persistent altered consciousness.[9] In the case described in this chapter, EEG was able to exclude non-convulsive seizures as the cause of delayed awakening after evacuation of an acute subdural haematoma.

cEEG is a resource intense technology requiring skilled personnel for interpretation. Technological advances have led to the introduction of user friendly processed EEG (pEEG) techniques, including automated seizure detection software. Telemedicine, which allows interpretation away from the bedside, may also increase the adoption of cEEG.

The bispectral index (BIS) monitor is a widely used pEEG device that was developed to monitor the depth of anaesthesia. The BIS monitor uses a proprietary algorithm to process frontal EEG signals and derive a number between 0 and 98. Values above 90 reflect a preponderance of higher frequency beta waves suggesting wakefulness. With progressive EEG suppression, BIS value approaches 0. There is no evidence to support the use of BIS monitoring to guide sedation or other interventions in the ICU. Its raw EEG display in association with the BIS value is sometimes used prior to definitive EEG monitoring in patients at risk of seizures or to guide sedation in status epilepticus but it should be emphasised that BIS does not replace formal EEG monitoring in these circumstances. There is some preliminary evidence that BIS value might have some prognostic significance in determining which patients will not recover from cardiac arrest-associated brain anoxia.

Multimodal Monitoring

Therapeutic targets and choice of therapy after ABI are best determined by monitoring more than one variable (multimodal monitoring). In current clinical practice this most commonly involves the simultaneous measurement of ICP, CPP and PtiO$_2$, as in this case. Other modalities, such as CA, CBF and EEG monitoring, are increasingly being adopted.[10] Multimodal monitoring can be used to guide patient-specific management after ABI, including the withholding of potentially dangerous therapy in those with no evidence of brain hypoxia-ischaemia.

Conclusion

Several techniques are available for global and regional brain monitoring which provide assessment of cerebral perfusion/ oxygenation, and early warning of impending brain hypoxia-ischaemia. Neuromonitoring allows an individually tailored, patient-specific approach to the management of ABI and identification of cerebral complications in critically ill patients without primary brain injury.

Key Learning Points

- Cerebral monitoring can be used to guide the management of acute brain injury and identify cerebral complications of critical illness in patients without primary brain injury.
- ICP and CPP-guided therapy is a standard of care after severe TBI but brain resuscitation guided by ICP and CPP monitoring alone does not prevent cerebral hypoxia-ischaemia in all patients.
- Monitoring brain tissue oxygenation provides an assessment of the balance between cerebral oxygen supply and demand, and the effectiveness of cerebral perfusion.

- Multimodal monitoring, including assessment of cerebral perfusion and oxygenation, allows early warning of impending brain hypoxia-ischaemia.
- EEG monitoring is recommended to rule out non-convulsive seizures in all comatose patients with unexplained and persistent altered consciousness.

References

1. Sharshar T, Citerio G, Andrews PJ, et al. Neurological examination of critically ill patients: a pragmatic approach. Report of an ESICM expert panel. *Intensive Care Med* 2014;40:484–95.

2. Kirkman MA, Smith M. Intracranial pressure monitoring, cerebral perfusion pressure estimation, and ICP/CPP-guided therapy: a standard of care or optional extra after brain injury? *Br J Anaesth* 2014;112:35–46.

3. Le Roux P, Menon DK, Citerio G, et al. Consensus summary statement of the International Multidisciplinary Consensus Conference on Multimodality Monitoring in Neurocritical Care: a statement for healthcare professionals from the Neurocritical Care Society and the European Society of Intensive Care Medicine. *Intensive Care Med* 2014;40:1189–209.

4. Chesnut RM, Temkin N, Carney N, et al. A trial of intracranial-pressure monitoring in traumatic brain injury. *N Engl J Med* 2012;367:2471–81.

5. Nangunoori R, Maloney-Wilensky E, Stiefel M, et al. Brain tissue oxygen-based therapy and outcome after severe traumatic brain injury: a systematic literature review. *Neurocrit Care* 2012;17:131–38.

6. Ghosh A, Elwell C, Smith M. Review article: cerebral near-infrared spectroscopy in adults: a work in progress. *Anesth Analg* 2012;115:1373–83.

7. Bouzat P, Oddo M, Payen JF. Transcranial Doppler after traumatic brain injury: is there a role? *Curr Opin Crit Care* 2014;20: 153–60.

8. Aries MJ, Czosnyka M, Budohoski KP, et al. Continuous determination of optimal cerebral perfusion pressure in traumatic brain injury. *Crit Care Med* 2012;40:2456–63.

9. Claassen J, Taccone FS, Horn P, et al. Recommendations on the use of EEG monitoring in critically ill patients: consensus statement from the neurointensive care section of the ESICM. *Intensive Care Med* 2013;39:1337–51.

10. Oddo M, Villa F, Citerio G. Brain multimodality monitoring: an update. *Curr Opin Crit Care* 2012;18:111–18.

Monitoring Cardiac Output

Tim Meekings

Introduction

One of the clinical challenges posed when managing a critically ill, unstable patient is that of measuring the patient's cardiac output, as this forms an important background to formulating a management plan to try to bring about a clinical improvement. The assessment of cardiac output in a critically ill patient can be made both clinically and using a variety of devices. The ideal method for monitoring cardiac output would be accurate, noninvasive, cheap, reproducible and portable. This monitoring system should also be reliable in accurately sensing rapid physiological changes in a timely fashion, as in real life conditions there are dynamic changes in stroke volume, systemic vascular resistance and heart rate and rhythm which alter the cardiac output on a beat-to-beat basis. Therapeutic interventions such as administration of a fluid bolus or vasoactive drugs and the subsequent effect on cardiac output would also have to be detectable and accurately measured. In truth, no single monitor of cardiac output available to date fulfills all these criteria: in the interim a variety of technologies are available that partially meet this requirement.[2]

This case discusses a patient with shock and considers the benefits of each of the tools for cardiac output assessment that can be integrated into patient care.

Clinical Case

A 77-year-old female was admitted to the intensive care unit with a combination of respiratory and cardiovascular failure. Earlier that day, she had attended the emergency department with a 3-day history of breathlessness and lethargy which had worsened in the preceding 24 hours, associated with a cough productive of green sputum. Past medical history for the patient included treated hypertension and type 2 diabetes mellitus. Investigations at admission revealed a raised white cell count with neutrophilia and left bundle branch block on a 12 lead ECG. An initial chest X-ray demonstrated widespread alveolar shadowing and blunting of both costophrenic angles. Initial management included high flow oxygen therapy via facemask, intravenous broad-spectrum antimicrobials and insertion of a radial arterial line to facilitate blood pressure monitoring and arterial blood gas analysis.

Following assessment in the emergency department, the patient was transferred to the intensive care unit for a trial of CPAP via a hood. Following two hours of CPAP therapy, she became increasingly hypoxaemic and agitated and thus underwent sedation, tracheal intubation and invasive ventilation. Subsequently, although the patient's oxygenation improved with invasive ventilation, this was associated with a rising lactate and a tachycardia of 140 beats per minute and persistent hypotension with both arterial and non-invasive blood pressure monitoring displaying a blood pressure of around 75/40 mmHg. A central venous catheter was inserted via the right internal jugular vein and an infusion of nor-adrenaline was commenced on the assumption that the cause of the hypotension was sepsis related. Despite this returning the blood pressure back to a more normal range, the patient's lactate remained elevated and urine output fell to less than 0.5 ml/kg/hr. There was concern that cardiogenic shock was an additional factor and use of pressors and inotropes needed careful assessment.

Case Discussion

In this situation, it would firstly be useful to establish whether the patient had sustained a myocardial infarction that was contributing to the shock. Serial cardiac enzyme measurement in addition to trying to compare the current 12 lead ECG with any previous recordings to confirm whether the left bundle branch block was a new occurrence is necessary. If myocardial ischaemia or infarction is confirmed, a specialist opinion should be sought as to whether further assessment in the form of percutaneous intervention is indicated; alongside this, secondary prevention measures such as antiplatelet agents, anticoagulation and statin therapy should also be considered.

Early transthoracic echocardiography would be clinically useful to both qualitatively assess cardiac output and also detect significant complications affecting cardiac output, such as valvular incompetence or left ventricular aneurysm. This information can then be combined with ongoing assessment of cardiac output to monitor trends in cardiac output and stroke volume in response to therapeutic interventions such as fluid resuscitation and the institution of vasopressor or inotropic therapy.

A number of methods are available to provide ongoing assessment of cardiac output.

Clinical Assessment of Cardiac Output

The simplest method of estimating a patient's cardiac output relies upon clinical examination and the interpretation of simple investigations in conjunction with the patient's medical history and clinical presentation. The clinical presentation of the patient may give some indication as to their cardiac output, for example in the early stages of sepsis a hyperdynamic circulation with raised cardiac output may be apparent. In contrast, a patient presenting following a myocardial infarction may demonstrate a low cardiac output state due to left ventricular failure. This presenting history is combined with clinical examination incorporating peripheral perfusion, capillary refill time, pulse rate, blood pressure, central venous pressure, urine output and skin perfusion to give some idea as to whether the patient's cardiac output is normal, increased or reduced. The addition of results from some simple blood tests including mixed venous oxygen saturation can provide additional information – for example a suspicion of a low cardiac output based on clinical examination and presenting history would be supported by the presence of a raised lactate and metabolic acidosis picture from an arterial blood gas. However the high degree of inter-observer variability, the problems of multiple pathologies giving a mixed picture as in this case, and the subjective nature of a purely clinical assessment of cardiac output make this an unreliable method for objectively assessing cardiac output with any degree of certainty.[1]

Multiple attempts have been made at developing systems to reliably measure cardiac output.

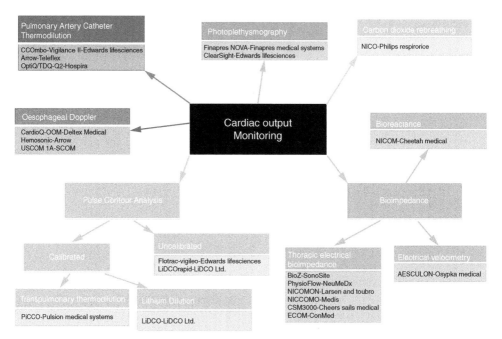

Figure 37.1 Cardiac output monitoring techniques and devices.

Pulmonary Artery Catheter Thermodilution

One of the earliest methods for cardiac output monitoring in the clinical setting utilised a thermodilution technique via a pulmonary artery catheter (PAC). An embedded heating filament in the PAC releases thermal pulses that are then detected at the tip of the catheter; the cardiac output is then derived from the area under the thermodilution curve.[3] This has the advantage of providing a near continuous measurement of cardiac output with a relatively high degree of reliability and reproducibility. This remains an invasive technique, which requires specific training and skill to institute. There are also significant complications with the use of PAC, which include but are not limited to pulmonary embolus and infarction, infection, arrhythmias and damage to the pulmonary valve.[2] To minimise or eliminate these risks, noninvasive techniques to measure cardiac output have subsequently been developed.

Oesophageal Doppler

The oesophageal Doppler probe is placed to measure blood flow in the descending aorta, and when this is combined with the calculated cross sectional area of the descending aorta, an algorithm based upon thermodilution data is then utilised to calculate the cardiac output.[4] Amongst the advantages of this technique are that it is relatively noninvasive and can also provide other indices such as corrected flow time and systolic volume variation. These may give some indication of cardiac preload and thus guide therapeutic interventions in the form of administration of fluid boluses.[2] This may explain why there is a good evidence base for the use of oesophageal Doppler perioperatively to guide fluid administration in surgery, resulting in improved outcomes and reduced morbidity. One of the disadvantages of oesophageal Doppler use relate to the fact that it cannot be used to directly measure cardiac output as 30 per cent of cardiac output is diverted proximal to the descending aorta.[4] In conjunction with the fact that the cardiac output displayed is often a derivation based upon a calculated aortic cross sectional area, this limits the accuracy of the measurement. Measurements may also be unreliable in turbulent flow conditions such as atrial fibrillation and the probe cannot be tolerated in a patient who is conscious or placed in a patient with an oesophageal disorder, e.g., recent surgery.[3] There are also practical issues with the use of the oesophageal Doppler probe in the intensive care unit as there is a degree of training required in its use to minimise inter-operator variability and there are considerable difficulties in maintaining the probe in a stable position whilst the patient is moved at regular intervals during the day for nursing and medical interventions.

Pulse Contour Analysis

Early attempts to use the area under the arterial pulse waveform to calculate the stroke volume were hampered by the fact that the compliance of the arterial tree is nonlinear. To measure the cardiac output with any degree of accuracy using this method therefore required another method to calibrate the system.[2] Consequently the initial systems utilised the area under the curve of the arterial waveform to calculate the stroke volume and thus cardiac output, relying upon a calibration when the monitoring is set up. The two commonly available methods use transpulmonary thermodilution and lithium dilution as calibration methods.

Transpulmonary Thermodilution

In this technique cold saline is injected via a central venous catheter and the subsequent thermodilution is measured in a proximally placed arterial line (femoral, brachial or axillary). When this is combined with pulse contour analysis, a continuous measurement of cardiac output can be performed.[5] Although this has the advantage of using a central venous catheter, which may already be in place for other therapeutic interventions, a specific arterial line has to be placed in a proximal artery with the attendant risks of thrombosis and arterial damage.

Lithium Dilution

Lithium is an ideal indicator for measuring cardiac output: it does not naturally occur in the plasma, is rapidly redistributed and does not undergo first pass loss from the circulation.[2] A bolus of lithium is administered either via a central or peripheral cannula and the resulting lithium concentration decay is then measured through a lithium-sensitive electrode attached to the patient's arterial line.[2,3] The concentration against time graph of lithium is then used to calculate cardiac output by integrating the area under the curve.[2] This method appears to compare favourably with thermodilution techniques in terms of accuracy[4] and has the advantage that once calibrated, this method provides truly continuous data rather than the intermittent nature found in thermodilution techniques.[6] The drawbacks of this method include repeated blood sampling for calibration and the need for recalibration, particularly during periods of haemodynamic instability.[3]

Pulse Contour Analysis - Uncalibrated

Further developments in pulse contour analysis have led to the introduction of uncalibrated systems. These devices use the arterial waveform to compute cardiac output continuously by multiplying heart rate by a calculated stroke volume. The stroke volume is estimated by multiplying arterial pulsatility by a constant. The arterial pulsatility is derived from the standard deviation of the pressure wave over a 20 second period. The constant is comprised of a combination of biometric measures (sex, age, height and weight) along with waveform characteristics that are measured every minute.[3] The advantages of this system include ease of use and provision of continuous data. These benefits are countered by the potential limitation of this device in the face of rapid changes in systemic vascular resistance, which may be encountered clinically, that may impair its accuracy in the absence of calibration.[3] Comparisons of pulse contour analysis devices seem to reveal that the calibrated systems outperform the uncalibrated systems, especially when faced with large changes in cardiac output during periods of haemodynamic instability.[4]

Bioimpedance

The use of thoracic bioimpedance cardiography to measure stroke volume and cardiac output has appeared to be an attractive prospect as it is noninvasive, continuous, operator-independent and cost effective.[7] This technology is based on the assumption that the electrical resistance of the thorax is related to intrathoracic blood volume and will therefore change as intrathoracic blood volume varies.[4] Electrodes are placed on either side of the patient's neck and across the lower thorax. The impedance of flow of current from the outermost to the innermost set of electrodes is measured; this value is indirectly proportional to the volume of intrathoracic fluid.[2] The initial models for this system utilised an algorithm describing the human thorax as a cylinder or cone to convert the change in impedance into a measurement of stroke volume and cardiac output. This model is described as thoracic electrical bioimpedance.

Electrical Velocimetry

To increase the accuracy of the original bioimpedance devices, a new technology called electrical velocimetry was introduced. Electrical velocimetry is based upon the effect which velocity of blood flow in the aorta has on conductivity rather than the intrathoracic blood volume.[4]

Bioreactance

A further refinement of bioimpedance technology, bioreactance describes the phase shift in voltage across the thorax.[5] The use of bioreactance is thought to reduce the signal-to-noise ratio of the bioimpedance signal and thus reduce the inaccuracies of bioimpedance measurements secondary to electrode positioning, body size, temperature and humidity.[4]

Bioimpedance is highly sensitive to electrode positioning, pulmonary oedema and electrical noise.[4] Furthermore, research has consistently demonstrated bioimpedance to be less accurate than thermodilution and Doppler-based techniques when measuring cardiac output in surgical and critically ill patients.[2] The combination of practical difficulties and inaccurate measurements has meant that to date bioimpedance has not yet found widespread use in the measurement of cardiac output in the clinical setting.

Carbon dioxide Rebreathing

The Fick principle has previously been used in the research setting to calculate cardiac output. The Fick principle states that the total uptake or release of a substance by an organ is the product of the blood flow to that organ multiplied by the arteriovenous concentration difference.[2] More recently, devices have been developed that use a partial rebreathing method to measure end tidal carbon dioxide and carbon dioxide elimination and from this estimate the cardiac output.[2] This technique has primarily been validated against thermo-dilution in animal studies to date.[4] There is a lack of clinical data to demonstrate this system to be reliable and accurate in the haemodynamically unstable patient. This is also combined with the drawbacks of a relatively long response time and the fact that this method only measures cardiac output and does not monitor intravascular volume status or fluid responsiveness.[2,4]

Photoplethysmography

The photoplethysmographic waveform is related to the arterial pressure waveform and consequently has a relationship to stroke volume.[4] The Penaz technique describes a combination of an infrared transmitter and receiver, the photoplethysmograph, and an inflatable finger bladder with a feedback control mechanism.[4] The photoplethysmograph detects the volume of arterial blood in the finger under the cuff at mean arterial pressure. Following this, the finger cuff is inflated or deflated as required to keep this measured blood volume constant. The finger pressure waveform can thus be transduced to give a peripheral arterial pressure waveform, which can then be used to estimate stroke volume. This technique has demonstrated reasonable agreement between the measured peripheral arterial pressure and invasive blood pressure monitoring, however there is limited data to also verify estimated stroke volume based upon photoplethysmography and this technique has not yet seen widespread use.[4]

Conclusion

Although there are a wide variety of monitoring devices available to attempt to measure cardiac output, none of these fulfil all of the criteria of an ideal system. A cross comparison of cardiac output trending accuracy of thermodilution and indicator dilution (both cali-brated and uncalibrated) devices with pulmonary artery catheters found that although they all showed similar mean cardiac output values, they often trended differently in response to therapy and had varying degrees of agreement between devices.[8] Doppler-based measure-ments seem to have similar accuracy to thermodilution pulmonary artery catheters with the advantage of being truly continuous monitors and less invasive.[4] However, the practical difficulties of using them in a real life intensive care setting are significant. Bioimpedance devices appear less accurate than either thermodilution or Doppler techniques and as yet there is insufficient evidence to verify that this is any better with the evolution of electrical velocimetry and bioreactance.[4]

As most forms of cardiac output monitoring described here are associated with meas-urement errors of up to 40 per cent,[1] perhaps the term estimating rather than measuring cardiac output should be used. If there were one system that reliably measured cardiac output, this would obviously negate the need for the plethora of systems based upon differing technologies currently available. Until an ideal system is either refined from the currently available devices or discovered anew, cardiac output monitoring systems are probably best used to monitor trends in cardiac output rather than to make decisions based upon absolute measurements of cardiac output or stroke volume.

Key Learning Points

- Estimation of cardiac output based purely on clinical assessment is unreliable.
- The use of thermodilution pulmonary artery catheters was amongst the first clinically widespread method of trying to measure cardiac output and although usage has declined, often remains the gold standard against which newer devices are measured.
- Oesophageal Doppler measurement of cardiac output is relatively noninvasive and has a good evidence base in certain surgical patient groups.
- Pulse contour analysis has gained widespread use: calibrated and uncalibrated systems for measuring cardiac output are available.
- Bioimpedance has the advantage of being noninvasive but is limited by practical difficulties with monitoring and concerns relating to accuracy in haemodynamic instability.
- Other technologies such as carbon dioxide rebreathing and photoplethysmography are available but are not in widespread use.

References

1. Imhoff M. Alea lacta Est: A New Approach to Cardiac Output Monitoring? *Anesth Analg* 2013;117:295–6.

2. Funk DJ, Moretti EW, Gan TJ. Minimally Invasive Cardiac Output Monitoring in the Perioperative Setting. *Anesth Analg* 2009; 108:887–97.

3. de Waal EEC, Wappler F, Buhre WF. Cardiac output monitoring. *Curr Opin Anaesthesiol* 2009;22:71–7.

4. Thiele RH, Bartels K., Gan TJ. Cardiac output monitoring: A contemporary assessment and review. *Crit Care Med* 2014. doi: 10.1097/CCM.0000000000000608 (Accessed October 13, 2014.)

5. Critchley LA, Lee A, Ho AM-H. A Critical Review of the Ability of Continuous Cardiac Output Monitors to Measure Trends in Cardiac Output. *Anesth Analg* 2010;111:1180–92.

6. Thiele RH, Durieux ME. Arterial Waveform Analysis for the Anesthesiologist: Past, *Present and Future Concepts. Anesth Analg* 2011;113:766–76.

7. Fellahi JL, Caille V, Charron C, et al. Noninvasive Assessment of Cardiac Index in Healthy Volunteers: A Comparison Between Thoracic Impedance Cardiography and Doppler Echocardiography. *Anesth Analg* 2009;108:1553–9.

8. Hadian M, Kim HK, Severyn D, et al. Cross-comparison of Cardiac Output Trending Accuracy of LiDCO, PiCCO, FloTrac and pulmonary artery catheters. Critical Care 2010;14:R212.

Chapter 38

The Surgical Patient on Critical Care

John Jameson

Introduction

This case describes the progress of a 64-year-old man admitted to critical care, 4 days after a laparoscopically assisted anterior resection for an upper rectal cancer. The patient had a 29-day stay on critical care and was discharged from hospital on the 56th post-operative day. The details of the case will be outlined and the points at which surgical management decisions were made will be explored in more detail to consider the options available to the clinical teams and the advantages and disadvantages of those options. This case has been chosen as an example of a situation where the evidence base for many of these decisions is not strong, and frequently is based on individual opinion and patient circumstances.

Case Description

A 64-year-old man was admitted electively for a laparoscopically assisted anterior resection for an upper rectal cancer. Surgery was uneventful and performed with curative intent. Prior to surgery the patient had been fit and well although five years previously he had developed a post-traumatic lower limb deep venous thrombosis that had been treated with 3 months of warfarin. The patient's body mass index (BMI) was 26.6.

Four days after surgery, he was referred to critical care with increasing hypoxia and deteriorating renal function. A contained anastomotic leak had been diagnosed on cross-sectional imaging earlier that day and the initial surgical decision was to treat the leak conservatively. The CT scan had also shown extensive bilateral lung consolidation for which the patient had been started on piperacillin/tazobactam.

The patient was admitted to the level 2 High Dependency Unit for CPAP and the following day, a decision was made to take the patient back to theatre for a laparotomy and Hartmann's procedure. At operation a contained leak with peritoneal soiling was confirmed, the anastomosis was taken down, a left iliac fossa end colostomy fashioned and the rectal stump closed. The abdomen was closed at the end of the procedure and a drain left in situ. It was decided not to extubate the patient due to his premorbid state and surgical findings, and he was returned to the level 3 intensive care unit.

Post-operatively, he experienced worsening hypoxia and deteriorating renal function, thought to be due to the abdominal sepsis. He was treated with fluids, vasopressors, antibiotics and bronchoscopy. Intra-abdominal pressure was monitored.

Over the next three days, he had signs of ongoing severe sepsis treated with antibiotics and antifungal agents, fluids and vasopressors. During daily sedation holds, he was noted to be not waking up well and having to be re-sedated for inappropriate responses. He was also not absorbing his nasogastric feed, as evidenced by high nasogastric aspirates and he was noted to have abdominal distention and a non-functioning stoma. Total parenteral nutrition (TPN) was therefore established.

Although concerns remained about abdominal distention and raised intra-abdominal pressures (19 mm Hg), he was extubated onto CPAP by day 8. He was also noted to be extremely oedematous.

Unfortunately the following day (day 9) he became more overtly septic with raised inflammatory markers and his abdominal wound was noted to have dehisced with pus exuding from it. Skin clips were removed from the lower end of the wound and some cellulitis around it was noted. Nasogastric feeding was still not successful so TPN was continued. At this point the patient was also noted to be becoming confused. Although nasogastric feeding did later become established and renal function improved, by day 11 enteral contents were noted to be coming from the abdominal wound. The patient remained confused and had bilateral pleural effusions. A CT scan was discussed although the patient was CPAP dependent at that point and so it was not arranged.

Oedema remained along with continued abdominal discharge, intermittent pyrexias and intermittent confusion. Little patient progress was occurring, and as time progressed, NG aspirates started to increase and stoma function decreased. A CT scan of the chest and abdomen was performed on day 18 which showed a small pleural effusion, basal lung consolidation and left-sided abdominal collections. The collections were therefore drained by means of ultrasound-guided percutaneous drainage. two left-sided abdominal collections were identified, one draining serous fluid, the other foul smelling bloodstained pus.

Although there was a slight overall improvement with the drains, no further progress occurred, as the patient remained confused, bowel function was variable and there was still a need for CPAP. On day 23 a further acute deterioration with more overt sepsis occurred. More of the wound had broken down and when the abdomen was pressed, pus oozed from the midline wound. The sepsis was still treated conservatively as a repeat CT scan showed the original collections were smaller and no further surgical intervention was therefore felt to be necessary.

Slow progress with treatment for ongoing sepsis was made but by day 29 the patient was able to be discharged to ward

Case Discussion

At a number of points surgical planning decisions were made in conjunction with the critical care team.

Decision to Take the Patient Back to Theatre after the Diagnosis of the Contained Leak

There is no robust evidence base to guide treatment of anastomotic leakage and standard treatment is re-operation, taking down of the anastomosis and stoma formation as in this case. This, however, is clearly a major insult for the patient who, assuming he or she survives the leak, will be facing a significant life change with the stoma and possible further major surgery to reverse it in the future. Indeed, many patients will never come to reversal. With the increased use of cross-sectional imaging in the post-operative phase and the ability to diagnose contained leaks more accurately, conservative management of this clinical situation has been recognised as being safe in selected cases.[1,2,3]

It does need to be understood that radiology cannot conclusively determine the extent of a leak. The decision to treat an anastomotic leak conservatively is a difficult one and depends on several factors, including the degree of physiological disturbance shown by the patient in response to the leak, the patient's existing co-morbidities and the extent of physiological support necessary; these aspects are best assessed by the critical care team and decision-making needs to be shared between them and the surgical team along with a clear plan as to where and how the patient will be managed.

Treating a contained leak conservatively does run the risk of the peri-anastomotic abscess perforating in the near future and patients undergoing conservative treatment need close supervision. It might have been reasonable to attempt to manage this patient conservatively in view of the fact that he had little pre-exisiting comorbidity if he was not deteriorating on the critical care unit.

Paradoxically patients with more co-morbidity could be treated more aggressively initially in an attempt to avoid further deterioration that they may not tolerate very well. Occasionally, when a patient is returned to theatre for a suspected leak, if there is minimal contamination and systemic upset, it may be possible to raise a defunctioning rather than an end stoma which has the advantage of making the reversal procedure much less of a risk to the patient.

At the end of a laparotomy, there are also further decisions to be made: first, whether the abdomen should be closed or not, as there is a risk of subsequent abdominal compartment syndrome. If the abdomen is not closed and the patient is managed with a laparostomy, this adds considerably to patient morbidity should he or she survive, and may require a further trip back to theatre in the interim if a decision is made to re-attempt closure. This again can be difficult and requires good communication between surgeon and the critical care team and joint decision-making.

Management When Pus Exuded from the Abdominal Wound on Day 9

At this stage the patient was more septic and the discharge of pus from the wound was an obvious indication of the site of the sepsis. The question at this stage is whether this was related to the wound alone or was an indication of more extensive intra-abdominal sepsis. The key to management at this stage is control of the sepsis in the least invasive way possible. Opening the wound is an appropriate way to do this and at this stage a decision should be made, if possible, as to whether the infection is confined to the superficial part of the wound or whether the abdominal muscle closure has given way. While a full thickness wound dehiscence may not need any different specific management from a superficial wound infection at this stage, the short term implication is that the patient has more extensive sepsis and that there is a greater risk of fistula formation together with the longer term consequences for the patient of significantly delayed wound healing and incisional hernia development. Furthermore, it is possible that the wound discharge is in fact the first manifestation of a fistula with the leakage of bowel contents only becoming obvious in a day or two. The use of CT scanning should be considered at this stage to help determine the extent of any collections unless it is obvious that the sepsis is confined to the superficial part of the wound and is controllable. If the later course is pursued and no rapid improvement in the patient's condition occurs, the plan will need revising.

Management When the Bowel Contents were Noted in the Abdominal Wound Day 11

Once it is apparent that an intestinal fistula has formed, the principles of management are to control the sepsis (s), to protect the skin (s), to establish nutrition (n), to determine the anatomy of the fistula (a) and when appropriate, to plan definitive management of the fistula (p). This can be remembered using the acronym SSNAP. Depending on the degree of the sepsis, further surgery may be necessary but in general, a further laparotomy should be avoided if possible at this time post-surgery as there will almost certainly be extensive dense adhesion formation in the abdomen and a further exploration can easily lead to further fistulation and a significant worsening of the situation. In general, CT scanning should be performed at this stage to help determine the extent of any collections and, if possible, to drain these percutaneously under radiological control. In terms of the anatomy of the fistula possible sources in this case are the small bowel (proximal or distal), colon or the rectal stump. Cross-sectional imaging may or may not help in determining the level of the fistula and other methods of clinical assessment may need to be used. The volume and appearance of the fistula contents can be a guide with a high volume fistula being more difficult to manage in terms of fluid and electrolyte imbalance, skin problems and the establishment and maintenance of nutrition. Distal small bowel and colonic fistulas are lower volume, skin care is generally less of a challenge and the enteral route can generally be used to maintain nutrition.

Management After the Second CT Scan on Day 23

For several days after day 20, the patient failed to make progress. At this stage specific management is concerned mainly with draining the sepsis as adequately as possible while not exposing the patient to undue risk. The disadvantage of draining the two left-sided collections with radiological drains is that those drains are relatively small bore. It is possible to improve drainage by accessing the collections by exploring the percutaneous drain track under general anaesthesia and inserting first a guarded sucker into the collection followed by a larger bore drain. Better drainage of the abdominal discharge can be achieved by exploration of the wound under general anaesthetic with a view to opening it adequately, debriding any dead tissue, washing the wound out and applying a suitable dressing. This does need to be done cautiously and the aim is not to explore the abdominal cavity any more than absolutely necessary, if at all, at this stage. Significant collections may accumulate in the defunctioned rectal stump and can lead to disruption of the stump with attendant pelvic and abdominal sepsis as was thought to have occurred in this case. The presence of a rectal stump collection can easily be determined by digital rectal examination and can be drained using a large bore Foley catheter inserted into the rectum. This development can be potentially avoided at the time of surgery by washing out the stump and leaving a Foley catheter in situ. Any pelvic collections can be drained and irrigated via a rectal catheter in the presence of a disrupted rectal closure.

General Points About the Use of CT Scanning in Critical Care Patients

Cross-sectional imaging of surgical patients can be useful but should not be used as a substitute for or to delay decision-making in critically unwell patients. The result of any CT should change management of the patient in order to arrange the investigation; if it is clear that a laparotomy or some other form of surgical intervention is needed on clinical grounds, a CT is not necessary. One way to consider the use of CTs is to say 'what finding in the CT scan will stop an operation being done'?

Conclusion

The management of surgical patients with significant abdominal sepsis on critical care can be difficult and effective communication and team working between the critical care and surgical teams is key to the successful management of the patient. All the involved teams need to be aware of the reasoning for any management plans and decisions, so they can be amended should the clinical picture change.

Key Learning Points

- Successful patient management requires good communication and joint decision-making between the critical care and surgical teams.
- Sepsis from any source should be actively sought and treated.
- Adequate control of sepsis should use the least invasive means possible.
- Cross-sectional imaging should be used in a selective manner and at the right time to allow for decision-making and planning. It should not result in a delay in decision-making.

References

1. Maggiori L, Bretagnol F, Lefevre JH, Ferron M, Vicaut E, Panis Y. Conservative management is associated with a decreased risk of definitive stoma after anastomotic leakage complicating sphincter-saving resection for rectal cancer. *Colorectal Disease* 2011;13(6):632–7.

2. Kanellos D. Anastomotic leakage after colonic resection. *Techniques in Coloproctology* 2010;14(Suppl 1):S43–4.

3. Kanellos D, Pramateftakis MG, Vrakas G et al. Anastomotic leakage following low anterior resection for rectal cancer. *Techniques in Coloproctology* 2010; 14(Suppl 1):S35–7.

Chapter 39

Delirium in the Intensive Care Unit

Richard Bourne

Introduction

Delirium is characterised by an acute change or fluctuation in mental status, inattention and disorganised thinking or an altered level of consciousness. It is common in critically ill patients, with European studies reporting a prevalence rate of approximately 30 to 45 per cent.[1] The rate is affected by patient factors such as the vulnerability of the patient (e.g., older age, dementia), acuity of illness (severe sepsis), need for mechanical ventilation and environmental factors (physical restraints) or unit specific practices (e.g., benzodiazepine-based sedation). Furthermore, the timing of delirium assessment in relation to the patient's sedation level or sedative exposure significantly affects the prevalence rates reported.[2] The development of delirium has significant implications for critically ill patients: it is associated with increased duration of intensive care and hospital length of stay, increased mortality and long-term cognitive impairment.[3]

There are three motoric subtypes of delirium: hyperactive (the person is agitated, may be a danger to themselves and staff), hypoactive (apathetic, lethargic, drowsy) or mixed (fluctuation between hyper- and hypo-active delirium). Hyperactive delirium is the easiest to identify, but is actually the least common in most prevalence studies. Without the use of a specific delirium screening tool, delirium may be missed or misdiagnosed, particularly in the case of patients with hypoactive delirium.[3] Delirium screening tools have been developed and validated for use in critical care patients to improve identification and monitoring of delirium. The most valid and reliable screening tools are the CAM-ICU (Confusion Assessment Method for the Intensive Care Unit) [Box 39.1] and ICDSC (Intensive Care Delirium Screening Checklist) [Box 39.2].[3] Although there are advantages and disadvantages with both these tools, the important aspect is that each hospital or unit chooses one that they can implement and routinely use in clinical practice. A wide range of terms are still used in some clinical practice to describe delirium symptoms (e.g., ICU psychosis, septic encephalopathy); however, using these

---

Box 39.1 Confusion Assessment Method for the Intensive Care unit (CAM-ICU)

Features and descriptions (absent/present as defined). The patient is delirium positive when features 1 and 2 and either feature 3 or 4 are present.
[Ely EW et al. *Critical Care Medicine* 2001; 29: 1370–79]

1. Acute onset or fluctuating course
2. Inattention
3. Disorganised thinking
4. Altered level of consciousness

Box 39.2   Intensive Care Delirium Screening Checklist (ICDSC)

The scale is completed based on information collected from each entire 8–h shift or from the previous 24 h. Each item has a definition. Obvious manifestation of an item = 1 point; no manifestation of an item or no assessment possible = 0 point. The score of each item is recorded as 0 or 1 and then totalled; the patient is delirium positive when he or she scores 4 or more points.

1. Altered level of consciousness
2. Inattention
3. Disorientation
4. Hallucination, delusion or psychosis
5. Psychomotor agitation or retardation
6. Inappropriate speech or mood
7. Sleep/wake cycle disturbance
8. Symptom fluctuation

[Bergeron N et al. *Intensive Care Medicine* 2001; 27: 859–64]

---

terms suggests that delirium is inevitable and may detract from attempts to correct modifiable factors[4]

Relatively little is known about the pathophysiology of delirium and it may be different for hyperactive and hypoactive subtypes. Recently it has been proposed that an acute illness or precipitating factor(s) triggers an inflammatory process which in turn may aggravate or drive a central neurotransmitter dysfunction and disturbances involving one or more of serotonin, dopamine, noradrenaline or acetylcholine.[5]

Case Description

A 60-year-old female presented for elective endonasal odontoid peg resection for basilar invagination/chiari malformation with decreased swallow, headaches, pain and abnormal sensation in the arms and an unsteady gait. Her pre-operative medications included quinine sulphate 300 mg nightly as required and ibuprofen 400 mg 8 hourly as required. Pregabalin 100 mg twice daily was started on admission for analgesia.

The patient was admitted to the level 2 high dependency unit (HDU) post-operatively, and then transferred to the ward where she had a fall on Day 7 that required her to wear a hard collar for an unstable neck injury. On day 8 she developed respiratory failure due to aspiration and was moved to critical care for elective intubation and respiratory support. On day 10 pharyngeal swelling was noted on direct observation and she was commenced on intravenous (IV) dexamethasone 4 mg 8 hourly.

She was subsequently given a tracheostomy to aid weaning from respiratory support. Candida was also cultured from an arterial line tip and she was started on IV fluconazole as treatment.

By day 11 she had become severely agitated. Medical review noted that she had a recent aspiration pneumonia and ongoing treatment for fungal line sepsis although sepsis markers were improving. Agitation was felt likely to be secondary to ongoing infection as no obvious organic focus or neurosurgical cause could be found. She was therefore given additional analgesia in the form of tramadol and prescribed haloperidol to be given if she became dangerously agitated.

Two subsequent doses of IV haloperidol were administered, which were reported to worsen her delirium symptoms and she removed her nasogastric (NG) feeding tube. A dose of parenteral olanzapine was subsequently given which had a sedating effect.

Later that day the nurses reported worsening delirium symptoms (scoring 7 on Intensive Care Delirium Screening Checklist (ICDSC)) and were concerned she needed further medication to control her agitation. Advice was sought from a pharmacist by telephone who recommended starting regular parenteral olanzapine based on the patient's poor response to haloperidol and the lack of enteral access limiting other treatment options. Clonidine infusion was not felt to be indicated at this stage as the patient had no significant alcohol history so low doses of IV midazolam (1 mg) were recommended for severe or dangerous agitation.

Over the next few days, nocturnal agitation remained a problem and zopiclone was added for night sedation but the patient remained delirious. On day 14, hyoscine butylbromide was also started as treatment for bladder spasm.

The next day, the neurosurgical ward round reviewed the patient and said she had 'ICU psychosis' which could last for months and planned to begin weaning the dexamethasone. A pharmacist reviewed the delirium management at the same time. It was noted that the woman remained delirium positive with poor nocturnal sleep and hallucinations the most notable symptoms. Although she was not distressed by them, there was a concern she might try to remove her tracheostomy. Neck pain was still a feature despite regular paracetamol (1 g 6 hourly), codeine phosphate 60 mg 6 hourly and pregabalin 100 mg twice daily since admission. Her last tramadol dose was three days previously. Although the hyoscine butylbromide had been started for bladder spasm, this was no longer a feature, and the dexamethasone started for pharyngeal swelling was still being administered 4 days after starting it and concurrent with fluconazole treatment for the Candida. The possibility of interaction between the two was noted.

A plan was therefore formulated to stop the hyoscine butylbromide, stop the codeine and convert to regular immediate release oxycodone 5 mg 6 hourly NG plus additional doses as needed to improve analgesia. The pro-serotonin effects of the tramadol were also thought undesirable so it was stopped and the dexamethasone converted to prednisolone 30 mg daily with a plan to reduce by 10 mg every three days to stop.

In addition night-time olanzapine was to continue at an increased dose of 7.5 mg and the zopiclone was to be stopped as it was a GABA-minergic agent.

The next day, the patient was reported to have slept well overnight, was pain-free and her ICDSC score had reduced to 2 (delirium negative). The patient remained delirium negative and the olanzapine was weaned off over 5 days and the prednisolone stopped a week later.

Case Discussion

Precipitating Factors

When reviewing a patient with delirium, it is paramount to exclude precipitating causes that require immediate treatment, e.g., hypoxia, hypoglycaemia, sepsis, electrolyte abnormalities. Since delirium causes are usually multifactorial, particularly in critical care patients, a review of all modifiable causes is required. This patient had no obvious predisposing factors, but a number of precipitating factors for developing delirium were present.[6,7]

Outside of critical care, older age is often reported as a risk factor, although in the absence of dementia, this may be less significant in critical care patients who are exposed to many other risk factors. This woman had no significant social history of smoking or alcohol dependency which are also known predisposing risk factors.[6,7] She did however, have a number of important precipitating factors including; infection (fungal line sepsis), polypharmacy including opioids, use of GABA-mimergic drugs (zopiclone), medicines with pro-serotonin effects (tramadol) or anticholinergic activity (codeine), significant pain, prolonged critical care stay and corticosteroid exposure.[6,7] The infection was being appropriately treated with fluconazole and sepsis markers were improving: this was reassuring as the potential for the patient to develop a candidaemia and risk of a CNS infection, particularly with the dexamethasone exposure, was another possibility.

Medication Review

Medication is often one of the most modifiable factors and this was certainly the case in this woman as her delirium symptoms resolved quickly once these were rationalised. Possibly the most important change was the planned dose reduction of dexamethasone by the neurosurgeons. Dexamethasone is a relatively long-acting glucocorticoid both in terms of its pharmacokinetic half-life, but also its biological half-life or pharmacodynamic effect. Such prolonged effects predispose to arousal and sleep disturbances and sometimes attempts to compensate by increasing the patient's nocturnal sleep quantity with the use of benzodiazepines or 'z-drugs' (e.g. zopiclone) paradoxically aggravate sleep disturbances by worsening delirium symptoms. There is some potential for the co-administration of fluconazole to have reduced the hepatic metabolism of dexamethasone by a minor degree and hence further increased the patient's dexamethasone exposure. This underlines the importance of considering drug–drug interactions or pharmacokinetic changes as a result of multi-organ failure on accumulation of medicines as a cause of delirium, e.g., penicillins in renal failure. The change to prednisolone probably had three benefits, a reduced half-life so less of a nocturnal arousal effect, the corticosteroid dose was further reduced when converted to the prednisolone dose and less potential for interaction with fluconazole.

Discontinuing medication with overt or covert anticholinergic activity or conversion to an alternative with less anticholinergic activity is an important intervention.[5] Although in this case the butylbromide salt of hyoscine has a low systemic bioavailability and is less likely to penetrate the CNS than the hydrobromide, it was no longer needed and it was appropriate to stop it. The codeine was also converted to oxycodone which also reduced the cumulative anticholinergic burden but possibly more importantly improved the patient's analgesia (acute on chronic neck pain) thereby improving sleep disturbances as well as delirium symptoms. Not all patients benefit from the analgesic effect of codeine which relies significantly on the hepatic conversion to morphine via Cytochrome P450 2D6, as up to 10 per cent of Caucasians have low levels of this isoenzyme. Although the pro-serotonin effects of tramadol may be beneficial in patients with an element of neuropathic pain, the patient did not describe neuropathic pain problems on assessment at this stage and was already established on pregabalin. Particularly in septic patients, the pro-serotonin effect of tramadol may potentially aggravate delirium symptoms[5] and so this was also stopped even though the patient's septic markers were unremarkable. Accumulation of GABA-pentinoids in renal failure increases the cognitive toxicity of these medicines. However, the patient had no signs of renal failure and had been established on pregabalin for some weeks prior to developing the delirium symptoms, so this was continued as was the regular paracetamol to optimise non-opioid analgesia.

Therapeutic Options

When deciding how to treat delirium symptoms it is important to identify if these are contributed to by agent withdrawal. Most notable of these are alcohol and opioid withdrawal states, but these can also occur with other drugs such as antidepressants. At times it can be difficult to identify whether withdrawal delirium is a factor in some patients, and it may be that withdrawal delirium needs to be covered in tandem with efforts to identify further modifiable causes. Intravenous thiamine replacement as well as benzodiazepine therapy is paramount to the effective treatment of the neuroexcitatory effects of glutamate. However, in patients in whom escalating doses of benzodiazepines appear to worsen delirium symptoms attributed to alcohol withdrawal, adjunctive sedatives such as alpha-2-agonists (e.g. clonidine, dexmedetomidine) may improve hyperactive delirium symptoms by reducing noradrenaline sympathetic activity. However, they must be used in combination with benzodiazepines (or other GABA-minergics e.g. propofol) to prevent alcohol withdrawal seizures.[8] Alpha-2-agonists may similarly assist with the symptomatic control of withdrawal symptoms for opioids and nicotine. As this patient did not have a history of alcohol excess, clonidine therapy was discounted earlier in their delirium course.

In the management of non-withdrawal delirium, non-pharmacological management is advocated first line. However in the critically ill patient, hyperactive delirium symptoms are often severe enough to endanger patients (removal of endotracheal tube or intravenous lines) and staff (risk of physical assault). Pharmacological management is frequently required and the most common medications used are haloperidol and benzodiazepines. Benzodiazepines themselves are a risk factor for developing or worsening delirium and therefore their use in non-withdrawal delirium is usually restricted to rapid sedation in dangerously agitated patients as in this case.

In recent years, a number of large randomised controlled trials have reported benefits of prophylactic haloperidol and olanzapine in the prevention of delirium or reduction of delirium symptoms and duration, in high risk patients undergoing elective procedures. Studies of prophylactic haloperidol in intensive care patients have not demonstrated any benefit over placebo in the incidence of delirium.[9,10] The evidence supporting the use of antipsychotics in the treatment of delirium is limited and extrapolated from a variety of patient groups (e.g., the elderly, palliative care). A small randomised controlled trial of quetiapine versus placebo in intensive care patients with delirium reported a faster resolution of delirium symptoms and less agitation with quetiapine.[11] Haloperidol was reported to worsen this patient's delirium symptoms and was converted to olanzapine, but the patient's delirium and sleep disturbances did not improve until the outlined changes were made.

Antipsychotics are not without safety concerns. Most notable is the IV use of haloperidol and regulatory warnings about risks of a prolonged QTc interval, although the HOPE study, did not report any safety concerns with IV haloperidol used in moderate doses.[10] Moreover these medications may increase the risk of some patients developing hypoactive delirium and there is controversy over how best to treat these patients. Hypoactive patients are generally best treated by discontinuing medication with CNS suppressing effects, although some patients with distressing paranoia or delusional symptoms may also warrant a trial of low dose antipsychotic treatment. Typical and atypical agents have also been associated with increased risk of cerebrovascular adverse events and mortality in patients when used long term for control of the behavioural and psychological symptoms of dementia. Consequently, antipsychotic medication should be used for the shortest period required and regularly reviewed with the delirium indication clearly identified. Unintended continuation of antipsychotics commenced for management of delirium symptoms is a risk on patient discharge from both the critical care unit and hospital.

Conclusion

The hyperactive delirium symptoms this patient developed in critical care are a relatively common occurrence. The causes were multifactorial and many of these related to modifiable medications. It was only when these were fully addressed that the patient's delirium symptoms resolved and discontinuation of antipsychotic therapy was achieved.

Key Learning Points

- Patients should be routinely screened for delirium with a recognised screening tool (the CAM-ICU or ICDSC) so that if delirium develops, a structured review of modifiable factors can be undertaken.
- Delirium should not be regarded as an inevitable consequence of acute care in any patient and left to resolve with time.
- Delirium causes are multifactorial and effective treatment of delirium usually requires prompt review and often multiple changes in therapy to correct these.
- Simply adding more sedative medicines to control a patient's delirium symptoms without tackling the likely causes will lead to prolongation or worsening of delirium symptoms.
- When prescribing medication, think about the patient's co-existing predisposing and precipitating factors for delirium.
- Antipsychotics commenced for the pharmacological management of delirium should be clearly indicated as such and reviewed regularly.

References

1. Gusmao-Flores D, Figueira Salluh JI, Chalhub RA, Quarantini LC. The confusion assessment method for the intensive care unit (CAM-ICU) and intensive care delirium screening checklist (ICDSC) for the diagnosis of delirium: a systematic review and meta-analysis of clinical studies. Crit Care 2012;16(4):R115.

2. Haenggi M, Blum S, Brechbuehl R, Brunello A, Jakob SM, Takala J. Effect of sedation level on the prevalence of delirium when assessed with CAM-ICU and ICDSC. Intensive Care Medicine 2013;39(12): 2171–9.

3. Barr J, Fraser GL, Puntillo K, et al. Clinical practice guidelines for the management of pain, agitation, and delirium in adult patients in the intensive care unit. Critical Care Medicine 2013;41(1):263–306.

4. Morandi A, Pandharipande P, Trabucchi M, et al. Understanding international differences in terminology for delirium and other types of acute brain dysfunction in critically ill patients. Intensive Care Medicine 2008;34(10):1907–15.

5. Cerejeira J, Firmino H, Vaz-Serra A, Mukaetova-Ladinska EB. The neuroinflammatory hypothesis of delirium. Acta neuropathologica 2010;119(6):737–54.

6. Van Rompaey B, Elseviers MM, Schuurmans MJ, Shortridge-Baggett LM, Truijen S, Bossaert L. Risk factors for delirium in intensive care patients: a prospective cohort study. *Critical Care* 2009;13(3):R77.

7. Van Rompaey B, Schuurmans MJ, Shortridge-Baggett LM, Truijen S, Bossaert L. Risk factors for intensive care delirium: a systematic review. *Intensive and Critical Care Nursing* 2008;24(2):98–107.

8. Sarff M, Gold JA. Alcohol withdrawal syndromes in the intensive care unit. *Critical Care Medicine* 2010;38(9): S494–S501.

9. Girard TD, Pandharipande PP, Carson SS, et al. Feasibility, efficacy, and safety of antipsychotics for intensive care unit delirium: the MIND randomized, placebo-controlled trial. *Critical Care Medicine* 2010;38(2):428.

10. Page VJ, Ely E, Gates S, et al. Effect of intravenous haloperidol on the duration of delirium and coma in critically ill patients (Hope-ICU): a randomised, double-blind, placebo-controlled trial. *The Lancet Respiratory Medicine* 2013;1(7):515–23.

11. Devlin JW, Roberts RJ, Fong JJ, et al. Efficacy and safety of quetiapine in critically ill patients with delirium: A prospective, multicenter, randomized, double-blind, placebo-controlled pilot study. *Critical Care Medicine* 2010;38(2): 419–27.

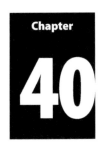

Chapter 40

Death and Organ Donation

Steven Lobaz and James Wigfull

Introduction

Organ transplantation can offer patients with end-stage disease the chance of improved quality of life and life expectancy.[1] It may revolutionise their medical management enabling some to become disease free. The majority of transplanted organs in the United Kingdom come from brain-stem dead donors. In addition to these, since 2008, there have been an increasing number coming from donations made after circulatory death.[2] Despite these efforts, a wide discrepancy continues to exist between the number of patients waiting for an organ and the number of organs available for transplant.[3] The case below illustrates the process of organ donation within critical care and highlights some of the key clinical, ethical and legal issues faced by clinicians.

Case Description

A 20-year-old man was hit by a car, sustaining significant head injuries. On arrival to the accident and emergency department (ED) at 00:30h, he was unconscious. His Glasgow coma score (GCS) was 3 out of 15, with bilaterally fixed and dilated pupils and no respiratory effort evident. Oxygen saturation on pulse-oximetry was 98 per cent on 15 litres oxygen with paramedic administered bag-mask ventilation. His airway was secured with an endotracheal tube after modified rapid-sequence induction, and main-tenance sedation with propofol was commenced. Trauma CT scan of the patient was urgently undertaken, revealing extensive traumatic brain injury with intra-cranial haem-orrhages, significant loss of grey-white matter differentiation and uncal herniation. No other injuries were identified except a right upper lobe contusion. Neurosurgical opinion was that this traumatic brain injury was un-survivable and not reversible with surgical intervention. The intensive care consultant therefore arranged for the patient to be transferred to the critical care unit, to allow the patient's family time to come to terms with the situation and importantly to allow a full and controlled assessment of the patient's suitability for organ donation.

On arrival to the intensive care unit, the patient was ventilated with pressure controlled ventilation. An adequate minute volume was achieved with an inspiratory pressure (Pinsp) of 10 cmH$_2$O and positive end-expiratory pressure (PEEP) 5 cmH$_2$O. Initial arterial blood gases with an inspiratory oxygen fraction (FiO2) of 0.5 showed: pH 7.25, PaCO$_2$ 6.04 kPa, PaO$_2$ 24.2 kPa, HCO$_3$ 19 mmol/L, BE-7 and lactate 2.7. A central venous catheter was inserted as low dose noradrenaline was required to treat hypotension. Sedation was stopped to allow prompt neurological assessment within 24 hours. The patient's family were updated and informed of the poor prognosis and the intention to undertake brain-stem death testing later in the day. The specialist nurse for organ-donation (SNOD) was informed about the case.

At 18:00, the patient's clinical condition remained unchanged. Sedation had now been off for over 17 hours with no neurological improvement observed. A multi-disciplinary team planning meeting was undertaken between intensive care consultant, SNOD, specialist registrar and staff nurse, with each individual's role being clarified prior to a decision to undertake brain stem death testing. The Academy of Medical Royal Colleges (2008) code of practice proforma was used to undertake brain-stem death testing (UK-standard) by the critical care team, independent of the SNOD.[4] Brain-stem death was confirmed at 21:00h and verified on immediate second testing.

At 21:10 h the family were approached by the clinical team and informed unequivocally that brain-stem death testing showed that their relative was dead. On acceptance of death by the family, the SNOD was introduced in a separate consultation in line with recommended best practice, and discussion about organ donation took place.[1, 5, 6] Following this discussion, the family consented to proceed with organ donation and preparations for organ donation were then instigated by the SNOD.

At 22:00h, the patient acutely deteriorated with a sudden desaturation. All ventilatory requirements increased (FiO2 from 0.3 to 1.0, Pinsp to 28 cmH$_2$O and PEEP to 10 cmH$_2$O). Inspiratory rate was increased from 12 to 18 breaths per minute. Tidal volumes achieved were 0.54 litres. Arterial blood gas analysis showed: pH 7.19, PaCO$_2$ 9.31kPa, PaO$_2$ 10.8kPa, HCO$_3$ 25.5mmol/L, BE-1.8, lactate 1.5. Due to worsening haemodynamic instability, noradrenaline requirements had also increased. Vasopressin (4 units/hr) was commenced with the aim of reducing the overall noradrenaline requirement. A triiodothyronine (liothyronine sodium, T3) 3 µg intravenous bolus was also given. Cardiological assessment with echocardiography was also requested by the transplant team and showed normal heart function and structure.

At 02:20 h, brief episodes of extreme hypotension were becoming more frequent (less than 75 mmHg systolic). Noradrenaline was increased to 0.8 µg/kg/min with vasopressin remaining at 4 units/hr. Occasional boluses of adrenaline (10 to 50 µg) were required. Urgent discussion with the transplant team took place, but the retrieval team were not available to undertake immediate retrieval at this time and advised maintenance of current management although they discouraged further use of adrenaline. Over the next hour, the patient's blood pressure stabilised.

At 04:43 h, a further deterioration occurred with persistent hypoxia and cardiovascular instability. Despite high ventilatory pressures (Pinsp 30 cmH$_2$O and PEEP 10 cmH$_2$O) and respiratory rate (18 breaths per minute), alveolar minute ventilation was inadequate. Arterial blood gases on FiO2 1.0: pH 7.13, PaCO$_2$ 10.3 kPa, PaO$_2$ 7.8 kPa, HCO$_3$ 24.4 mmol/L, BE-3.8, lactate 2.7. Noradrenaline was increased to 1.0 µg/kg/min, with continued vasopressin 4 units/hr and T3 3 µg/hr. Right basal crepitations were present on auscultation. Further increases in PEEP were not tolerated due to worsening blood pressure. Cardiovascular stability improved on reducing PEEP to zero. Dexamethasone 8mg was given on advice from the retrieval team and as a last resort, the patient was turned into the prone position. This change in position improved respiratory parameters almost immediately, stabilising the situation.

At 09:00 h, the retrieval team arrived. The patient was transferred to theatre in the prone position, with the plan to proceed to donation after circulatory death if the patient arrested on turning to the supine position. In the event of turning supine, the patient remained stable to allow successful organ donation including heart retrieval.

Case Discussion

Since the first renal transplant in the United Kingdom by Sir Michael Woodruff in 1960, the concept of donating organs after death has become widely accepted.[2] The case for organ transplantation is well established in terms of improvement in quality of life, reduced mortality and economic benefit to healthcare providers and the country as a whole.

Since 1960, the numbers of patients waiting for organ transplantation has consistently exceeded availability of suitable organs.[3] Currently, approximately 10,000 patients are waiting for a solid organ transplant in the United Kingdom. Of these, around 1,000 will die each year whilst waiting for a suitable organ to become available, despite a slow but steady increase in the rates of organ donation after death and from live related donors.[6,7] In 2013/14, there were 4,655 organ transplants undertaken within the United Kingdom. [3]

A major factor in the United Kingdom that limits donation after death is a very high refusal rate, with over 40 per cent of families of potential donors refusing permission for donation. Refusal occurs even when the patient has expressed a previous wish to relatives to donate or by joining the organ donor register. Compared to similar European nations, this refusal rate is significantly higher and is in contrast to repeated surveys of public opinion, which suggests the vast majority of adults in the United Kingdom agree with the principle of organ donation. It is therefore incumbent on all clinical staff working with potential donors to ensure that all cases are discussed with families in an environment that allows the wishes of the donor to be fully considered.

Creating an environment for relatives and friends to consider the patient's wishes when they are in a state of emotional turmoil is difficult and time consuming. Training required to achieve this is not something that doctors working in critical care are likely to have received. They are even less likely to have the necessary time to devote to this one issue, whilst looking after the rest of the intensive care unit. Specialist nurses in organ donation (SNOD) have the time and training that a potential donor's family needs. Despite this, some consultants feel that because they have been dealing with the family throughout the patient's stay in critical care, it is more appropriate for them to bring up such a sensitive issue. It would therefore be expected that a consultant-only approach to family would yield a higher consent rate than when a multidisciplinary approach is used, as in this case. However consultant-only approaches to family consistently result in much lower consent rates.[1,5,6] In the case of brainstem dead patients, a consultant only approach yields a consent rate of approximately 50 percent compared to approximately 70 percent when a multidisciplinary approach is used. The equivalent figures for donation after circulatory death are approximately 35 percent and 65 percent respectively. The message here is to involve the specialist organ donation nurses as recommended by NHS Blood and Transplant, as they are more likely to achieve the donors' wishes.[1,3,7]

Organ donation can be emotionally draining for all staff involved, as well as for the family and friends of the patient. In addition, it is ethically complex. A clear understanding of the ethical framework surrounding organ donation can alleviate much of this stress. The Academy of Medical Royal Colleges formed the UK Donor Ethics Committee which published 'An Ethical Framework for Controlled Donation after Circulatory Death (DCD)' in 2011.[6] Many of the issues raised in this document are equally relevant to donation after brainstem death (DBD). Whilst a full discussion of all aspects of organ donation is beyond the scope of this article, certain aspects that are well illustrated by this case and which have been considered controversial or poorly understood by some are discussed below.

Consent for Organ Donation

In the case study above the word 'consent' has been used deliberately. The legal standing of the family's decision to donate, particularly if the patient is not on the organ donation register, is frequently confused.

Under UK law it is generally recognised that individuals cannot give consent for a procedure to be done to another adult who lacks capacity to consent themselves. In an urgent or emergency situation, doctors may seek 'assent' from relatives if a treatment is deemed urgent and medically necessary for that person. It is recognised that assent has no standing in law but seeking it helps to inform the family of the reasons for the medical team's treatment plans and maintain their trust with the medical team.

For organ donation matters the situation is different, because the legislation that applies is the Human Tissue Act 2004 (HTA), which specifically uses the term 'consent'.[6] In Scotland, the equivalent legislation is the Human Tissue Act (Scotland) 2006, which uses the term 'authorisation'. This difference has led to many publications that apply to the United Kingdom as a whole either avoiding both terms altogether or joining them together, leaving many to wonder what a 'consent/authorisation' might be. In all parts of the United Kingdom, the decision by family and friends to proceed with donation does have legal standing based on an Act of Parliament. Whilst most families will reach a decision collectively, the person who will actually give consent is defined by HTA as one who is in a 'qualifying relationship'. A hierarchy of qualifying relationships is defined from spouse or partner at the top, to a friend of long standing at the bottom. This ensures that for almost all potential donors, the person who knows their wishes, values and beliefs the best, can give legal consent for donation to occur.

Definition of Death

There is no universally accepted definition of death.[8] In the United Kingdom, the Academy of Medical Royal colleges has defined death as the process whereby the patient has 'irreversible loss in the capacity for consciousness and irreversible loss in the ability to breathe'.[4] Both consciousness and respiration are dependent upon brainstem function. Brainstem death occurs within five minutes of cardiorespiratory arrest without resuscitation. Organ retrieval can therefore occur after neurological diagnosis of brainstem death or five minutes after cardiorespiratory arrest without cardiopulmonary resuscitation.[4,6]

Maastricht Classification of Donation after Circulatory Death

This classification system was developed to allow comparison in practice between nations that have applied donation after circulatory death (DCD) to patients dying in different circumstances. It was initially limited to four categories, the fifth was added in 2000:[2]

1. Dead on arrival to hospital
2. Unsuccessful cardiopulmonary resuscitation
3. Cardiac arrest follows planned withdrawal of life sustaining treatments
4. Cardiac arrest in a patient who is brainstem dead
5. In-hospital cardiac arrest

Only categories 3 and 4 are considered controlled deaths. A programme of uncontrolled donation is currently being assessed in Scotland. In the rest of the United Kingdom, controlled deaths only are considered for organ donation after circulatory death. In practice, this is almost exclusively after withdrawal of invasive positive pressure ventilation. Tissue donation is not as time dependant as for solid organs, and tissue can be removed in the mortuary several hours later. All Maastricht categories of potential donor are suitable for tissue donation.

Organ Optimisation before Retrieval

In this case study, there was a significant escalation in care and several new interventions begun, after a diagnosis of brain stem death had been made. These interventions could not be considered to be directly in the patient's best interests, if best interests are only considered in the context of clinical outcome, because the patient was already brain dead. Without these additional interventions, it is very unlikely that any organs could have been successfully transplanted because the retrieval team could not assemble at such short notice. This situation represents an apparent ethical dilemma for some clinicians, since this could be interpreted as an intervention imposed on one patient for the benefit of others. This ethical consideration has been clarified by the UK Donor Ethics Committee (UKDEC).[6] If consent is given, successful donation is considered to be in the patient's best interests because it complies with their wishes. This is true even if the patient has never expressed an opinion about organ donation because, as part of the consent process the specialist nurse will have discussed their wishes, values and beliefs with the family and others in a qualifying relationship. The UKDEC states that 'caring for the patient during the dying process in such a way as to maintain the organs in the best possible condition for donation does not represent a conflict of interest on the part of the treating clinician'. They go on to say that such interventions are likely to be of overall benefit to the donor, unless they cause or risk harm or distress. The concepts of 'harm and distress' in this context are not defined, leaving clinicians to make decisions based on their own experience. Both terms can be interpreted in the psychological sense as well as the physical. A conscious patient clearly has a greater capacity for psychological distress than the unconscious patient and there is an absolute requirement to treat the dying patient with utmost dignity and respect. Whilst clinicians used to dealing with critically ill patients may feel they are achieving this, the family may well interpret things differently. Relatives' distress can be minimised with regular and sensitively delivered information; however, if they object to an intervention, clinicians would be most unwise to proceed.

Conclusions

The gift of organ donation can have a huge impact on the lives of recipients. For grieving families, the donation process may allow something positive to come out of an often sudden and devastating situation. For medical staff involved in the identification of potential donors and their care, through to the successful retrieval of organs in theatre, the process can be long and arduous. Medical teams have a duty of care to ensure that patients are given the opportunity to be organ donors, with consideration being made and discussed in any palliative situation in accordance with GMC guidance.[9] Organ donation raises many ethical and emotional issues requiring education and support for staff.[10] Once successful transplantation has taken place, it is valuable to reflect on the donation process and the difficulties it raised in the context of saving or transforming so many lives.

Key Learning Points

- The number of organs available for transplant does not meet the growing demand for transplantation. Many patients die whilst waiting for a transplant.
- The process of organ donation can be time consuming and complex. Busy clinical teams must be resourced and educated appropriately to ensure that those who wish to donate organs do so successfully.
- A multidisciplinary approach to relatives increases the consent rate for organ donation substantially in comparison to doctors attempting this process alone.
- The care of organ donors during the final stages of their lives is governed by Parliamentary legislation and backed up by numerous guidance documents published by national bodies such as NICE, UKDEC and NHSBT.
- The ethical debate regarding organ optimisation prior to donation has received much attention and is considered acceptable when it does not cause harm or distress to the patient.

References

1. National Institute of Health and Clinical Excellence (NICE). Organ donation for transplantation. NICE Clinical Guideline 135. www.nice.org.uk. 2011.

2. Department of Health. Organs for transplant: A report from the organ donation taskforce. 2008.

3. NHS Blood and Transplant. Organ donation statistics. www.organdonation .nhs.uk/statistics/latest_statistics/?dm_t= 0,0,0,0,0. 2014.

4. Academy of Medical Royal Colleges. A code of practice for the diagnosis and confirmation of death. www.aomrc.org.uk/ doc_view/42-a-code-of-practice-for-the-diagnosis-and-confirmation-of-death. 2008.

5. Vincent A, Logan L. Consent for organ donation. *British Journal of Anaesthesia* 2012;108(S1):i80–i7.

6. UK Donation Ethics Committee (UKDEC) & Academy of Medical Royal Colleges. An ethical framework for controlled donation after circulatory death. www.aomrc.org.uk/ doc_view/9425-an-ethical-framework-for-controlled-donation-after-circulatory-death. 2011.

7. The British Transplantation Society (BTS). Transplantation from donors after deceased circulatory death. www.bts.org.uk. 2013.

8. Gardiner D, Shemie S, Manara A, Opdam H. International perspective on the diagnosis of death. *British Journal of Anaesthesia* 2012;108(S1):i14–i28.

9. General Medical Council (GMC). Treatment and care towards the end of life: good practice in decision making. www.gmc-uk.org/end_of_life .pdf_32486688.pdf32486688pdf. 2010.

10. D L. Organ Donation. Practicalities and ethical conundrums. *American Journal of Critical Care* 2014;23:81–4.

Chapter 41

Managing the Acutely Ill Child Prior to Transfer

David Rowney

Introduction

Invasive meningococcal disease is an important cause of mortality and morbidity in children. Cases present to a wide variety of acute hospital settings and children require seamless escalation of care from initial resuscitation and stabilisation, through interhospital transportation (retrieval) to a paediatric intensive care unit (PICU).

This case presented features of severe septic shock. We describe the specific clinical management, the logistics of undertaking retrieval and discuss the evidence behind currently recommended practice and organisation of paediatric retrieval services.

Case Description

A 3-year-old girl with no past medical history of note and fully vaccinated, presented to the accident and emergency department (ED) of a large district general hospital at 11 pm as a 'stand-by' call from the ambulance service. The girl had been seen by a GP at the evening surgery with a 12-hour history of being non-specifically unwell, irritable, feverish and with poor oral intake and had received treatment and advice for a presumed viral illness. Having deteriorated, she presented again several hours later with a non-blanching rash to the out-of-hours GP surgery. The GP administered intramuscular benzylpenicillin and organised an emergency ambulance. The ambulance paramedic administered facial oxygen and expedited transfer to hospital.

On examination, she was crying irritably. Respiratory rate was 50 to 60 breaths/minute with signs of increased work of breathing (suprasternal and subcostal indrawing and moderate sternal recession). Her chest was clear on auscultation. SpO_2 was 98 per cent on 15 l/min O_2 via a non-rebreathing face mask (89 percent when she pulled the face mask off). She had cardiovascular parameters consistent with severe decompensated shock: marked tachycardia (160 to 170 bpm), hypotension (non-invasive blood pressure was initially reading intermittently at around 65/40 mmHg) and prolonged capillary refill time (CRT) of 8 seconds. She was 'stone cold' to the touch and her skin was mottled up to the knees and elbows with a widespread petechial rash. Pupils were normal size and reactive. She was irritable and combative unless cuddled by her mother, but no neck stiffness could be demonstrated. Central temperature was 38.9°C and toe skin temperature 29.5°C. Blood glucometer reading was 5.2 mmol/l. Other examination was unremarkable.

Initial investigations were markedly abnormal; raised WCC (24.0×10^9/l with marked neutrophilia), elevated CRP (210 mg/l), low platelets (89×10^9/l), deranged coagulation screen (PT 18, APTT 61). The remaining full blood count, liver function tests, urea, creatinine and electrolytes were within normal ranges. Capillary blood gases (CBG) showed a profound metabolic acidosis: pH 7.19 Base Excess (BE) −15 mmol/l, lactate 5.9 mmol/l, $PaCO_2$ 4.9 kPa and PaO_2 5.4 kPa on 15 l/minute via a non-rebreathing face mask.

A 22G cannula was inserted into the left antecubital fossa vein and a 16G IO (intraosseous) needle inserted into the left tibia. Cefotaxime and a first fluid bolus (20 ml/kg, 0.9% saline over 5 to 10 minutes) were administered.

There was no obvious clinical improvement after this and a subsequent fluid bolus, so additional staff (paediatrician and intensivist) were requested to attend. At the third fluid bolus, an adrenaline infusion was made up and preparation for intubation and ventilation commenced.

On re-assessment following the third fluid bolus (cumulative total; 60 ml/kg, 0.9 percent saline over 45 minutes) it was clear that the shock was not resolving, and the child was quieter and now tolerating CPAP (100 percent O_2, 6 l/minute via a tight-fitting facemask using a Mapleson-F anaesthesia circuit) to maintain SpO_2 at 97 per cent. A second CBG was worse (pH 7.03, BE -19 mmol/l, lactate 7.6 mmol/l) and so the adrenaline infusion was started at 0.5 mcq/kg/min and quickly increased to 1.0 mcq/kg/min. Rapid sequence induction of anaesthesia (with fentanyl, ketamine and suxamethonium) and tracheal intubation with a micro-cuffed tube were performed, followed by controlled ventilation and sedation with morphine and midazolam infusions, increased slowly to target rates as tolerated. A chest X-ray was done to assess any degree of pulmonary oedema and check the tracheal tube position.

At this point a referral call was made to the regional paediatric retrieval service who provided ongoing clinical advice whilst mobilising a retrieval team to transfer her to the regional PICU.

During the subsequent 60 minutes before they arrived, stable ventilation settings were established and a further two fluid boluses were administered (cumulative total; 100 ml/kg 0.9 percent saline). A urinary catheter was inserted and a femoral venous triple lumen central line and a right radial arterial were inserted and monitored. Despite this, the tachycardia persisted (170 to 180 bpm) and she remained hypotensive (invasive blood pressure 65/25 to 80/35) and oliguric. The adrenaline infusion was increased to 1.5 mcq/kg/min and noradrenaline also commenced at 0.5 mcq/kg/min. Sodium bicarbonate was administered to correct the acidosis, and calcium gluconate administered to treat a low ionised Ca^{2+} of 0.7 mmol/l. Her measured blood glucose was 3.6 mmol/l and so she was given dextrose along with hydrocortisone 2 mg/kg for refractory shock, on the advice of the retrieval service.

Her parents were updated regularly and the need for retrieval explained so they could give consent. A retrieval service/PICU information leaflet was also provided. The transfer to PICU was uneventful.

Following admission to PICU, all ongoing treatment modalities were continued. CVVH was begun (via a femoral venous haemofiltration line) initially aiming for neutral hourly fluid balances and progressing to negative hourly balances as the shock resolved. A further 80 ml/kg of fluid boluses were administered over the first 24 hours in PICU (cumulative total: 180 ml/kg 0.9 percent saline). Milrinone (0.7 mcq/kg/min) was started to off-load the left ventricle, increase cardiac output and promote global oxygen delivery. The shock steadily resolved; noradrenaline was weaned and discontinued by 24 hours and adrenaline was discontinued by 72 hours after PICU admission. Repeated review by the paediatric plastic surgery team was required to observe the evolving marked purpuric rash, for concerns about ischaemia to a hand and both feet and to monitor for compartment syndrome. Enteral tube feeding was started and reached the target rate by 48 hours.

She was extubated onto high flow humidified nasal oxygen therapy on 5 days after arrival on PICU. Milrinone was discontinued on day 6 and she was discharged to the paediatric ward for rehabilitation on day 7 on antibiotics, weaning regimens of hydrocortisone and sedation.

Polymerase chain reaction testing for Neisseria meningitidis returned positive results although the case was notified to Public Health on the first day of admission, resulting in chemoprophylaxis being administered to the parents and four staff members.

Case Discussion

Invasive meningococcal disease is a common cause of septic shock in children. This case exemplifies many of the features of severe bacterial septic shock in children, including the requirement for rapid and seamless escalation of care using specific treatment interventions for paediatric septic shock 'bundled' together into an 'Early Goal Directed Therapy' regimen to minimise mortality and morbidity.[1]

The pathophysiology of paediatric septic shock is often referred to as 'Cold Shock' with the predominant clinical features resulting from myocardial failure, hypovolaemia and profound compensatory peripheral vasoconstriction giving the typical 'stone-cold' appearance.[2] Unlike adults, in the majority of cases of paediatric septic shock, mortality is associated with severe hypovolaemia and low cardiac output, and tissue oxygen delivery in children, not oxygen extraction, is the major determinant of oxygen consumption.[1]

Available international guidelines outline rapid, stepwise interventions in the first hour. Further haemodynamic optimisation using metabolic endpoints to treat global tissue hypoxia are recommended when practical.[1,3] (Table 41.1) Inclusion of $ScvO_2$ in the goal-directed therapy bundle has been shown to result in administration of more fluid, red blood cells and inotropic support during the first 6 hours of resuscitation in paediatric septic shock, with a resulting 3.3-fold reduction in mortality.[4]

Aggressive early fluid resuscitation – 20 ml/kg bolus of isotonic intravenous fluid over 5 to 10 minutes repeated up to 3 times in the first hour until haemodynamic goals are reached or there is evidence of developing fluid overload (basal lung crepitations, increased work of breathing, worsening hypoxaemia and hepatomegaly) – is the cornerstone of shock management.[1,3] There are few trials looking solely at fluid therapy or types of fluid in paediatric shock. The authors of a recent systematic review concluded that due to the considerable limitations in the existing studies, there was insufficient evidence to inform the preferential use of either colloids or crystalloids for treating paediatric shock.[5] Booy and colleagues reported a reduction in mortality to 5 per cent with the exclusive use of albumin

Table 41.1 Resuscitation goals

Clinical parameter	Haemodynamic parameters
age-appropriate HR & BP	superior vena cava oxygen saturation (ScvO$_2$) ≥70%
no differential between peripheral and central pulses	cardiac index >3.3 and <6.0 l/min/m^2
warm extremities	
urine output >1 ml/kg/h	
normal mental status	

as part of a 'bundle' for treatment of meningococcal septic shock.[6] However, the Paediatric Intensive Care Society – Study Group (PICS-SG) recently reported that albumin was used only one sixth of the time in the United Kingdom for the early treatment paediatric septic shock.[7] De Oliveira reported improved survival with the addition of a treatment target of $ScvO_2$ greater than or equal to 70 percent to the 2002 American College of Critical Care Medicine-Pediatric Advanced Life Support (ACCM-PALS) guidelines.[4] The achievement of the additional target required blood administration. While conservative goals for blood administration are widely used in paediatric intensive care, the various guidelines for treatment of septic shock include transfusion to a target haemoglobin of 100g/L (to achieve Scvo2 greater than or equal to 70 percent) in the acute resuscitation phase of septic shock[1] Profound capillary leak as part of the sepsis/SIRS response can remain for 48 hours or more requiring ongoing fluid resuscitation (up to 200 ml/kg) over this period leading to the development of clinically significant tissue oedema and secondary organ dysfunction. This fluid should be excreted (using diuretics) or removed using CVVH as soon as tolerated following shock reversal and stabilisation of the patient.[3]

Ninis and colleagues examined the factors leading to death in children presenting with meningococcal disease. Failure of staff to administer adequate inotropes was found to be independently associated with increased risk of death.[8] The fundamental requirement for early inotrope administration in fluid refractory shock (after 60 ml/kg) was emphasised in the 2007 revision of the ACCM-PALS guidelines (subsequently adopted by the Surviving Sepsis Campaign guidelines 2012) with a new recommendation to administer peripheral / intraosseous inotropes pending subsequent placement of a central venous line.[1,3]

The haemodynamic response of children with septic shock to vasoactive drugs is variable reflecting the complex pharmacokinetics and pharmacodynamics in paediatric septic shock. Fluid refractory (after 60 ml/kg) septic shock should be immediately treated with an inotrope, e.g. adrenaline, via peripheral, intraosseous or central venous vascular access.[1,3]

Following attainment of a satisfactory blood pressure (and usually after admission to PICU), 'Cold Shock' will require cautious addition of a vasodilator agent to reduce left ventricular afterload, resulting in improved cardiac output and global oxygen delivery. A popular choice is a type 3 phosphodiesterase inhibiter such as milrinone, as used here.

'Warm Shock', which is similar to the prevalent form of adult septic shock, with high/ normal cardiac output and reduced systemic vascular resistance, has been reported as being more common in hospital-acquired paediatric septic shock caused by central venous line infection.[2] This can quickly progress towards 'Cold Shock' as myocardial function and cardiac output deteriorate. Management of 'Warm Shock' centres around the use of vasoconstrictor agents typically noradrenaline, in most cases as an addition to inotropic agents, e.g., adrenaline.[1,3]

Knowing when to proceed to intubation and ventilation is challenging. It is now common practice to have administered 60 ml/kg of fluid resuscitation rapidly, and started an inotrope, e.g., adrenaline, prior to administering drugs for intubation as in this case. Benefits of intubation and ventilation are reduction in the work of breathing (which can account for 40 percent of cardiac output and oxygen consumption), diverting oxygen delivery to other vital organs, reduction in left ventricular afterload (beneficial in 'Cold Shock') and facilitation of temperature control measures (reducing global oxygen consumption). Facial CPAP (100 percent O_2, 6 to 8 l/minute via a tight-fitting facemask using a Mapleson-F anaesthesia circuit) will significantly reduce the work of breathing and off-load the left ventricle and is recommended as a temporising measure while preparing for intubation and ventilation.[3]

Early antibiotic administration is fundamental to reducing mortality in septic shock.[1,3] Empirical use of cefotaxime (or ceftriaxone) with the addition of ampicillin or amoxicillin to cover for Listeria is widely recommended.

All of the available guidelines share almost identical 'goals' and treatment recommendations. An ever-increasing number of studies have reported earlier resolution of shock and improved survival with the use of these guidelines.[6,7,8] However, the UK Paediatric Intensive Care Society Study Group undertook an observational study on 200 children with septic shock accepted for PICU admission within 12 hours of admission to hospital (from 17 UK PICUs and 2 Regional Retrieval Services). Those who had shock reversed prior to PICU admission had better outcomes than those in whom shock was not reversed. In only 38 per cent of children were accepted guidelines followed for fluid and inotrope therapy prior to PICU admission; in the remainder shock was under appreciated or under treated.[7]

Centralisation of paediatric intensive care services into PICUs located in specialist children's hospitals rather than in multiple 'general' intensive care units has led to improved survival for critically ill children. As a result, approximately 5000 critically ill children per year present to a DGH and then require subsequent inter-hospital transport to the regional PICU (www.picanet.org.uk). The majority of these transfers are now undertaken by specialist (regional) retrieval services. The remainder, usually for time critical conditions e.g. intracranial emergencies needing neurosurgical intervention, are carried out by referring hospital staff. Intensivists are expected to play a major role in the resuscitation and stabilisation of critically ill or injured children and commence intensive care pending transfer to a regional PICU.[9] This case highlights the importance of seamless escalation in care including commencement of intensive care level management, often before the retrieval team arrives. Studies have shown that, despite concerns to the contrary, core skills of intubation and insertion of central and arterial lines by referring hospital staff in these cases has increased in recent years.[10] The establishment of close links between the regional retrieval service/PICU and referring sites facilitates the provision of ongoing support, education and training, guidelines, protocols, drug monographs and clinical governance review. Retrieval services provide booklets for parents and most have web sites with useful information to inform the parents about the need for transfer and what to expect when they arrive in the PICU. It is becoming normal practice to get informed consent from parents for the transfer as in this case. Parents often want to accompany their child during transportation and the possibility of this should be discussed early in the referral process with the retrieval team so the parents can be counselled appropriately.

Referrals to PICU should be made as soon as it is evident that the child is critically ill and will require transportation to a regional PICU. Children often compensate and appear 'well' in the early stages of critical illness, then rapidly deteriorate when their compensatory mechanisms start to fail. An organ system failure (physiological) approach to criteria for PICU referral is outlined in Table 41.2.

Conclusion

Invasive meningococcal disease is a common cause of septic shock in children, which if not managed aggressively with a seamless escalation to intensive care level support, will result in significant levels of preventable mortality and morbidity. Fundamental components of

Table 41.2 Criteria for PICU referral

Compromised airway	Chest wall recession 'See-saw' breathing Stridor
Respiratory distress / failure	Rate >60 min/1 Chest wall recession SaO_2 <94% or PaO_2 <8 kPa $PaCO_2$ >6 or <3.5 kPa Exhaustion
Shock	HR >180 or <80 (<5yrs), HR >160 or <60 (>5yrs) Absent peripheral pulses Capillary refill >2 sec Cold peripheries Systolic BP <70+(age in years x2) mmHg
Deteriorating level of consciousness	
Recurrent or resistant seizures	
Burns >10%	
Multiple trauma	
Metabolic acidosis of unknown origin	

management within the first hour of presentation include; early antibiotic administration, up to 60 ml/kg of isotonic fluid boluses and commencement of an inotrope infusion via an IO needle or peripheral cannula pending placement of a central venous line. Intubation and ventilation will commonly be undertaken before arrival of the retrieval team. Paediatric intensive care services and the associated regional retrieval services have become centralised to optimise the care provided. Maintenance of close links with these services and early referral of cases will result in the best outcomes for these children.

Key Learning Points

- Intensivists are expected to play a major role in the resuscitation and stabilisation of critically ill or injured children and commence intensive care level support pending transfer to a regional PICU.
- Early referral to, and ongoing communication with, the centralised paediatric intensive care services and associated regional retrieval services is key to achieving the seamless escalation in care required to minimise mortality and morbidity.
- Septic shock in children often presents as 'Cold Shock' and mortality is associated with severe hypovolaemia and low cardiac output. Adequate resuscitation prior to transfer is extremely important in producing a good outcome.
- Guidelines are available from a variety of sources outlining the fundamental components of early management (within the first hour of presentation) which include; early antibiotic administration, up to 60 ml/kg of isotonic fluid boluses and commencement of an inotrope infusion via an IO needle or peripheral cannula pending placement of a central venous line.

References

1. Brierley J, Carcillo JA, Choong K. Clinical practice parameters for hemodynamic support of pediatric and neonatal septic shock: 2007 update from the American College of Critical Care Medicine. *Crit Care Med* 2009;37:666–88.

2. Brierley J, Peters MJ. Distinct hemodynamic patterns of septic shock at presentation to pediatric intensive care. *Pediatrics* 2008;122:752–9.

3. Dellinger RP, Levy MM, Rhodes A. et al. Surviving Sepsis Campaign: international guidelines for management of severe sepsis and septic shock: 2012. *Crit Care Med* 2013;41:580–637.

4. de Oliveira CF, de Oliveira DS, Gottschald AF, et al. ACCM/PALS haemodynamic support guidelines for paediatric septic shock: An outcomes comparison with and without monitoring central venous oxygen saturation. *Intensive Care Med* 2008;34:1065–75.

5. Akech S, Ledermann H, Maitland K. Choice of fluids for resuscitation in children with severe infection and shock: systematic review. *BMJ* 2010;341:c4416.

6. Booy R, Habibi P, Nadel S, et al. Meningococcal Research Group: Reduction in case fatality rate from meningococcal disease associated with improved healthcare delivery. *Arch Dis Child* 2001;85:386–90.

7. Inwald DP, Tasker RC, Peters MJ, et al. Emergency management of children with severe sepsis in the United Kingdom: the results of the Paediatric Intensive Care Society sepsis audit on behalf of the Paediatric Intensive Care Society Study Group (PICS-SG). *Arch Dis Child* 2009; 94:348–53.

8. Ninis N, Phillips C, Bailey L, et al. The role of healthcare delivery on outcome of meningococcal disease in children: Case control study of fatal and non-fatal cases. *BMJ* 2005;330:1475.

9. The Department of Health Working Group. *The Acutely or Critically Sick or Injured Child in the District General Hospital: A Team Response.* London: Department of Health, 2006.

10. Lampariello S, Clement M, Aralihond AP, et al. Stabilisation of critically ill children at the district general hospital prior to intensive care retrieval: a snapshot of current practice. *Arch Dis Child* 2010;95:681–5.

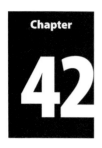

Chapter 42

Who to Admit to Critical Care?

Daniele Bryden

Introduction

One of the greatest difficulties in dealing with the newly referred critically ill deteriorating patient is the uncertainty of knowing whether the deterioration is recoverable or will turn out to be a terminal event for the person at that time. Practice in such situations sometimes requires balancing the rights and wishes of the patient with the expectations of their family and carers in addition to clinical impressions as to whether any escalations of treatment are likely to produce overall benefit to a patient.[1] There is also a potential conflict in the GMC duty of care to treat the patient in front of us and a wider duty to use limited resources in a way that is mindful of the needs of the patients we don't see or care for.[2] This can make decision-making regarding escalations of treatment or admission to critical care very difficult to judge on occasion.

Clinical Case

An 89-year-old woman was referred to critical care in the middle of the night with evidence of type 1 respiratory failure due to a presumed community-acquired pneumonia. She had suffered a hip fracture 5 months previously and spent a total of 6 weeks in acute hospital and community rehabilitation. She had re-presented to hospital acutely from her own home with a 2-week history of shortness of breath, fever and cough. Prior to her hip fracture, she was said to have been playing 18 holes of golf regularly despite an apparent diagnosis of interstitial pneumonitis. The admitting ward team had set up a 'Do Not Attempt Resuscitation' (DNAR) order at her request but referred her to critical care for consideration for continuous positive airway pressure (CPAP) as her oxygen saturations were 82 percent on 15 litres of oxygen.

As her husband was not available for consultation and the patient was unable to give any further history due to breathlessness, the critical care team considered the options and felt that on balance as this was a relatively acute presentation, it would be appropriate to attempt a trial of CPAP therapy, pending provision of more information to enable them to decide on the appropriateness of further therapy and escalations of treatment. It was not felt that the DNAR discussions had covered consideration of CPAP and so the patient's wishes were not known.

CPAP was started on the critical care unit with a clinical improvement and an objective improvement in oxygen saturations enabling the inspired oxygen concentration to be reduced gradually, monitored by means of an arterial line. Antimicrobial therapy of co-amoxiclav and clarithromycin was continued along with DVT prophylaxis and attention to nutrition: there was a plan to insert a nasogastric tube if elemental sip feeds and oral intake were insufficient.

By the following afternoon, the lady was feeling much better in the CPAP hood although still desaturating to less than 90 per cent when it was briefly removed. Discussion with the family indicated that although she had been at home since her surgery, her husband estimated that she was only performing at about 60 to 70 per cent of her previous levels of function and health. Her diagnosis of interstitial pneumonitis was made from a CT scan report at the time of her hip fracture, and an outpatient appointment with a respiratory physician was still awaited.

Although the patient had not expressed any prior wishes to her family regarding critical care admission and organ support, she had informed her husband prior to admission that she felt that she would probably need additional nursing care at home if she recovered from the pneumonia.

After discussion with the family, as the patient was still unable to engage in conversation and judged to lack capacity, the critical care team set a ceiling of treatment consistent with the provision of non-invasive respiratory support, They established that invasive ventilation, renal support or cardiopulmonary resuscitation would not either be consistent with previously expressed patient wishes or if required, would indicate the failure of the current management plan and a probable end of life situation for this lady.

Over the next 72 hours, she gradually improved, such that after a further 72 hours, she was no longer desaturating off the CPAP and maintaining saturations greater than 90 percent on low flow oxygen. She was discharged to continue further care on the ward with her DNAR still in place.

Discussion

Guidance on Admission

The Intensive Care National Audit and Research Centre (ICNARC) has estimated that ICU requirements will double in the next 20 years based on growth in demand from those over 60 years of age. Of note, one third of rapid response calls to medical emergency teams relate to patients at the end of their life which reflects the difficulties in identifying who will benefit from critical care, particularly in an age group that may be nearing the end of their lives.[3]

Several international professional bodies have attempted to produce guidelines to assist with admission decisions but they are limited in their usefulness. The European Society of Intensive Care Medicine guidelines produced in 1994 lack sensitivity to enable stratification of acute hospital inpatients as they suggest admitting patients in an 'unstable condition' or 'at risk of developing severe complications' using an objective parameters/diagnostic model.[3] Subsequent American College of Critical Care Medicine guidelines from 1999 use a model more consistent with pressured resources and that prioritises those who it's felt would benefit most from admission over those who would benefit least.[4] In contrast, the American Thoracic Society has attempted to address issues of equity in its statement that 'The duty of health care providers to benefit an individual patient has limits when doing so unfairly compromises the availability of resources needed by others'.[5]

Moreover survival to hospital discharge is clearly not reflective of the ongoing morbidity and burden of illness: young (median age 45 years) patients surviving after mechanical ventilation for acute respiratory distress syndrome have significant reported extrapulmonary disability one year after discharge spending 74 per cent of their days alive since discharge receiving hospital or home care.[6] Estimates as to the duration of the disability after critical care vary, but have been reported in some groups lasting for up to 15 years.[7]

Isolated factors such as increased age or the presence of premorbid cancer are not reliable markers of poor outcome[8] although age is a significant factor in terms of mortality for emergency admissions whether medical or surgical, with quoted hospital mortality rates of up to 60 per cent. ICU scoring systems, e.g., APACHE, are accurate for cohort mortality not individuals, having been developed for audit and benchmarking purposes.

Typical published ICU admission review criteria, as in this lady's case may include severity of illness on presentation, co-morbidities, frailty and disability, the expected impact of treatment on the outcome, expressed wishes regarding 'Do Not Attempt Resuscitation' orders, and the availability of beds. There is also evidence that a form 'ageism' can influence decisions. In one French study, despite the existence of criteria indicating ICU admission was appropriate, only 40 per cent of patients older than 80 years of age were referred by the emergency medicine department doctor and only half then admitted to the ICU.[5] ICU care itself is also not without risks of delaying recovery (nosocomial infection) or impairing recovery (iatrogenic injury from invasive procedures) in addition to the effect that developing de novo conditions such as delirium can have on overall mortality.[6] Although evidence regarding longer term outcomes from intensive care can be conflicting, a retrospective study of over 35,000 survivors from ICU over the age of 65 demonstrated an excess mortality over a 3-year period when compared to matched controls, which was greatest in those who had required mechanical ventilation whilst on ICU.[9]

This means that a practical approach in terms of trying to define criteria for identifying who will benefit from admission aligned to clearly outlining the potential benefits and burdens of treatment to patients and relatives is often the only strategy that can be adopted. This sort of approach has also been advocated by National Confidential Enquiry into Patient Outcome and Death (NCEPOD) which has suggested factors like frailty are factored into routine assessment of peri-operative needs in the elderly.[7]

Assessment of Frailty

The frailty phenotype of pre-morbid function, co=morbid illnesses and disability are not routinely considered in many intensive-care risk assessment scores. Frailty can be defined as a 'multidimensional syndrome with loss of physical and cognitive reserve predisposing to accumulation of deficits and adverse events'[11] or simply a 'global decrement in physiological systems'. It is thought to represent maladaptive inflammatory processes affecting metabolism, sarcopenia and chronic undernutrition. Diminishing physiologic reserves are needed to maintain homeostasis, and the ability to respond to even small physiological insults – e.g., urinary tract infection, falls, etc. – is impaired and there is further loss of health.

Validation of frailty scoring in the ICU environment is needed to identify the best instrument to assess it, although both Canadian and UK researchers report the use of the validated Clinical Frailty Scale.[10]

Frailty is highly predictive of risk of mortality and adverse outcomes in elderly people living in the general community, and there is now emerging data on frailty assessment in a more critically unwell population.[13] Studies report that frail patients are more likely to have their treatment withdrawn or limited on critical care (as in this case) and survivors were also likely to have a longer stay on ICU and in hospital.[13,14] Assessment of the frail state in individuals referred to critical care when combined with local audit of outcomes should facilitate better decision making between clinicians, patients and families regarding the likely survival and functional impact of critical care treatment.

Clinical Frailty Scale*

 I   **Very Fit** – People who are robust, active, energetic and motivated. These people commonly exercise regularly. They are among the fittest for their age.

 2   **Well** – People who have **no active disease symptoms** but are less fit than category 1. Often, they exercise or are very **active occasionally**, e.g. seasonally.

 3   **Managing Well** – People whose **medical problems are well controlled**, but are **not regularly active** beyond routine walking.

 4   **Vulnerable** – While **not dependent** on others for daily help, often **symptoms limit activities**. A common complaint is being "slowed up", and/or being tired during the day.

 5   **Mildly Frail** – These people often have **more evident slowing**, and need help in **high order IADLs** (finances, transportation, heavy housework, medications). Typically, mild frailty progressively impairs shopping and walking outside alone, meal preparation and housework.

 6   **Moderately Frail** – People need help with **all outside activities** and with **keeping house**. Inside, they often have problems with stairs and need **help with bathing** and might need minimal assistance (cuing, standby) with dressing.

 7   **Severely Frail** – **Completely dependent for personal care**, from whatever cause (physical or cognitive). Even so, they seem stable and not at high risk of dying (within ~ 6 months).

 8   **Very Severely Frail** – Completely dependent, approaching the end of life. Typically, they could not recover even from a minor illness.

9. **Terminally Ill** - Approaching the end of life. This category applies to people with **a life expectancy <6 months**, who are **not otherwise evidently frail**.

Scoring frailty in people with dementia

The degree of frailty corresponds to the degree of dementia. Common **symptoms in mild dementia** include forgetting the details of a recent event, though still remembering the event itself, repeating the same question/story and social withdrawal.

In **moderate dementia**, recent memory is very impaired, even though they seemingly can remember their past life events well. They can do personal care with prompting.

In **severe dementia**, they cannot do personal care without help.

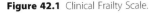

Figure 42.1 Clinical Frailty Scale.

Limitations of Treatment

Advancing age increases the acquisition of frailties and co-morbidities, but age alone is rarely sufficient reason by itself to restrict or continue treatment. The issue of treatment withdrawal or limitation however is frequently one of opinion and many clinicians may be uncomfortable making a definitive decision, if the supporting evidence for their decision is absent. There should always be a presumption of capacity in any patient presenting for critical care treatment (as occurred in the decision to admit this lady here), and clinicians should always attempt to consult the patient about their wishes regarding therapy. The Mental Capacity Act 2010 (similar but not identical legislation operates in Scotland) requires health care professionals to consult family or significant other persons who may be able to provide information as to the person's previously expressed wishes if the patient cannot. In this lady's case, it was fortunate that her views on resuscitation were at least known, as this could be used to guide decisions on invasive organ supports at a time when she was unable to take part in discussions and family opinions were not able to be assessed as to her wishes.

UK General Medical Council (GMC) guidance reinforces the ethical presumption to provide treatment to prolong life and also the legal presumption that an adult has the capacity to make decisions regarding their care.[15] However it also recognises that there are occasions when a person may lack capacity to make a decision and that the benefits of providing a life-saving treatment like invasive ventilation must be weighed against the burdens of such treatment as in this case. It therefore recommends that 'if an adult patient lacks capacity to decide, the decisions you or others make on the patient's behalf must be based on whether treatment would be of overall benefit to the patient'.[15] This is helpful as it shifts the focus for the decision back onto considering the circumstances of the individual patient, and is less about the 'experience' or otherwise of the decision makers. It therefore attempts a degree of objectivity that considers the burdens and benefits of treatment for an individual patient in a way that is not reflected in conventional critical care scoring systems but is starting to be explored in research looking at the impact of frailty in the critical care population.

Conclusion

In many groups of patients, the need for critical care organ supports, particularly the need for mechanical ventilation may mark the end point of a chronic disease/ condition(s) even if not previously identified as such. In survivors, an episode of critical illness and its treatment may shorten life expectancy regardless of patient age.

Use of screening tools such as frailty assessments and being mindful of GMC guidance of the need to consider the 'overall benefit' of a proposed treatment strategy for a patient can be helpful in discussions with patients, families and clinical teams regarding the difficult decision as to which organs to support and for how long.

Key Learning Points

- There is a growing demand for critical care therapies from an increasingly elderly population: doubling of critical care beds is expected by 2020 mostly from those over 60 years of age.
- Guidelines produced by professional bodies to facilitate decision-making are contradictory and of limited practical use in day-to-day decision-making.
- Although yet to be fully evaluated, functional and physiological assessments such as frailty assessment are likely to be of better use in deciding on treatments for individual patients than reliance on age alone.
- There is a UK-wide legal presumption that adult patients have capacity to make their own decisions regarding their treatment and an ethical imperative to prolong life if possible.
- GMC professional guidance recognises that on occasion, when a patient lacks capacity to make his or her own decision, the benefits and burdens of treatments must be considered in terms of the 'overall benefit' to the patient and may result in a decision to limit or withdraw treatment.

References

1. General Medical Council, *Treatment and Care Towards the End of Life: Good Practice in Decision Making*, GMC 2010, at www.gmc-uk.org/guidance/ethical_ guidance/end_of_life_care.asp

2. General Medical Council, *Good Medical Practice*, GMC 2013, updated April 2014 at www.gmc-uk.org/guidance/good_medical_ practice.asp

3. Cardona-Morrell M, Hillman K. Development of a tool for defining and identifying the dying patient in hospital: Criteria for Screening and Triaging to Appropriate aLternative care (CriSTAL). *BMJ Supportive & Palliative Care* 2015;0:1–13.

4. American College of Critical Care Medicine, Guidelines for ICU admission, discharge, and triage. *Crit Care Med* 1999;27:633–8.

5. American Thoracic Society, Fair allocation of intensive care unit resources. *Am J Resp Crit Care Med* 1997;156:1282–301.

6. Herridge MS, Cheung AM, Tansey CM et al. One year outcomes in survivors of the acute respiratory distress syndrome. *N Engl J Med* 2003;348(8):683–93.

7. Williams TA, Dobb GJ, Finn JC et al. Determinants of long term survival after intensive care. *Critical Care Medicine* 2008;36(5):1523–30.

8. Nguyen YL, Angus DC, Boumendil A et al. The challenge of admitting the very elderly to intensive care. *Annals of Intensive Care* 2011;1:29.

9. Wunsch H, Guerra C, Barnato AE et al. Three year outcomes for medicare beneficiaries who survive intensive care. *JAMA* 2010;303(9):849–56.

10. McDermid RC, Stelfox HT, Bagshaw S. Frailty in the critically ill: a novel concept. *Critical Care* 2011;15:301.

11. Fried LP, Tangen CM, Walston J. Frailty in older adults: evidence for a phenotype. *J Gerontol A Biol Sci Med Sci* 2001;56(3): M146–56.

12. Clegg A, Young J, Iliffe S et al. Frailty in elderly people. *Lancet* 2013;381(9868): 752–62.

13. Bagshaw SM, Stelfox HT, McDermid RC et al, Association between frailty and short- and long-term outcomes among critically ill patients: a multicentre prospective cohort study. CMAJ 2013. doi:10.1503/cmaj.130639

14. Le Maguet P, Roquilly A, Lasocki S et al. Prevalence and impact of frailty on mortality in elderly ICU patients: a prospective, multicenter, observational study. *Intensive Care Med.* 2014;40: 674–82.

15. General Medical Council. Treatment and care towards the end of life: good practice in decision-making. 2010.

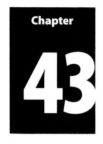

Clearing the Cervical Spine in the Unconscious Patient in the Intensive Care Unit

Michael Athanassacopoulos and Neil Chiverton

Introduction

The reported incidence of cervical spine injury in trauma patients with altered conscious level is known to be 7 to 8 per cent and significantly higher in the unconscious trauma patient. A missed unstable cervical spine injury can have serious potential consequences; significant morbidity for the patient, cost to the healthcare system and society, and anxiety to the clinician.

'Clearing' the cervical spine is the process of ensuring to the best of one's ability that there is no significant injury that will necessitate cervical spine precautions such as protective immobilisation. Following clearance of the cervical spine, a patient will be nursed without any collar or restrictions.

The advantages of early clearance and removal of the cervical collar include more effective airway management, improvement of respiratory FRC and FEV1, decreased intracranial pressure, and decreased risk of aspiration, thrombosis and decubitus ulceration. Prolonged immobilisation is also associated with increased nursing input.[1] Ideally the cervical spine should be cleared within the first 48 to 72 hours of admission in an unconscious patient, as following this time frame, the morbidity and mortality of spinal precautions become quite significant

The process of clearing the cervical spine is well established for the alert patient whilst in the unconscious patient the process has been less standardised. A level 1 Trauma Centre should have a protocol in place to aid the clearance process involving decisions based on clinical and radiological examinations that are performed and reported by several specialised personnel.

It is our aim through this case presentation to highlight the high index of suspicion for injury that should be maintained and to describe our protocol for cervical spine clearance in the ICU of our institution.

Case

A 38-year-old man was a passenger in a car involved in a road traffic collision. It was reported that it required more than 30 minutes to extricate him from the vehicle. On arrival in the accident and emergency department he was hypotensive with a Glasgow coma scale of 6/15. He had bilateral pneumothoraces which were decompressed, an open fracture to his left femur and tibia, and a closed ankle fracture. He also had a possible compartment syndrome of the right leg following intra-osseous fluid administration at the scene of the accident. He was reported to have had a GCS of 14 at the accident scene and was observed moving all four limbs. Past medical history was of asthma and intravenous drug use, and he was now on methadone.

He was intubated and resuscitated while maintaining spinal immobilisation. He was then transferred to the CT scanner for a trauma series from which a small subdural haematoma was diagnosed and there was suspicion of a widened C1–2 interarticular distance although no bony cervical injuries were identified (Figure 43.1).

Subsequently a spinal surgeon was consulted who noted the increased distance on imaging and requested an MRI scan to assess the soft tissues. The patient's neck remained immobilised in a rigid Aspen collar. The external fixator initially applied to stabilise the left tibial fracture was changed to an MRI compatible version, and an MRI was performed four days post admission whilst he was still sedated and ventilated. This verified a ligamentous injury at the craniocervical junction with widening of the atlanto – occipital and atlanto – axial facet joints with extensive soft tissue oedema (Figure 43.2). The injury was considered unstable and the patient underwent a C0–C3 instrumented fusion.

(a)

(b)

(c)

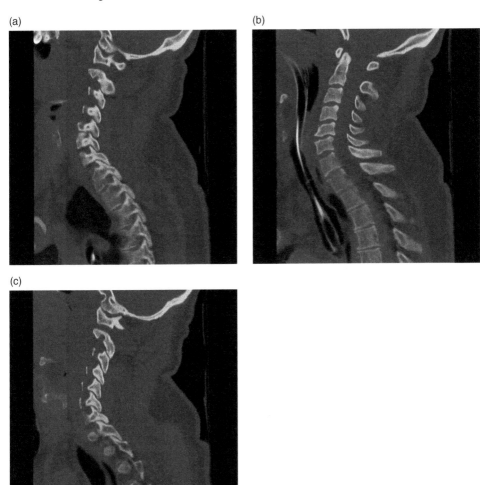

Figure 43.1 Sagittal sections of the patient's cervical spine CT through the right, centre and left facet plane. There is widening of the C1–2 interarticular distance.

Discussion

With an unconscious patient, there are two strategies for clearing the cervical spine. First, prolonged immobilisation and delayed examination when the patient is able to co-operate with a clinical examination when consciousness is recovered. In some cases, when combined with relevant imaging, this is the most effective way of ruling out any injuries, especially ligamentous injuries. The disadvantage of this approach is that the risks of prolonged immobilisation discussed earlier are significant.

The second strategy is to follow a protocol for early cervical spine clearance by sole reliance on cervical CT imaging. It has been argued that this approach carries a risk of missing significant injuries, particularly ligamentous ones, however several recent studies have shown a very small false negative rate.[1]

(a)
(b)
(c)

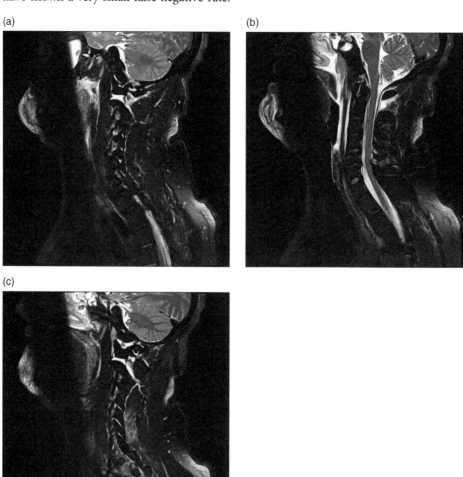

Figure 43.2 T2 weighted MRI sagittal sections of the patient's cervical spine through the mid sagittal plane and the facets showing increased signal in the joints between the occipital condyles and C1 and C1–2, the anterior longitudinal ligament and the posterior complex.

In a recent study, only 57 per cent of level 1 trauma centres in the United States of America had a written cervical spine clearance protocol and nearly 30 per cent did not have a specific management plan for the obtunded patient. Amongst those who did there was no consensus regarding the appropriate screening technique with 13 different approaches.[2] It is therefore necessary to have a protocol in situ, but there is however great debate with no consensus on what imaging modalities should be performed and in what order or which specialties should be consulted.

In our institution we have a protocol in place that is based on the 2008 recommendations of the British Orthopaedic Association's Standards for Trauma (BOAST 2: Spinal Clearance in the Trauma Patient)[3] with some modifications. The on-call spinal surgeon is consulted to review the CT scan following a report by a senior radiologist even if the scan has been reported as having no obvious pathologies: a 2010 study noted that spinal surgeons identified injuries on 20 per cent of trauma CT scans reported as normal.[4] If there is doubt after this review, then a musculoskeletal radiologist can be consulted or further imaging requested. A recent study performed with a similar protocol in the United States showed no significant cervical spine injuries were missed in 197 obtunded patients.[5]

X-ray scans alone (antero-posterior, lateral and open mouth odontoid views) have a sensitivity of 64 to 84 percent and have false negative rate at 15 to 17 percent. Adding

---

Box 43.1[3]

BOAST 2 Standards for Practice Audit:

1. A protocol for protection of the entire spine must be in place in all hospitals managing trauma patients at risk of spinal injury. This protection must be maintained from arrival until appropriate examination or investigations are completed and the spine cleared of injury.
2. Documentation of the neurological status must be made in all at-risk patients; any sign of spinal cord injury mandates urgent scanning.
3. A clinical examination of the whole spine should be documented.
4. If it is anticipated a patient will remain unconscious, un-assessable or unreliable for clinical examination for more than 48 hours, radiological spinal clearance imaging should be undertaken.
5. For the cervical spine, the appropriate standard is a thin slice (2–3mm) helical CT scan from the base of the skull to at least T1 with both sagittal and coronal reconstructions; extending that scan to T4/5 overcomes the difficulties of imaging the upper thoracic spine.
6. It is recommended that this cervical spine CT scan be undertaken as a routine with the first CT brain scan in all head-injured patients who have an altered level of consciousness.
7. The remaining thoracic and lumbar spine may be adequately imaged either by AP and lateral plain radiographs or by sagittal and coronal reformatting of helical CT scans of the chest, abdomen and pelvis undertaken as part of a modern CT trauma series (<5mm slices).
8. A senior radiologist must report spinal clearance images prior to withdrawal of spinal protection precautions.
9. If a spinal injury is detected, a neurological assessment must be made, even if incomplete, and repeated regularly prior to urgent transfer to an appropriate spinal injury service.
10. MRI is the urgent investigation of choice for spinal cord injury.

flexion extension views has not shown a significant change to this rate. X-ray imaging combined with a CT scan has a false negative rate of less than 1%.[6] More specifically, there is a 0.7% incidence of purely ligamentous injury that will not show on a CT scan. However these injuries when identified by later MRI scanning are not usually associated with instability and can be treated in most cases by either a collar or with no support at all.[8]

An MRI is the examination of choice for identification of injuries to the disco-ligamentous complex (as in this case) or the spinal cord. It does have a high false-positive rate, with reported identification of 'injury' in 25 to 40 percent of patients but where significant injuries were present in only 2 to 6 percent of patients. An MRI with fluoro-scopic views also has a false-negative rate similar to that of a CT scan.

CT scanning is faster, available in more centres, more economic and does not require removal of metallic objects which in a trauma/ITU setting may be impractical or at least an otherwise unnecessary undertaking. The sensitivity of helical CT of the cervical spine in unstable injuries is very close to 100 per cent.[7] Sections should be 2 to 3 mm and extend from the base of the skull to at least T1 with both sagittal and coronal reconstructions.

Furthermore, it has been shown that transportation to and performance of an MRI is associated with increased risk of traumatic brain insult to the head injured patient from increases in their intracerebral pressure while lying supine for prolonged periods of time.

A recent review concluded that CT scanning of the whole cervical spine, with sagittal and coronal reconstructions, should be the first imaging modality in an unconscious trauma patient.[8] If this is normal, then cervical immobilisation should be discontinued and the patient re-evaluated when they have recovered sufficiently to cooperate with clinical examination. Although there is a small risk that an isolated ligamentous injury will be overlooked by this strategy, such injuries are rare and very unlikely to require surgical intervention. These conclusions have been reinforced by meta-analysis of 14327 obtunded intubated trauma patients in 17 studies. This concluded that only in 1 in 4776 cases would a CT miss a clinically relevant cervical spinal injury whilst the incidence of complications attributed to cervical immobilization is 6.8 to 64 percent.[9]

For these reasons it is unlikely that MRI will become the routine screening modality for trauma patients. Although there are several studies that have shown a significant detection rate of injuries from MRI imaging when the cervical spine CT scan was negative, in most instances the management of the patient was not changed since these were not deemed clinically significant.[10] Only in a few studies and in a very small percentage of cases did MRI examination lead to further significant findings which altered clinical management. Although an MRI may not be necessary in most instances and is not appropriate for screening, it is the definitive standard for clearing the cervical spine in the unconscious patient.[11] The American College of Radiology suggests that a CT and an MRI are the appropriate modalities for assessment of the cervical spine in an unconscious patient. It also suggests that an MRI is obtained if the neurological status of the patient cannot be assessed within 48 hours post injury, even with a normal CT. This is a higher standard of practice than is recommended by current BOAST2 standards.

In this case simple cervical spine X-rays would not have identified any injury and it is possible that CT scanning may have been declared normal if the scan was reported by a trainee out of hours or even by a consultant radiologist without spinal expertise. However, use of a protocol ensured that the injury was detected and appropriate management followed. If the protocol was not followed the injury may have been missed and it is our recommendation that such protocols are implemented in trauma centres. We also recommend that patients should be examined and re-evaluated off sedation when clinically possible.

Conclusion

It is necessary to clear the cervical spine in the obtunded intubated patient as soon as possible in order to avoid the potential complications of unnecessary cervical immobilisation. The most appropriate initial imaging modality is a cervical CT scan. The formation and adherence to a specific protocol that includes imaging review by both a consultant musculoskeletal radiologist and a spinal surgeon will minimize the chances of missing a potentially unstable injury to an acceptable level.

Key Learning Points

- Early clearance of the cervical spine in an unconscious patient has significant benefits to the patient in reducing morbidity.
- Trauma centres are recommended to formulate and adhere to a protocol for imaging and clearing the cervical spine.
- Helical cervical spine CT scanning is the first line imaging modality of choice. Sections should be 2 to 3 mm and extend from the base of the skull to at least T1 with both sagittal and coronal reconstructions.
- Review of imaging by a senior radiologist (preferably musculoskeletal) and spinal surgeon provides the appropriate levels of expertise to detect abnormalities.
- An MRI should be performed if uncertainty remains or there are signs of neurological deficit.
- Patients should be examined and re-evaluated off sedation when clinically possible.

References

1. Morris CG, McCoy EP, Lavery GG. Spinal immobilisation for unconscious patients with multiple injuries. *BMJ* 2004;329(11): 495–9.

2. Alexander A. Theologis, Robert Dionisio, BS, Robert Mackersie, MD, Robert Trigg McClellan, MD, Murat Pekmezci, MD. Cervical Spine Clearance Protocols in Level 1 Trauma Centers in the United States. *SPINE* 2014;39(5):356–61.

3. British Orthopaedic Association Standards for Trauma (BOAST) November 2008. BOAST 2: Spinal Clearance in the Trauma Patient. Accessible at www.boa.ac.uk/publications/boa-standards-trauma-boasts

4. Simon JB, Schoenfeld AJ, Katz JN et al. Are "normal" multidetector computed tomographic scans sufficient to allow collar removal in the trauma patient? *J Trauma* 2010;68:103–8.

5. Como JJ, Leukhardt WH, Anderson JS, et al.Computed tomography alone may clear the cervical spine in obtunded blunt trauma patients: a prospective evaluation of a revised protocol. *J Trauma* 2011;70:345–9.

6. EAST Ad Hoc Committee on Practice Management Guideline Development. Practice management guidelines for trauma from the Eastern Association for the Surgery of Trauma. *J Trauma* 1998;44:941–6.

7. Brohi K, Healy M, Fotheringham T, et al. Helical computed tomographic scanning for the evaluation of the cervical spine in the unconscious, intubated trauma patient. *J Trauma* 2005;58:897–901.

8. Blackham J, Benger J. 'Clearing' the cervical spine in the unconscious trauma patient. *Trauma* 2011;13:65–79.

9. Panczykowski D, Tomycz N, Okonkwo D. Comparative effectiveness of using computed tomography alone with cervical spine injuries in obtunded or intubated patients: meta-analysis of 14,327 patients with blunt trauma. *J Neurosurg* / 17 May, 2011.

10. Stelfox, HT. Getting Computed tomography for early and safe discontinuation of cervical spine immobilization in obtunded multiply injured patients. *J Trauma* 2007; 63:630–6.

11. Muchow RD, Resnick DK, Abdel MP, Munoz A, Anderson PA. Magnetic resonance imaging (MRI) in the clearance of the cervical spine in blunt trauma: A meta-analysis. *J Trauma* 2008;64:179–89.

12. Daffner RH, Hackney DB. ACR Appropriateness Criteria on suspected spine trauma. *J Am Coll Radiol* 2007;4:762–75.

Alcohol Related Liver Disease (Whom to Admit to Critical Care, When to Refer to a Specialist Centre)

James Beck and Phil Jackson

Introduction

Alcoholic Liver Disease (ALD) is a significant and increasing healthcare burden in the United Kingdom. The alcohol-related death rate is increasing, of which ALD makes up the majority. intensive care unit (ICU) admissions with ALD have tripled between 1996 and 2005 with an estimated annual cost of £14.7 million.[1]

Patients with ALD presenting for ICU admission have traditionally been considered to have poor outcomes.[1] This case study aims to summarise the limited evidence to help guide admission decisions based on identifying patients with potential for recovery and a brief section suggesting who to transfer to a specialist centre.

Case Report

A 48-year-old male patient presented to the emergency department (ED) with a massive haematemesis. He was referred to the ICU team by the gastroenterology registrar for assistance with stabilisation, endoscopy and subsequent management on ICU.

The patient had a 15-year history of excessive alcohol consumption and he admitted to still drinking heavily. He had been unwell for 24 hours prior to admission with jaundice and confusion and had been found by his ex-wife that morning.

His initial haemodynamic instability responded to fluid challenges but he was non-compliant and agitated. He was transferred to theatre where he underwent endoscopy under general anaesthetic. Variceal bleeding was identified but not controllable with banding; consequently a Sengstaken tube was placed and he was transferred to the ICU for continued sedation and airway support.

On his arrival to ICU he was oxygenating well on 35 percent oxygen. He was haemo-dynamically stable having received 2 litres of crystalloid and 2 units of blood. Urine output was approximately 1 ml/kg/hr. He was sedated with an infusion of propofol, and alfentanil. Terlipressin, lactulose and prophylactic antibiotics were prescribed as per local policy, as well as routine ICU prescriptions.

He remained stable and underwent removal of the Sengstaken tube and repeat endos-copy on ICU the following day without complication. Further variceal bands were placed. He was then successfully extubated following a sedation hold. Alcohol withdrawal was managed with chlordiazepoxide and he was discharged to the gastroenterology ward later on that evening.

Five days later he was re-referred to ICU by the outreach team. He had markedly deteriorated since discharge with escalating oxygen requirements, hypotension and oliguria. On review by the ICU doctor he was saturating at 93 per cent on 15 litres/minute of oxygen, he had a blood pressure of 80/40 mmHg despite fluid therapy and he had not passed urine for 12 hours. His blood tests revealed worsening liver function and an acute kidney injury. He was confused and had a liver flap on examination. A diagnosis of sepsis due to hospital acquired pneumonia (HAP) was made. Extensive discussion between the gastroenterology and ICU team occurred due to the severity of his presentation. However, in view of his first presentation to hospital with symptoms of ALD, it was agreed with the gastroenterology team and family that he would be admitted for supportive care and reviewed at 48 hours with a decision regarding ongoing care made at that time.

He was readmitted to ICU where he underwent intubation, mechanical ventilation and insertion of invasive arterial monitoring, central venous access and a urinary catheter. Despite further fluid resuscitation, inotropic support with noradrenaline and antibiotics, he deteriorated rapidly during the subsequent 24 hours, with escalating inotropic and oxygen requirements, anuria and a worsening metabolic acidosis. In view of the worsening multi-organ failure a decision was made, with the understanding of the family, that initiating renal replacement therapy was inappropriate and that palliation was now the most appropriate strategy. Support was withdrawn approximately 30 hours after ICU admission and the patient died.

Discussion

ALD consists of a spectrum of histological and clinical disease from steatosis through to cirrhosis. Patients with ALD can present to hospital with a variety of acute-on-chronic complications such as haematemesis, encephalopathy, ascites, hepatorenal syndrome (HRS) and spontaneous bacterial peritonitis (SBP). The majority of these are managed outside the ICU by gastroenterology or hepatology teams. It is usually only when these patients deteriorate to the point of needing organ supports that they present to the ICU.

The management of these patients includes a routine 'ABCDE' approach to stabilisation and resuscitation, routine ICU supportive measures, treatments for alcohol withdrawal and nutritional deficiency and specific therapies based upon the concurrent ALD complications such as steroids or pentoxifylline for alcoholic hepatitis and lactulose for encephalopathy. A full discussion of these is beyond the scope of this review, though summaries are available elsewhere.[2,3]

As this case study aims to consider which patients could benefit from ICU it is first necessary to determine a baseline for ALD mortality from ICU. A recent systematic review of patients with alcoholic liver disease admitted to the ICU found reported unit mortality ranging from 34 to 63 percent but acknowledged the difficulty in comparing data sets and the limitations of the evidence base being largely retrospective observational studies.[1] Overall, it concluded that the unit mortality for this group is between 40 to 50 percent, higher than the 27 percent national average for critically ill medical patients.[1]

In order to benefit from Critical Care, patients must have a reversible component to their condition and the potential for survival from their physiological derangement. Therefore, information on the factors that determine ICU outcome in this patient cohort will help to guide decisions about appropriateness for ICU in subsequent patients. These factors can be broadly divided into reason for ICU admission, severity of illness, and 'first presentation' ALD.

Reason for ICU Admission

Studies of cirrhotic patients stratified by admitting diagnosis frequently demonstrate a better outcome for those patients presenting to ICU with GI bleeding (mortality 51 percent,[4]

39 percent,[5] 48 percent[6]) and encephalopathy (mortality 46 percent,[4] 14 percent[6]) than for those patients presenting with acute renal failure (mortality 87.5 percent,[4] 92 percent,[5] 75 percent[6]) or sepsis (90.6 percent,[4] 83 percent,[5] 78 percent[6]). However, the majority of these studies used mixed background cohorts (i.e., not just ALD patients)[4,5] and the one study that looked exclusively at ALD patients[6] only had 7 patients in the encephalopathy group and a high mortality in this group at 12 months.[1]

Similarly, studies that have stratified patients according to which organ requires supportive treatment have demonstrated better outcome with a requirement for respiratory support (mortality 31 percent[6]) when compared to a requirement for cardiovascular support e.g. inotropes (mortality 86 percent[1,6]) or renal support (mortality 89 percent,[6] 100 percent[1]).

Severity of Illness

Irrespective of which organ system has failed, the number of failing organs seems to be consistently related to mortality across the literature[3] ranging from 33 to 45 percent for single organ failure, 65 to 75 percent for two organ failures and 90 to 100 percent for three organ failures.[1]

As well as the absolute number of organs failing, more specific severity of illness scoring systems have been evaluated in ALD patients for mortality prediction. Attempts at stratifying patients according to scoring systems have usually concluded that the liver specific scoring systems such as the Child Pugh Score (CPS) and Model for End-stage Liver Disease (MELD) are less prognostically accurate than the physiology-based scoring systems such as the Acute Physiology and Chronic Health Evaluation (APACHE) and Severity of Organ Failure Assessment (SOFA) scores,[3] with SOFA appearing to be the most consistently predictive.[1,3] This is perhaps logical considering that the majority of ALD patients will be in liver failure with CPS grade C at presentation to ICU[1] and their outcome is related to the number of other organ systems failing beyond the existing liver failure, a feature CPS will not pick out. New scoring systems may further improve accuracy in future.[3]

Table 44.1 Child Pugh and MELD Scoring

	Child–Pugh Score		
Criterion	1 point	2 points	3 points
Bilirubin (micromol/litre)	<34	34–50	>50
Albumin (g/litre)	>35	28–35	<28
INR	<1.7	1.7–2.2	>2.2
Ascites	None	Controlled	Refractory
Encephalopathy	None	I–II or controlled	III–IV or refractory

Note: Scores 5–6=class A; Scores 7–9=class B; Scores 10–15=class C
Model for End-Stage Liver Disease (MELD)
$3.8 \times \log_e bilirubin(mg/dl) + 11.2 \times \log_e INR + 9.6 \times \log_e creatinine (mg/dl)$
Note: maximum score is 40; values of <1 are given values of 1; recent dialysis requires a creatinine value of 4.0

Analysis of data collected from over 80 ALD admissions to our own ICU confirmed the superiority of SOFA compared to CPS and indicated that a SOFA score greater than 10 on admission to ICU was associated with 97 per cent mortality (unpublished data).

Additionally, there is some evidence[1,3] that assessment later on in the course of the ICU stay is more discriminatory than the initial scores. This is further evidenced by a comparison of two studies. The Mackle study,[6] a retrospective cohort study of ALD patients on ICU found that those patients who needed only mechanical ventilation during their ICU stay had a 4 per cent ICU mortality. However, a retrospective observational study of intubated cirrhotics of mixed aetiology by Rabe[7] found that even the cohort intubated for airway protection alone had a 54 per cent mortality because the majority developed MOF during the course of their ICU stay. This implies that the development of additional organ failures during the ICU admission will worsen mortality over and above that of the admitting diagnosis.

First Presentation

One feature frequently cited as a reason for ICU admission irrespective of severity of illness is the 'first hospital presentation with ALD'. From a physiological perspective ALD requires many years of alcohol intake to develop;[2] therefore decompensation represents an acute-on-chronic (AoC) flare up rather than a new diagnosis. This is borne out by a study of liver biopsies in patients with first presentation disease[8] that found evidence of cirrhosis in over 70 percent of cases and evidence of fibrosis in 100 percent. Our local ALD data also demonstrates an 87 percent mortality in first presentation cases (compared to 67 percent overall) suggesting this is less relevant in predicting outcome.

Recently, two large retrospective cohort studies have suggested that mortality in cirrhotic patients is decreasing (60.7 to 54.6 percent[9]), even in those with sepsis (73.8 to 65.5 percent[10]). This is encouraging but again, these studies represent a mixed aetiology cohort of cirrhotics. Also, it is difficult to ascertain whether this mortality improvement is due to improved outcomes as a result of surviving sepsis interventions and other improvements in ICU care, or a survival bias due to more stringent refusal of ICU admission to ALD patients in recent years.[9]

Specialist Referral and Transplant

The majority of care for the ALD patient is supportive therapy and routine ICU interventions[2] therefore not requiring specialist intervention. The exceptions to this are need for transjugular portosystemic shunt (TIPS) or consideration for transplant.

Occasionally, patients with refractory variceal bleeding may be considered for TIPS,[3] which would require discussion with a tertiary centre (see Gastrointestinal Bleeding case). This may become a more utilised therapy in future.[3]

Outcomes in patients transplanted for ALD are as good as for patients with other liver disease.[11] However, in most circumstances patients must have demonstrated a period of abstinence and be assessed by a substance misuse team.[12] Critically ill patients presenting with an acute ICU admission with ALD whilst still drinking are therefore unlikely to be considered and even if abstinent they are likely to have to recover from their acute ICU admission and undergo assessment before they would be appropriate for transplant. Furthermore ALD is not an indication for super-urgent listing in the United Kingdom.[12]

Conclusions

Decision-making in relation to ALD patients is difficult due to the variety of possible presentations, the spectrum of background liver disease and the vagaries of the terminology. This is compounded by the paucity of evidence in the Critical Care literature. What evidence exists is often in other subspeciality literature, and frequently involves cohorts of patients with a variety of AoC liver diseases, not specifically ALD. Additionally, variations in the mortality statistic (ICU mortality vs hospital mortality vs 1 year mortality) make comparisons between studies difficult. Consequently, guidance and evidence must be inferred or extrapolated.

Key Learning Points

- A diagnosis of ALD should not exclude critical care, nor should a 'first presentation' guarantee it.
- No single factor out of presenting diagnosis, severity of illness or requirement for organ support can determine survivors from non-survivors. A pragmatic approach would seem to be assessing potential benefit of ICU based upon a combination of presenting diagnosis and severity of illness. For example, a patient with an acute GI bleed with single organ failure may potentially benefit from ICU, whereas a patient with severe sepsis and multiorgan failure may not.
- SOFA score is probably the most accurate scoring system for use in ALD patients. Reassessment and rescoring at 24 to 48 hours may further improve prognostication. New scoring systems may supersede SOFA in due course.
- Irrespective of admitting diagnosis and severity, in those patients developing worsening and/or new organ failure following admission careful consideration of the appropriateness of ongoing treatment is needed.
- The majority of cases can be managed with supportive care and simple specific treatments (such as terlipressin) on a general ICU. Refractory variceal bleeding or patients who are undergoing transplant assessment should be discussed with tertiary centres.
- Despite improvements in ICU care and a suggestion of reducing mortality in ALD in recent years this is still a high risk group with unit mortality of 50 per cent. Appreciation of this will allow realistic goal setting for the MDT and family.

References

1. Flood S, Bodenham A, Jackson P. Mortality of patients with alcoholic liver disease admitted to critical care: a systematic review. *JICS* 2012;13(2):130–5.

2. Jackson P, Gleeson D. Alcoholic Liver Disease. *Contin Educ Anaesth Crit Care Pain* 2010;10(3):66–71.

3. Karvellas CJ, Bagshaw SM. Advances in management and prognostication in critically ill cirrhotic patients. *Curr Opin Crit Care* 2014;20(2):210–17.

4. YP Ho et al. Outcome prediction for critically ill cirrhotic patients: a comparison of APACHE II and Child-Pugh scoring systems. *J Intensive Care Med* 2004;19:105–10.

5. Cholongitas E, Senzolo M, Patch D et al. Risk factors, sequential organ failure assessment and model for end-stage liver disease scores for predicting short term mortality in cirrhotic patients admitted to intensive care unit. *Aliment Pharmacol Ther* 2006;23: 883–93.

6. Mackle IJ, Swann DG, Cook B. One year outcome of intensive care patients with decompensated alcoholic liver disease. *Br J Anaesth* 2006;97:496–8.

7. Rabe C, Schmitz V, Paashaus M et al. Does intubation really equal death in cirrhotic patients? Factors influencing outcome in patients with liver cirrhosis requiring mechanical ventilation. *Intensive Care Med* 2004;30:564–71.

8. Elphick DA, Dube AK, McFarlane E, Jones J, Gleeson D. Spectrum of liver histology in presumed decompensated alcoholic liver disease. *Am J Gastroenterol* 2007;102(4): 780–8.

9. O'Brien AJ, Welch CA, Singer M, Harrison D. Prevalence and outcome of cirrhosis patients admitted to UK intensive care: a comparison against dialysis-dependent chronic renal failure patients. *Intensive Care Med* 2012;38:991–1000.

10. Galbois A, Aegerter P, Martel-Samb P et al. Improved Prognosis of Septic Shock Patients With Cirrhosis: A Multicentre Study. *Crit Care Med* 2014;42(7): 1666–75.

11. Lucey MR, Schaubel DE, Guidinger MK et al. Effects of alcoholic liver disease and hepatitis C infection on waiting list and post transplant mortality and transplant survival benefit. *Hepatology* 2009;50: 400–6.

12. NHSBT. Liver Transplantation: Selection Criteria and Recipient Registration (POL195/2). www.odt.nhs.uk/pdf/liver_ selection_policy.pdf (accessed 22 July 2014)

Hyperpyrexia

Sarah Irving

Introduction

MDMA (3,4-methylenedioxymethamphetamine), or 'ecstasy' is an amphetamine analogue with stimulant and hallucinogenic effects. It is a potent releasor and re-uptake inhibitor of serotonin (5-HT), dopamine (DA) and norepinephrine (NE). It causes a state of euphoria, so is often used as a recreational drug.[1]

Over 16 related compounds have been identified. These include its 'sister' drug 3,4-methylenedioxyethamphetamine, MDEA, 'Eve' and their common metabolite 3,4-methylenedioxyamphetamine, MDA, 'Ice'. Compounds sold as ecstasy have been found to contain varying amounts of MDMA, MDMA-related compounds and a variety of other drugs including amphetamine, methamphetamine, novel psychoactive drugs, caffeine, ketamine and acetaminophen (paracetamol).[2,3]

In 2012 the National Crime Survey for England and Wales found 2.9 per cent of young adults had used ecstasy within the previous year.[4] Although relatively few people suffer adverse side effects, in 2012 there were 31 deaths reported from its use.[3]

Toxic effects are similar to those of the other amphetamines but are less common. However, significant, life-threatening symptoms such as hyperthermia, centrally mediated hyponatremia and the serotonin syndrome can occur.[2]

Those presenting acutely with toxicity may give little history, or a history of mixed drug and alcohol use. Management requires prompt recognition of the condition and a focus on supportive care as well as controlling hyperpyrexia, cardiac arrhythmias and electrolyte abnormalities.

Case Description

A 21-year-old man was reviewed in the emergency department. He was usually fit and well and did not take any regular medications. According to acquaintances, he had consumed large quantities of alcohol with ecstasy tablets. On arrival, he was dangerously agitated and covered in bruises from punching and kicking a wall outside a nightclub. In order to assess him, the emergency doctors had administered a total of 14 mg of diazepam. He was moving all four limbs, but was drowsy, sweating (diaphoretic), still agitated and not oriented to time, place or person. He required intubation to facilitate proper assessment.

Observations post-intubation showed him to be tachycardic, hypertensive, but with good gas exchange and minimal oxygen requirements. He was pyrexial at 42.5°C. The 12 lead ECG showed sinus tachycardia and a prolonged QTc of 570 ms. CT of the head was normal. Blood gases showed a significant metabolic acidosis, with a bicarbonate of 14 mmols/l, Base Excess −12 mmols/l and lactate 5 mmols/l. WCC was slightly raised, but with a CRP of 15 mg/l. A review of the biochemistry showed that he had an acute kidney injury, with a creatinine of 150 μmols/l and sodium was 128 mmols/l. CPK was raised at 60,000 U/l as were transaminases, with AST 900 IU/l and ALT 340 IU/l. ALP, GGT and bilirubin were normal. Paracetamol and salicylate levels, and a urine and plasma drug screen were requested. Advice was taken from the poisons advice service.

Two litres of cold Hartmanns solution were infused and simple external measures were used in the ED prior to transfer to the ICU. Sodium bicarbonate at 1.4 per cent was infused to improve his acidosis and to correct the prolonged QTc. Once he was in ICU, his temperature remained at 42°C despite external cooling. He became oliguric after fluid resuscitation and so a decision was made to commence renal replacement therapy with a view to temperature reduction, limiting renal damage from rhabdomyolysis, correcting acid base disturbance and to replace renal function. Whilst he was deeply sedated, but once paralysis had worn off, repeated clinical examination was performed. There was increased tone and inducible clonus, especially in the lower limbs. Advice from the Poisons Service (NPIS) indicated possible serotonin syndrome. Cryptoheptadine was therefore started with a view to reducing temperature further.

Over the next 6 hours, his temperature reduced and tachycardia settled. Renal support was stopped after 24 hours and a sedation hold was performed, leading to successful extubation at 48 hours. Transaminases peaked at 24 hours, whilst bilirubin remained normal. He was discharged to the ward after a 4-day critical care stay.

Discussion

Pharmacology of Ecstasy

MDMA is mainly sold as a pill, but can be found in a powder to be snorted or smoked. Oral effects begin within 1 hour and typically last 3 to 6 hours. The half-life is around 8 hours.[1] A clear correlation between dose and severity of outcome has not been demonstrated. This suggests environmental influences and idiosyncratic reactions.[2]

MDMA causes the release of serotonin, dopamine and norepinephrine in the central nervous system, as well as binding and inhibiting their reuptake transporters at the synapse. The acute increase in the intra-synaptic concentration of these transmitters, leads to a period of depletion.[1,2]

In addition to control of mood, these neurotransmitters play a role in thermoregulation and control of sleep, appetite, reward and the autonomic nervous system.[1,2] Following MDMA administration, an increase also occurs in cortisol, prolactin, adrenocorticotropic hormone (ACTH), dehydro-epiandrosterone and antidiuretic hormone (ADH).[1,2]

MDMA has slight monoamine oxidase (MAO) inhibiting activity and some direct activity at several receptor types (5-HT_2, M_1-muscarinic, H_1-histamine and α_2-adrenergic), the significance of which is not known.[1,2]

Metabolism involves two main pathways. Both Cytochrome P450 isoenzyme CYP2D6 and catechol-O-methyltransferase (COMT) play a role in one pathway. This means that slow metabolisers may be at a higher risk of acute MDMA toxicity. COMT polymorphism may also contribute to inter-individual differences in ADH release after MDMA.[1]

Presentation of MDMA Toxicity

The immediate effects of Ecstasy vary from common minor symptoms to those that are rare but potentially fatal. Minor side-effects include trismus, tachycardia and teeth grinding.

Patients may present with acute delirium. Panic states and acute behavioural disturbances are common.[2]

More severe effects include hyperpyrexia, rhabdomyolysis, cardiovascular instability and multi-organ failure as in this case, serotonin syndrome, an acute panic disorder and hyponatraemia with cerebral oedema. Hepatic failure has been reported both as part of a picture of multi-organ failure and as isolated liver failure. Hypertension/tachycardia can be present, due to autonomic dysfunction. Hypotension and poor cardiac output states are possible due to cardiac effects of amphetamine like substances, or the development of organ dysfunction. Long QTc interval has been reported in association with MDMA toxicity and this may be the cause of cases of sudden death reported in users.[2]

Although difficult to quantify, trauma related injuries are probably increased in users. Cerebral haemorrhage, cerebral venous sinus thrombosis and aplastic anaemia have been reported as have pneumothorax and pneumomediastinum.[2]

Dilutional hyponatraemia leading to cerebral oedema has caused deaths in MDMA users. Patients present with confusion, delirium and convulsions and can rapidly progress to coma and death as a result of 'coning' (cerebral oedema, hypoxia and uncal herniation). The practice of drinking large amounts of water, or sugared/carbonated drinks, appears to be a major contributory factor. An increase in ADH release due to MDMA has been found.[2] Genetic polymorphism as discussed previously, puts some individuals at increased risk.

Hyperpyrexia Due to MDMA Toxicity

Patients present with hyperpyrexia, muscle rigidity and hyper-reflexia. Impaired consciousness, disseminated intravascular coagulation (DIC), rhabdomyolysis and multi-organ failure can follow. The degree and duration of hyperpyrexia are indicators of the risk of mortality. Temperatures over 41°C may be fatal. There are few survivors if the peak core temperature exceeds 42°C, although a survivor presenting with a temperature of 42.9°C has been reported. Rhabdomyolysis can be pronounced, with peak creatine phosphokinase (CPK) levels in the region of 30,000 to 100,000 IU/L. The highest recorded peak CPK in a survivor is 555,000 IU/L.[2]

The exact mechanism of MDMA related hyperthermia remains unclear and is likely due to several different mechanisms. Most cases appear to be associated with euphoric effects of the drug leading to excessive exertion with inadequate fluid replacement to maintain thermoregulation. Studies have shown that the temperature rise due to MDMA can be exaggerated by both a warmer environment and by being in more populous places.[5]

Both 5-HT and dopamine are involved in central control of thermoregulation and so MDMA can lead to the activation of mechanisms that conserve and generate heat.[2] Hyperpyrexia can present as part of serotonin syndrome and those taking regular serotonergic agents are at increased risk. However, life threatening temperature rises occur without features of serotonin toxicity. Another suggested mechanism is the uncoupling of oxidative phosphorylation in skeletal muscle mitochondria and peripheral vasoconstriction due to activation of β-3 and α-1-adrenoceptors.[6]

There is overlap in clinical features between MDMA-induced hyperthermia, neuroleptic malignant syndrome, serotonergic syndrome and MH. It has been suggested they share a final common pathway.[2] (See Table 45.1).

The connection with malignant hyperpyrexia, has led to the use of dantrolene in MDMA induced hyperpyrexia and several case reports. A systematic review (with only

Table 45.1 Differentiation of hyperpyrexic syndromes due to pharmacological agents

Syndrome	Trigger	Cardinal features	Key points
MDMA Toxicity	MDMA	Delirium, dysautonomia, pyrexia	May present with serotonin syndrome
Serotonin syndrome (SS)	SSRI, MAOI, psychoactive drug, tramadol etc	Triad of mental status change, dysautonomia + neuromuscular abnormalities Meets hunters criteria	Less rigidity than MH and NMS Onset in hours Prodrome (nausea, vomiting, diarrhoea)
Malignant hyperthermia	Anaesthetic agent	Pyrexia, rigidity, dysautonomia	Onset within minutes Can be fulminant
Neuroleptic malignant syndrome	Neuroleptic/ Antipsychotic agents started or dose increased Parkinsons drugs reduced	Tetrad of mental status change, muscular rigidity, hyperthermia and autonomic instability	Less shivering, hyperreflexia, myoclonus, ataxia than SS Onset in 1–3 days
Central anticholinergic syndrome	Anticholinergics	Flushing, mydriasis, dry mucous membranes, bladder distension Confusion/ encephalopathy	No rigidity, diaphoresis, raised CPK

small numbers) found that of the 13 patients who had a temperature of greater than 42°C and who received dantrolene, 8 survived (62 per cent). None of the 4 patients with a temperature greater than 42°C who did not receive dantrolene survived.[7] However, without evidence from a randomised controlled trial, controversy regarding its use continues.

Other agents, such as carvedilol have been shown experimentally to reduce the hyperpyrexia, but are unproven in critically ill patients.[8]

Serotonin Syndrome

Serotonin is a neurotransmitter involved in control of mood, appetite and sleep regulation; cognition; perception; motor activity; temperature regulation; pain control; sexual behaviour and hormone secretion. Serotonin syndrome is a potentially life-threatening condition due to increased serotonergic activity in the central nervous system. It is seen with therapeutic medication use, especially selective serotonin reuptake inhibitor (SSRI) antidepressant agents and inadvertent interactions between drugs, including psychoactive drugs of abuse. A particular risk is to those taking MAO inhibitors and serotonin reuptake inhibitors.[9]

Serotonin syndrome consists of a triad of mental status changes, autonomic hyperactivity and neuromuscular abnormalities. The diagnosis is made solely on clinical grounds. The Hunter Toxicity Criteria Decision Tool is the most validated tool[9] (see Figure 45.1).

Following a change or initiation of a drug most cases present within 6 and at most 24 hours. Typical signs include tachycardia and hypertension. Severe cases may develop hyperthermia and rapid, severe autonomic instability. Physical examination findings include:

hyperthermia, agitation, ocular clonus, tremor, akathisia, deep tendon hyperreflexia, inducible or spontaneous clonus, muscle rigidity, dilated pupils, dry mucus membranes, increased bowel sounds, flushed skin and diaphoresis. Neuromuscular findings are typically more pronounced in the lower limbs. In severe cases, rhabdomyolysis with acidosis and frank renal failure may subsequently result.[9]

Central to the management of the syndrome is discontinuation of all serotonergic agents, supportive care, sedation to control agitation and dysautonomia and administration of serotonin antagonists. Management of autonomic instability can be difficult. Beta-blockers used in isolation may be associated with increased hypertension due to loss of β-mediated vasodilatation. Nitrates and esmolol are useful short acting agents. For hypotension from monoamine oxidase inhibitors (MAOIs) treatment should be with low doses of direct-acting sympathomimetic amines and avoidance of indirect agents.[9]

Control of hyperthermia is critical and involves eliminating excessive muscle activity. Antipyretic agents are ineffective. Standard treatments for hyperthermia should be implemented. Patients whose temperature is above 41.1°C may need prompt sedation, paralysis and tracheal intubation.[9]

If supportive care fails to improve signs, treatment with cyproheptadine, an oral histamine-1 receptor antagonist, is suggested. Chlorpromazine is an alternative intravenous agent.[9]

Management of MDMA Toxicity

Initial management is supportive, following an A,B,C approach. Routine lab investigations, CPK, blood sugar and urine toxicology screens should be sent. When unknown substances are ingested, the differential includes novel psychoactive substances. Discussion with toxicologists will ensure the correct immunoassay drug screens are performed.

The use of activated charcoal is recommended up to 1 hour post-ingestion. Benzodiazepines may be required for agitation and increased sympathetic drive. They will also ease increased tone contributing to hyperpyrexia.

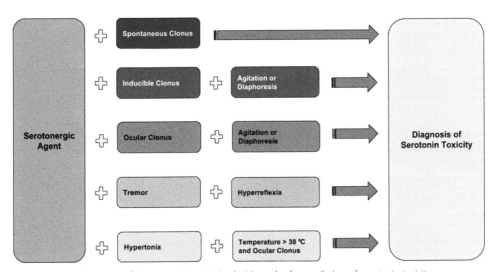

Figure 45.1. Adaptation of Hunter toxicity criteria decision rules for prediction of serotonin toxicity.

Urgent fluid replacement is essential in the patient with marked hypotension and tachycardia from intravascular volume depletion. Invasive monitoring and vasopressor support should be established early if multi-organ dysfunction develops. Metabolic acidosis should be corrected with sodium bicarbonate if prolonged QTc is present on the ECG.[2] Adequate fluid is also important to protect the kidneys from injury due to myoglobinuria. Urinary alkalinisation has been used,[2] but in theory could reduce MDMA clearance.

Treatment of tachycardia and hypertension secondary to the sympathomimetic effects of MDMA may be required. The treatment rationale is similar to that for serotonin toxicity. As well as esmolol or nitrates, labetalol may be considered as it has both alpha and beta blocking effects.[2]

It is also important to correct hypovolaemia and thus enable thermoregulation. Patients with core temperatures greater than 39.0°C should be treated aggressively. Early rapid measures include patient exposure, iced-water sponging, strategic ice placement and infusion of cold fluids. Specialist external cooling devices are available and in resistant cases, bladder or gastric lavage with cooled fluids have been described. With all of these methods, shivering can be problematic.[2] Continuous renal support can manage the effects of organ dysfunction and rhabdomyolysis, whilst simultaneously controlling hyperthermia.

Any patient with a significantly impaired level of consciousness, seizures or established hyperpyrexia above 41°C, should be sedated and ventilated to break the cycle of heat generation. For critically ill patients, discussion with the National Poisons Information Service (NPIS) should occur and consideration be given to using dantrolene, or centrally acting serotonin antagonists for those meeting criteria for toxicity.[2]

MDMA associated hyponatraemia will usually correct automatically, so fluid restriction is appropriate if asymptomatic. For significant neurological impairment, including seizures, hypertonic saline may be required to correct sodium to a level where symptoms subside.

In hypovolaemic patients, isotonic saline may be more appropriate. Rapid correction of hyponatraemia can lead to central pontine myelinolysis (CPM). However, those risks are less if the initial fall in sodium is within 48 hours. Hence risks and benefits must be carefully considered, experienced clinicians involved and correction be no greater than 10 to 12 mmols/l in 24 hrs and 18 mmols/l in 48 hrs[10] (See Table 45.2).

Conclusion

MDMA remains in wide use as a substance of misuse. Although it rarely causes harm, in a small subset of people it can cause life threatening complications. In many of those cases hyperpyrexia is central and this should be promptly managed within a critical care environment to prevent a cycle resulting in rhabdomyolysis, multiorgan failure, hyponatraemia and death.

In those cases not responding to benzodiazepines and simple cooling measures, early sedation and ventilation is key and more invasive measures of cooling and renal replacement therapy should be instituted. Discussion with the NPIS is important, in resistant cases. Dantrolene may be useful, but consideration should be given to the contribution of serotonin syndrome when cyproheptadine or chlorpromazine can be used.

Table 45.2 Management of MDMA toxicity

Problem	First line treatment	Second line
Clearance	Activated charcoal within 1 hour	
Anxiety/ Agitation	Benzodiazepines	Sedation and ventilation
Reduced GCS	Intubation if GCS <9	Consider alternate diagnosis or co-ingestion CT head
Autonomic instability	Labetalol or esmolol if hypertensive/tachycardic Avoid other beta blockers Alpha agonists for hypotension	Sodium bicarbonate if prolonged QTc
Hyperpyrexia	Benzodiazepines Simple measures External cooling devices	Sedation+ventilation Dantrolene Consider serotonin syndrome RRT
Serotonin syndrome (SS)	Benzodiazepines Labetolol or esmolol if hypertensive/tachycardic Avoid other beta blockers Avoid indirect acting sympathomimetic agents Cooling measures	Sedation+ventilation early Cyproheptadine or chlorpromazine
Hyponatraemia	Fluid restrict If acute and severe neuro signs correct with hypertonic saline until symptoms subside	Expert advice early
Rhabdomyolysis	Check CPK Rehydrate Consider alkalinisation urine	Renal replacement therapy

Key Learning Points

- Ecstasy toxicity causes hyperthermia, associated MODS, rhabdomyolysis and hyponatraemia.
- Hyperthermia is multifactorial and can be due to serotonin syndrome.
- Aggressive temperature management is key.
- Consider sedation and ventilation early to facilitate temperature management.
- Hyponatraemia should be carefully corrected to prevent central pontine myelinolysis.
- Discussion with the NPIS is important.
- Dantrolene may be useful for hyperpyrexia.
- Serotonin syndrome is a clinical diagnosis based on the Hunters Criteria.
- Cyproheptadine or chlorpromazine can be used for associated serotonin syndrome.

References

1. de la Torre R, Farré M, Roset PN, et al. Human pharmacology of MDMA: pharmacokinetics, metabolism, and disposition. *Ther Drug Monit* 2004 Apr; 26(2):137–44 Review.

2. Hall AP, Henry JA. Acute toxic effects of 'Ecstasy' (MDMA) and related compounds: overview of pathophysiology and clinical management. *Br J Anaesth* 2006 Jun; 96(6):678–85. Epub 2006 Apr 4.

3. Office for National Statistics. Deaths Related to Drug Poisoning in England and Wales, www.ons.gov.uk/ons/rel/ subnational-health3/deaths-related-to-drug-poisoning/2012/index.html (Accessed 15 July 2014).

4. Drug misuse findings from the 2012 to 2013 Crime Survey for England and Wales. *Home Office*. Published 25 July 2013. www.gov.uk/government/publications/ drug-misuse-findings-from-the-2012-to-2013-csew (Accessed 6 June 2014).

5. Green AR, O'Shea E, Colado MI. A review of the mechanisms involved in the acute MDMA (ecstasy)-induced hyperthermic response. *Eur J Pharmacol* 2004 Oct 1; 500(1–3):3–13.

6. Rusyniak DE, Tandy SL, Hekmatyar SK, et al. The role of mitochondrial uncoupling in 3,4-methylenedioxymethamphetamine-mediated skeletal muscle hyperthermia and rhabdomyolysis. *J Pharmacol Exp Ther* 2005 May; 313(2):629–39.

7. Grunau BE, Wiens MO, Brubacher JR. Dantrolene in the treatment of MDMA-related hyperpyrexia: a systematic review. *CJEM* 2010 Sep; 12(5):435–42.

8. Hysek C, Schmid Y, Rickli A, et al. Carvedilol inhibits the cardiostimulant and thermogenic effects of MDMA in humans. *Br J Pharmacol* 2012 Aug; 166(8):2277–88.

9. Boyer EW. Serotonin syndrome. In: *UpToDate*, S Traub (Ed) (Accessed 6 June 2014).

10. Vaidya C, Ho W, Freda BJ. Management of hyponatremia: providing treatment and avoiding harm. *Cleve Clin J Med* 2010 Oct;77(10):715–26.

Index

BV - #0092 - 130323 - C8 - 234/156/22 - PB - 9781107423374 - Gloss Lamination